THE ROLE OF OSTEOTOMY IN THE CORRECTION OF CONGENITAL AND ACQUIRED DISORDERS OF THE SKELETON

Edited by **James P. Waddell**

The Role of Osteotomy in the Correction of Congenital and Acquired Disorders of the Skeleton
Edited by James P. Waddell

Published by InTech
Janeza Trdine 9, 51000 Rijeka, Croatia

Publishing Process Manager Martina Durovic

Technical Editor Teodora Smiljanic

Cover Designer InTech Design Team

Additional hard copies can be obtained from orders@intechopen.com

The Role of Osteotomy in the Correction of
Congenital and Acquired Disorders of the Skeleton, Edited by James P. Waddell
p. cm.
ISBN 978-953-51-0495-7

For EU product safety concerns:
IN TECH d.o.o., Prolaz Marije Krucifikse Kozulić 3, 51000 Rijeka, Croatia,
info@intechopen.com or visit our website at intechopen.com.

Meet the editor

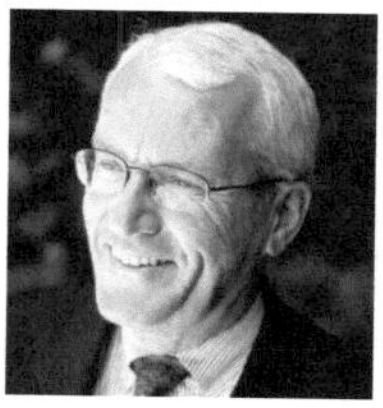

Dr. James P. Waddell was born in Alberta and graduated from the University of Alberta Medical School in 1967. He did his postgraduate training in orthopaedic surgery at the University of Toronto and assumed a staff position at St. Michael's Hospital in 1973. He has occupied a number of positions at St. Michael's Hospital including Surgeon-in-Chief and Medical Director of the Trauma Program; he completed 10 years as the Professor & Chairman, Division of Orthopaedic Surgery at University of Toronto in June of 2006. He has also occupied a number of positions in the Canadian Orthopaedic Association including President. He has completed a 10 year term as the Co-Editor of the Canadian Journal of Surgery. He is currently the Chair of the Expert Panel for Orthopaedic Surgery for the Province of Ontario and the Coordinator for the National Action Network for the Bone & Joint Decade in Canada. He also is the Co-Chair of the National Hip and Knee Knowledge Translation Network and the Board Chair for the Canadian Orthopaedic Foundation.

Contents

Preface

It is a pleasure for me to edit this book on osteotomy. I would like to thank all of the authors for their contributions, Ana Skalamera for her help in assisting me in editing this book and my secretary Cathy Smith.

Osteotomy is an ancient surgical skill recognized for centuries as a surgical technique that could address deformity thereby improving function or appearance.

In this text we have attempted to demonstrate various osteotomy techniques for correction of deformity, closure of bone defects, preservation of joint function and improved cosmesis.

The techniques presented have in common the need for appropriate imaging – if necessary three-dimensional imaging – as well as carefully thought out and executed surgical plan. Pre-operative planning is essential in the performance of osteotomy and the chapters in this book clearly outline the need for careful physical examination and imaging prior to the procedure.

The ubiquitous nature of joint replacement surgery has eclipsed osteotomy as the common tool for management of lower limb arthritis but increasingly it is apparent that in the younger patient population carefully planned and executed osteotomy can preserve the patient's own joint and avoid the need for joint replacement surgery for years or even decades.

It's a pleasure for me to be associated with a book that re-affirms the importance of this recently neglected surgical technique and I am proud to have been asked to perform the role of Editor.

I hope you enjoy the book and you find it of benefit to you in your work.

James P. Waddell, MD, FRCSC
Professor, Division of Orthopaedic Surgery
University of Toronto
Canada
JPW/cs

Part 1

Face and Skull

1

Surgery of the Bony and Cartilaginous Vault in Rhinoplasty

Pavel Dolezal
Slovak Medical University, Department of Otorhinolaryngology, University Hospital Bratislava, Bratislava, Slovakia

1. Introduction

An osteotomy must be performed in almost all types of external nose correction. By mobilising the bony skeleton, the nose may be sculpted into the desired shape and position. The osteotomy is carried out as gently as possible in an effort to minimize postoperative swelling and soft tissue bleeding. Finger and sharp chisels are used. Nasal bones are accessed through a short intercartilaginous incision above the lateral nasal cartilage. The outer periosteum is pushed to the side, then an osteotome is placed about 2mm paramedially and, using rhythmic taps of a metal mallet, a medial osteotomy is performed. The position of the osteotome is checked by finger palpation on the nasal dorsum. The osteotome is worked through the bone up to the level of the frontal bone. Before removal, the resilience of the nasal bone is checked by turning the instrument laterally.

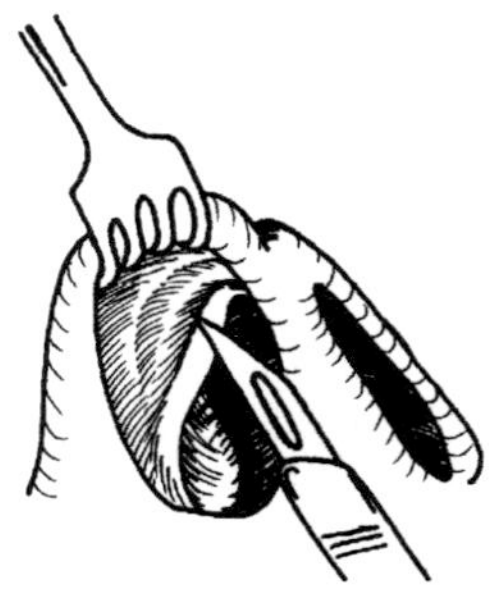

Fig. 1. Short intercartilaginous incision for a medial osteotomy

A lateral osteotomy is carried out through an ancillary vestibular incision in front of the head of the inferior turbinate. The incision is extended to the piriform aperture very close to the maxillary edge in order to obviate needless bleeding. A raspatory is used on the bony edge through a 1 cm long incision, and the anterior periosteum of maxilla and part of the nasal bone are prepared up to the middle canthus. In fact, a subperiostal tunnel is formed. An identical tunnel is created on the inner side, in the nasal cavity. An osteotome is applied to the bony edge and a lateral osteotomy is performed in the direction outlined in the picture. Cranially, the osteotome is turned towards the cranial end of the previous medial osteotomy. The nasal bone is broken on one side by lateral rotation of the osteotome and is checked by palpation.

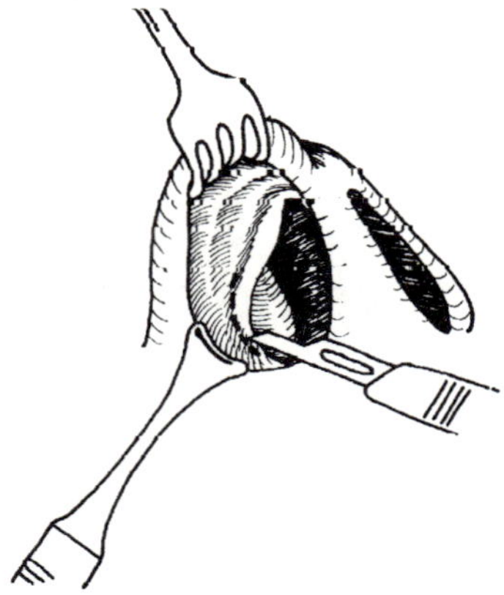

Fig. 2. Short lateral incision for lateral osteotomy

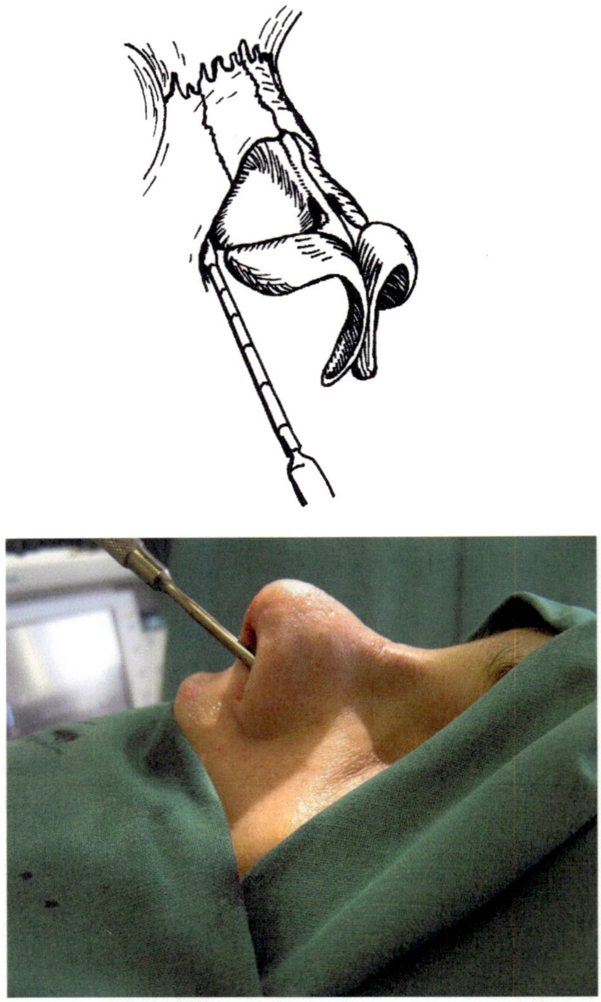

Fig. 3. Creation of a medial tunnel for a lateral osteotomy using a raspatory

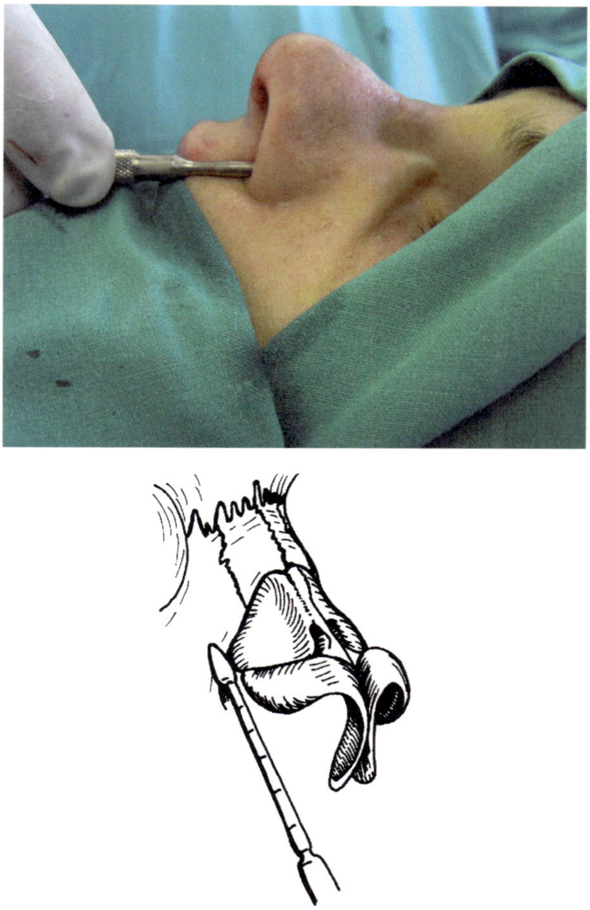

Fig. 4. Creation of a lateral tunnel for a lateral osteotomy

Thorough mobilisation of the nasal skeleton is the most important element in achieving the appropriate cosmetic effect. Sometimes this mobilisation is not sufficient even after a quadruple osteotomy. The transversal part of the osteotomy is sometimes questionable when a straight chisel is used. It can be done using a curved osteotome, following the line of lateral osteotomy slantwise upwards, aiming from the middle canthus to the frontal bone. However, an osteotomy performed using an osteotome, which is a rather thick instrument, is less precise and destroys more surrounding soft tissue than an osteotomy done using a sharp chisel.

If sufficient mobilisation was not obtained, a transversal osteotomy through the skin of the nasal root must be performed. In a skin fold on the nasal root a small incision to the bone surface is made with blade No.15. A 2-3mm wide chisel is put into the incision and, using rhythmic taps, a fixed section of the nasal bone is cut off. Care is taken with all bone fragments. A splinter can easily be pressed inward towards the nasal cavity. If a large fragment is broken, it must be elevated and redressed in the nasal vault line. Irregularities in the nasal skeleton are hidden by edema and hematoma after an osteotomy, but after absorption of edema and decomposition of hematoma all irregularities of the nasal vault become evident. Therefore, maximum care must be taken when performing an osteotomy. In using the closed technique, the progress of the operation must be confirmed by repeated palpation.

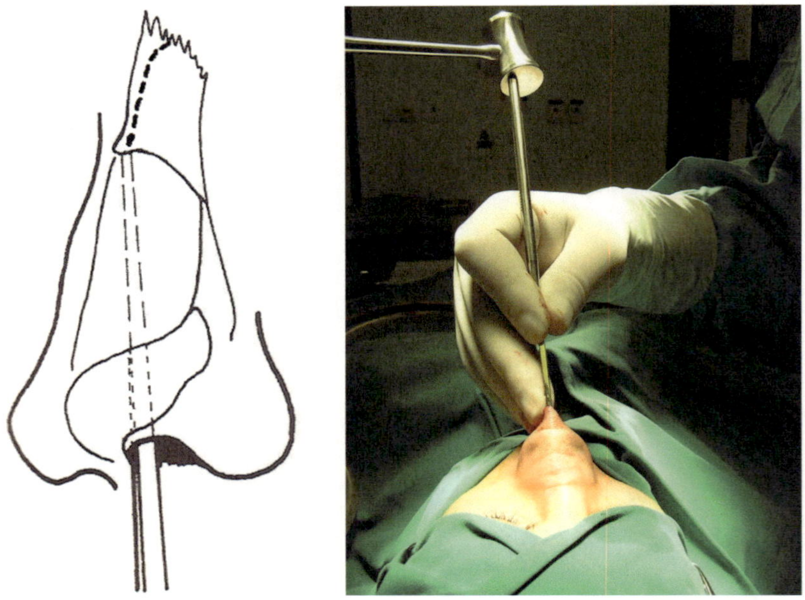

Fig. 5. Medial osteotomy. Osteotome or sharp straight chisel is worked paramedially along the upper edge of the nasal septum to the level of the frontal bone

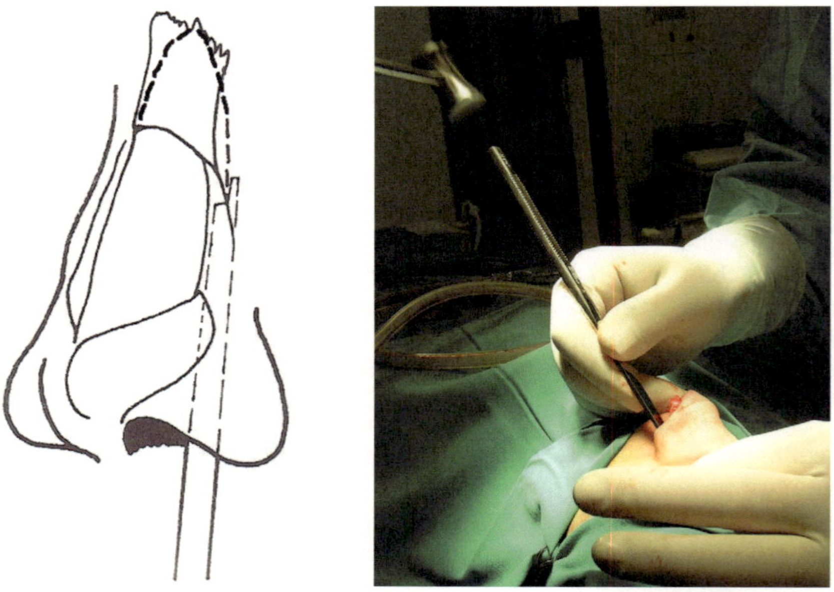

Fig. 6. Lateral osteotomy. Osteotome or chisel is directed across the frontal process of maxilla towards the nasal root and then turned upwards to the line of medial osteotomy. This procedure is also called transversal osteotomy.

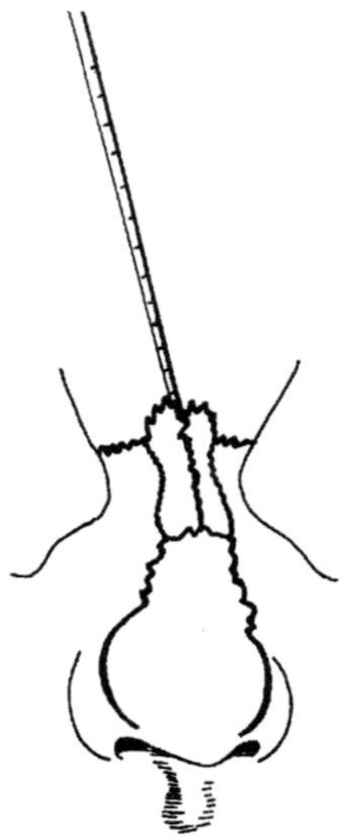

Fig. 7. Transversal transcutaneous osteotomy of nasal bones

In certain cases, the nasofrontal angle can be corrected using this approach. The so-called mini-osteotomy is another method of skeletal mobilisation. It consists of a multiple splitting of the the nasal bones in the line of medial and lateral osteotomy, gaining access through the skin. A narrow chisel can reach under the skin to the region of the frontal process of maxilla. The osteotomy is finished using an endonasal approach. Nasal bones are broken in the proposed line. As well, a mini-osteotomy can be performed through the skin using more incisions. This procedure is more precise, but small scars remain on the lateral nasal wall and mainly on the nasal slope.

2. Resection of a nasal hump

Resection of a nasal hump in the cartilaginous and bony part of the skeleton is a frequent procedure in rhinoplasty. Sometimes there is no real gibbus to correct, it is only necessary to lessen the projection of the nasal dorsum slightly overlapping the line from nasion to nasal tip. A nasal hump may be more developed in the cartilaginous area, where it is formed by septal and lateral cartilage. In the bony part, it is formed by prominent nasal bones. In almost all cases a hump is formed by both parts, therefore they should be reduced together. Several procedures are described in the literature (1-4). In a resection, scissors are used in the beginning to cut the cartilage to the level of resection. Septal cartilage and both prominent lateral cartilages are resected up to the level of the nasal bones. A sharp chisel is inserted under the resected cartilage and the resection of the bony hump is completed. In a successful case, a cartilaginous and bony hump is extracted in one piece using forceps. This piece is oval in shape and symmetric. After a resection, sharp edges are trimmed using a rasp. After each hump removal, a flat nose remains which must be narrowed and the defect in the nasal roof should be closed. A medial osteotomy must be performed and then a lateral osteotomy using the method desscribed in the previous chapter. When the nasal skeleton is mobilised, the bones are narrowed and the external nose is formed in the medial line.

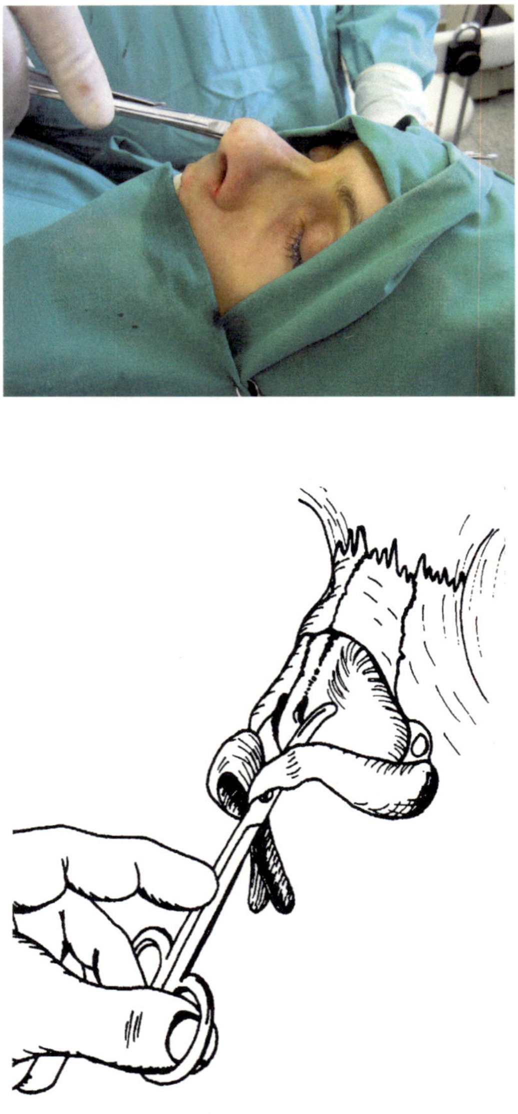

Fig. 8. Preparation of the upper part of the nasal pyramid. Using an intercartilaginous approach, scissors are inserted under the skin. Following the surface of the nasal hump, soft tissues are mobilised.

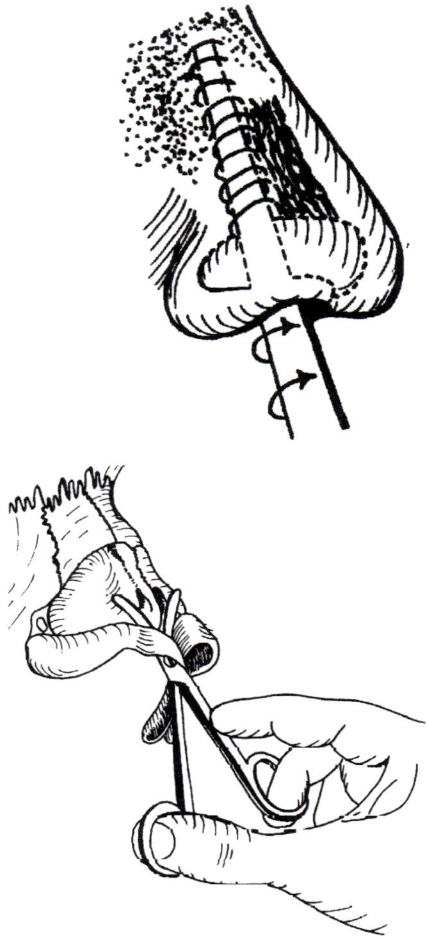

Fig. 9. Soft tissue mobilisation of the nasal pyramid using a raspatory

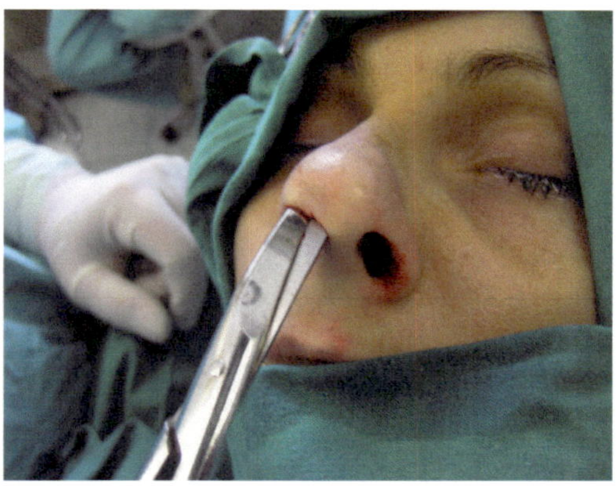

Fig. 10. Cutting the nasal septal cartilage that creates the caudal margin of a cartilaginous and bony hump. After accessing the margin of the nasal bones using scissors, the resection is completed using a straight chisel.

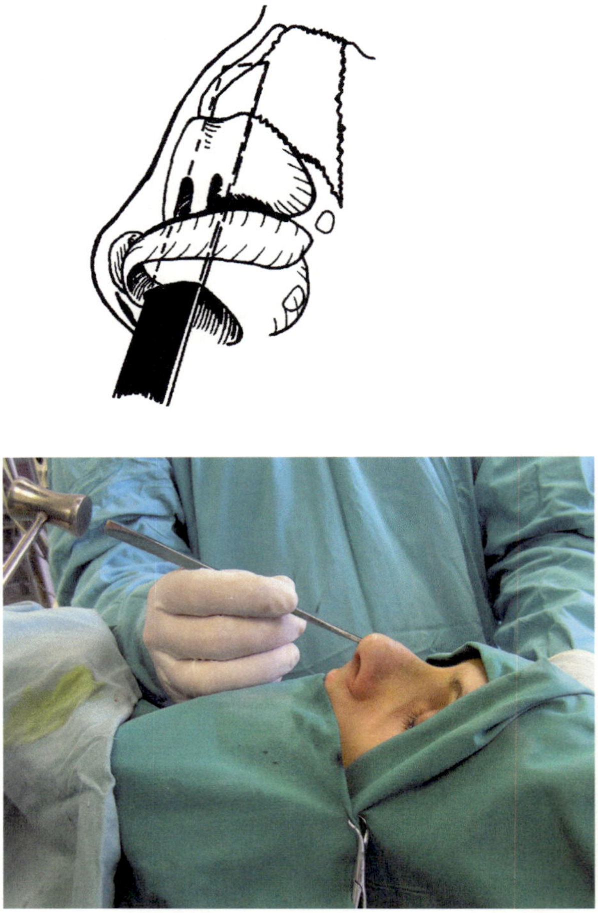

Fig. 11. Resection of cartilaginous and bony hump using a wide chisel

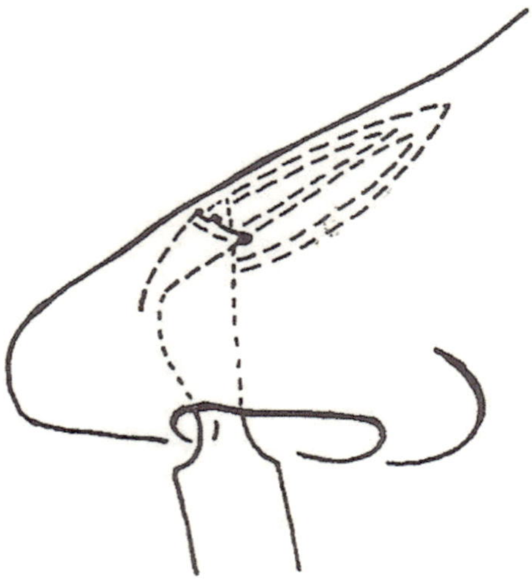

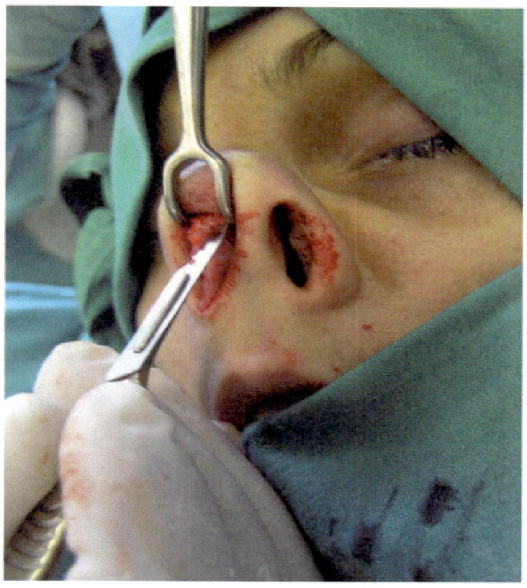

Fig. 12. Alignment of prominent cartilage using a scalpel

The lower, cartilaginous part of the hump may be cut off using a scalpel or sharp scissors. It is better to do so after retracting the skin and cutting under direct vision (figure 12).

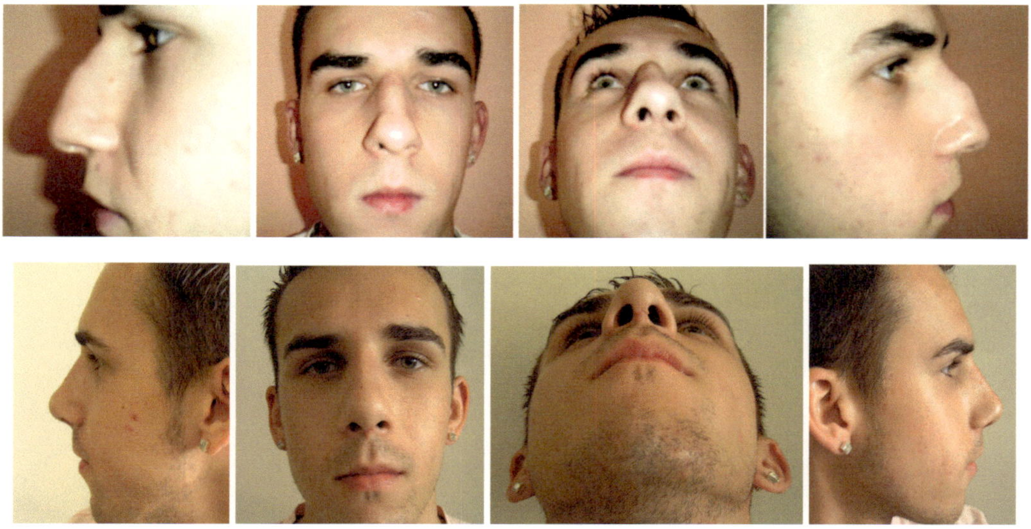

Fig. 13. Patient with a nasal hump, slight deviation to the right side and wide tip (upper pisctures). After resection of the hump, osteotomies and interdomal tip suture (lower pictures)

3. Osteotomy in external nose deviation

Fixed elderly external nose deviation causes asymmetry not only of nasal shape but also in the length of the lateral nasal wall. Osteotomy alone is usually not sufficient to align the nasal skeleton into the medial plane because on the opposite side of the deviation, the lateral nasal wall is larger. In this case a "wedge resection" is planned. On the larger side, part of the nasal bone is shaped into a wedge or triangle with its base inverted and the caudal bone is resected (figure 14). The surgeon has to be experienced and must make an adequate approach to the margin of maxilla and the nasal bone on the side of the resection. Subperiosteal tunnels are made as in a lateral osteotomy. The tunnels must be a little bit wider in order to insert long nasal forceps into them. After extending the branches margin of the pirifom aperture, the frontal process of maxilla and nasal bone are more visible. An assessment must be made of the width of the piece of bone to be removed. The first osteotomy is performed close to the nasal bone. A subsequent osteotomy is localized behind this line so that the two lines converge at the level of the inner canthus.The resected bone should therefore be in the shape of a triangle. If the bone is not removed in one piece, all remnants and fragments must be definitely eliminated, best done under direct vision. The lines of fracture should be straight and smooth in order not to hinder the reformation of the nasal skeleton in the new position. Usually a strip of cartilage and bone from the nasal septum must be removed at its base (figure 15).

Deviation may be corrected by outfracture of the nasal bone on the side of the deviation and by infracture on the opposite side. This procedure compensates for curvature optically because it redresses the length of both slopes of the nasal pyramid. Septal mobilisation and thoroughgoing osteotomy is necessary (figure 15)

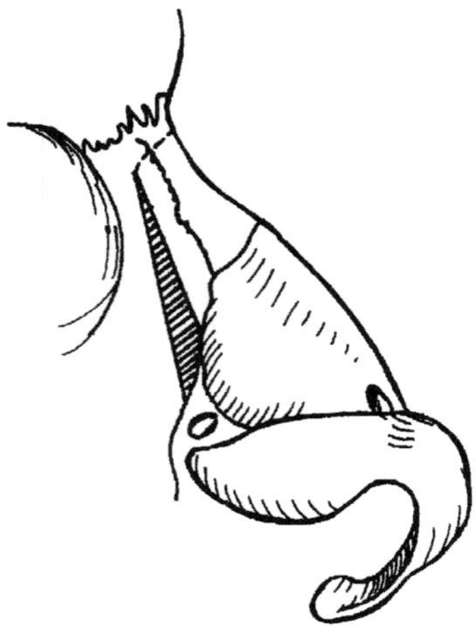

Fig. 14. Wedge resection of maxilla on the side opposite to the deviation

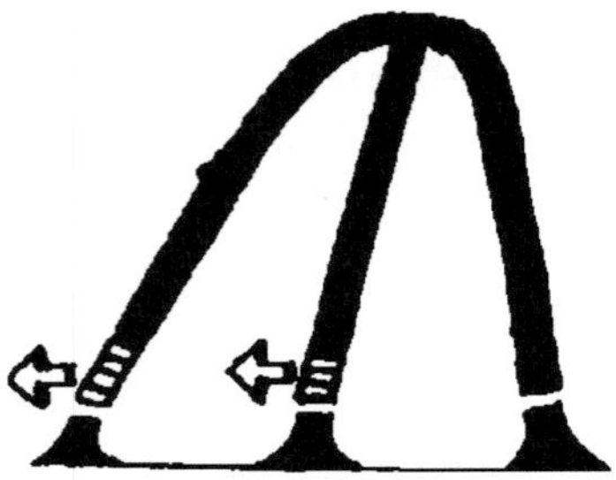

Fig. 15. Bony wedge resected from the frontal process of maxilla on the contralateral side of the deviation and resection of a basal strip of the nasal septum. Schematic picture of nasal pyramid in axial plane

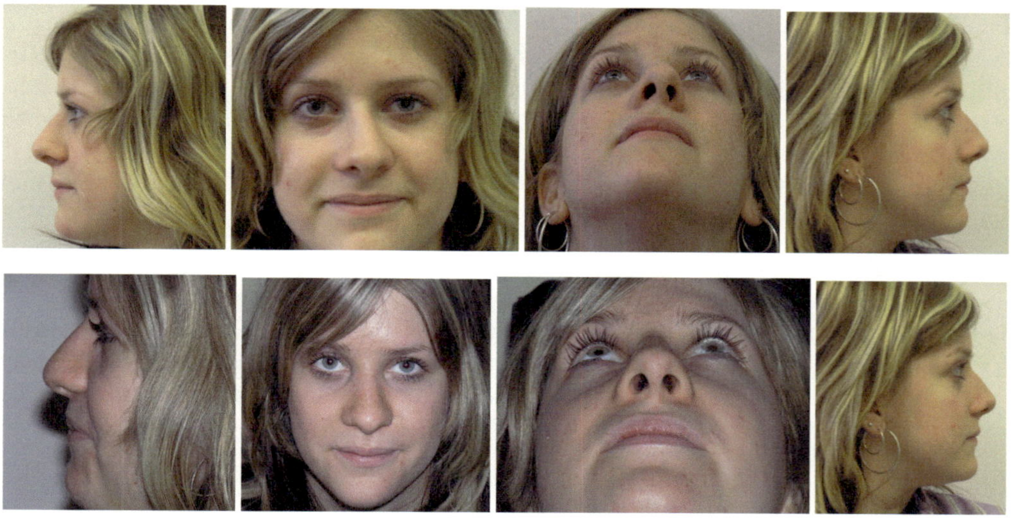

Fig. 16. Patient with external nasal deviation to the left side (upper pictures). After wedge resection on her right side, osteotomies and remodelation of nose to the medial plane (lower pictures)

4. Osteotomy in wide nasal vault

Medial and lateral osteotomy is unsufficient in the case of wide and flat nasal dorsum. Nasal bones create a wide arc even after their separation from septum and maxilla (figure 17) Thorough mobilisation would therefore not allow to narrow nasal vault in desired extend. It is neccesarry to think of it before and to perform multiple osteotomy. First is medial, then intermedial a finally lateral osteotomy. Originally wide nasal vault will divide to several bony fragments. They are elevated and narrowed in desirable shape.

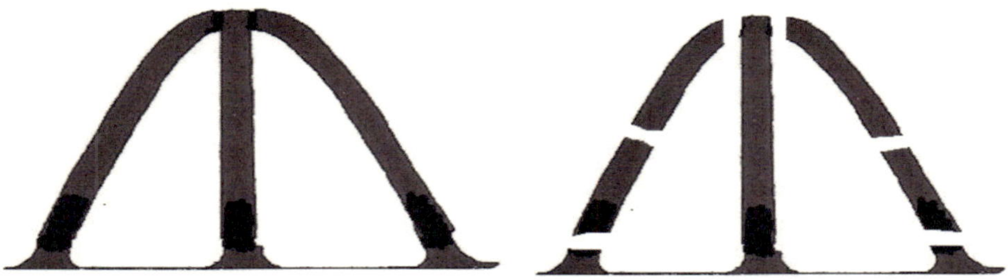

Fig. 17. Wide bony pyramid in axial plane. Medial, intermedial and laterál osteotomies are performed.

5. Correction of external saddle nose deformity

Severe saddle nose deformity of the external nose results after strong blow directly to the nasal dorsum. The nasal bones are smashed and moved in a lateral and dorsal direction. Viewed from the front, the nose is short, wide and unsightly because the nasal tip is retracted upwards. From a lateral view, the loss of the dorsal nasal vault becomes evident. The outcome of an injury to the nasal septum may be luxation or cartilage aposition with manifold spines and crests. In a mild saddle nose deformity, a cartilaginous or osseous graft is inserted into a prepared subcutaneous tunnel and this is sufficient to straighten the line from nasion to nasal tip. There is no need to use the open approach. On the contrary, if it is necessary to replace the nasal dorsum and columella and at the same time to correct the alar cartilages and the nasal tip, or alternatively the nasal septum with lateral cartilages, then the open approach and reconstruction of the whole nasal skeleton under direct vision is more convenient.

After external nasal skin withdrawal, the nasal septum is reconstructed using some of the techniques described previously. Then a quadruple osteotomy is done. Care is taken to keep the osteotome lateral enough because the nasal bones are usually wider and flatter in this type of deformity. Mobile bones should be elevated. Usually a sufficient nasal dorsal shape is not achieved using this procedure and it is therefore necessary to apply an autograft. It is more advantageous to use bone rather than cartilage.

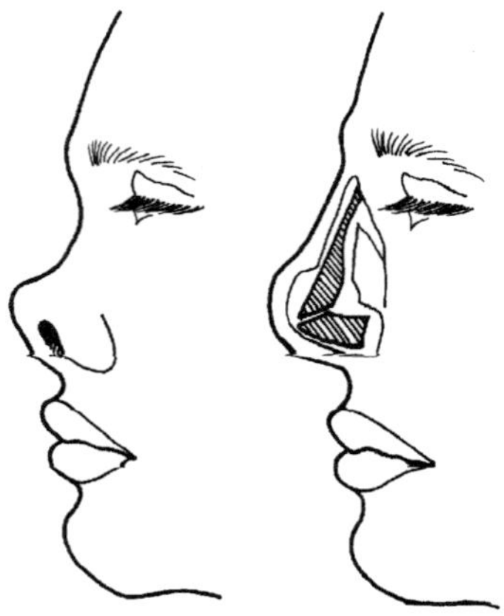

Fig. 18. Basic principle of saddle nose deformity correction using an "L"-shaped osseal or cartilaginous graft

5.1 Technique of harvesting an osseal graft

A bony graft is harvested from the pelvic bone shovel, from the area of the anterior superior iliac spine. Its anterior margin is accessed through an approximately 5cm long cut above the pelvic bone crest (figure 19). It is the case in which a rotary saw is used. Shorter incision is performed if the bony graft is removed by a chisel.

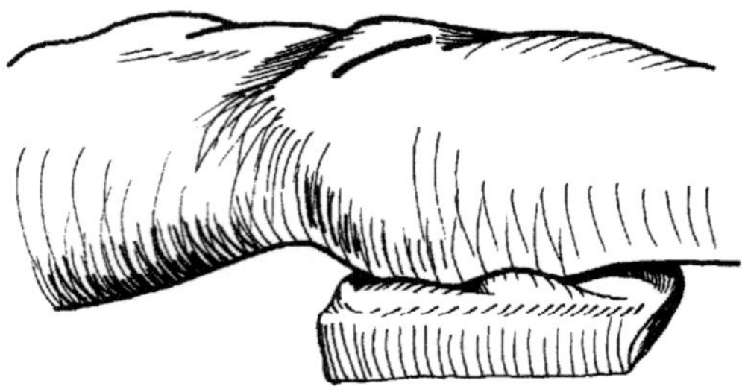

Fig. 19. Bony graft harvesting

The periosteum is torn and the bone surface is exposed. Medially, there are muscular tendons, therefore only the necessary bone area is disclosed. Resection lines are denoted by coloured pencil and from both sides the margins are partially cut using a sharp chisel, then the graft is cut off from top to bottom using a wide chisel. After harvesting the graft, bleeding from the donor site is controlled by bony wax or gel foam. Preserved periosteum is sutured in midplane. In greater part of patiens the postoperative pain is severe. Postoperative scar may cause an esthetic problem mainly in young women, therefore in such patient we predominantly use a cartilagineous graft from auricle

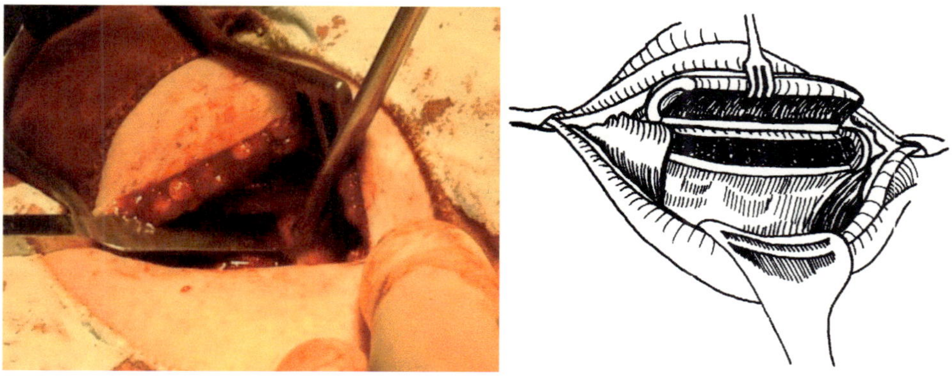

Fig. 20. Resection of bone of necessary size

The "L"-shaped graft is prepared from harvested bone material. After insertion into the prepared setting, both pieces of bone graft are sutured together in the correct angle, thereby ensuring a stable position. (figures 21 - 22)

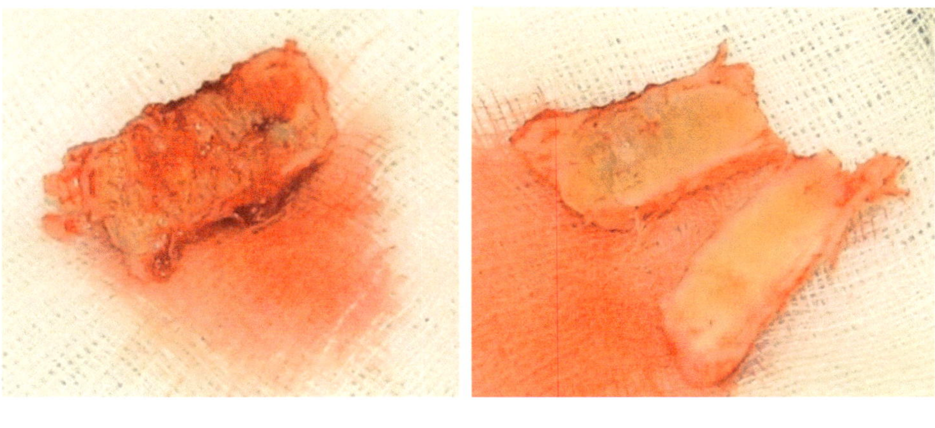

Fig. 21. Bony graft divided in two pieces

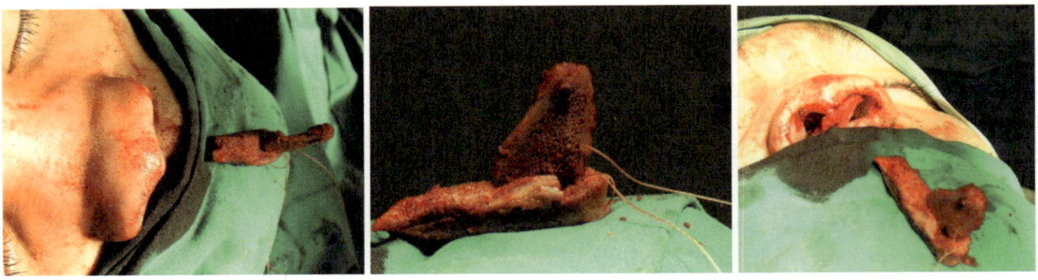

Fig. 22. Cantilever „L" shaped bony graft prepared for insertion

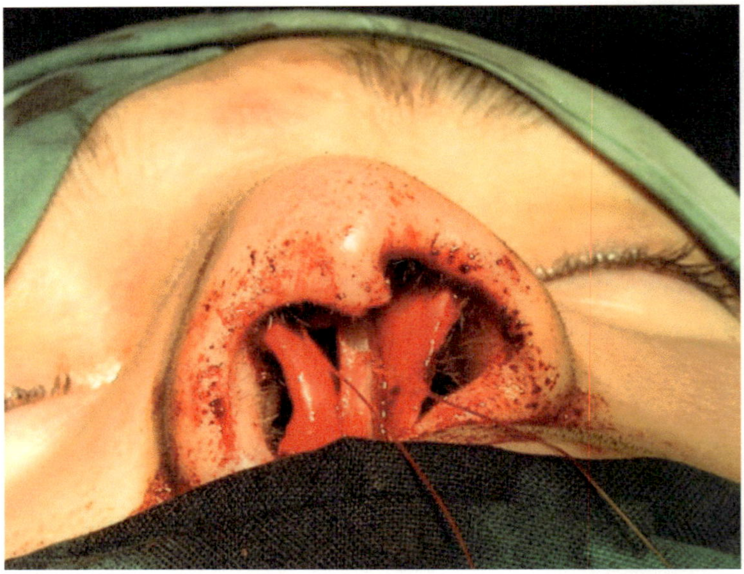

Fig. 23. Graft inserted in the nose

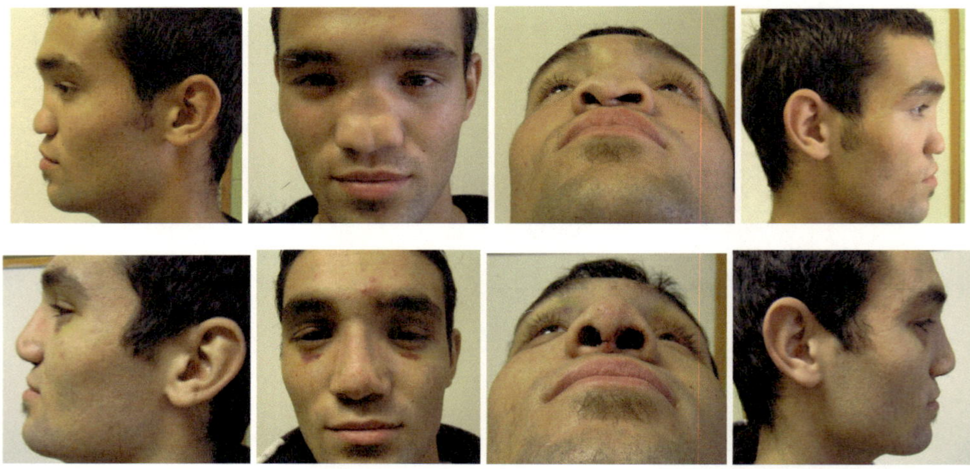

Fig. 24. Patient with sadle nose deformity (upper pictures). One week after the operation (lower pictures)

5.2 Technique of harvesting a chondral graft

A chondral graft is harvested from the cartilage by which ribs are joined to the sternum. In men, the skin incision and cartilage excision is usually localized between the sternal and parasternal line. In women, it is more convenient to plan the incision between the parasternal and mamillar lines at the lower border of the breast because the scar is then less visible.

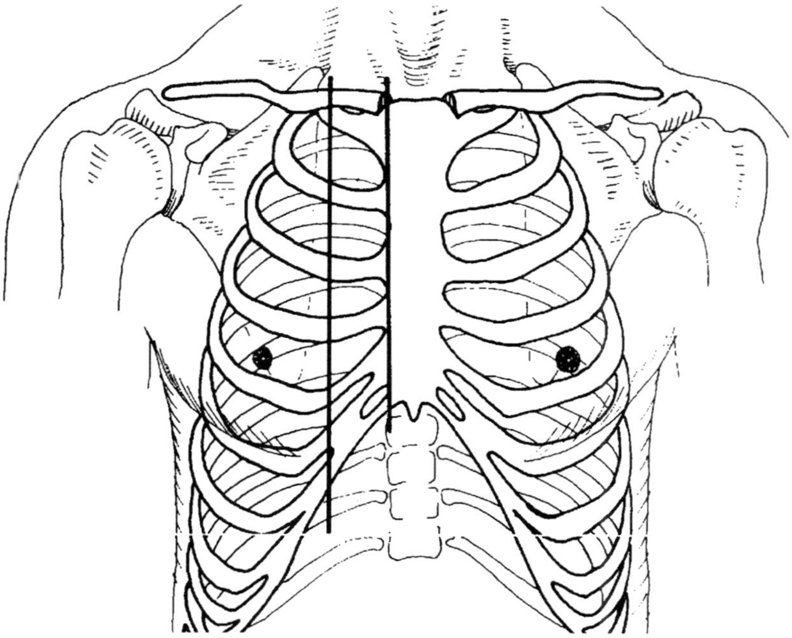

Fig. 25. Site of chondral graft harvesting

The graft can be taken from the fifth rib in cases where a combined chondro-osseous block is needed. A larger amount of cartilage occurs near the seventh and eighth ribs where the ribs are connected to one another and the cartilage is wider. An oblique skin incision about 4cm long is led downwards along the lower border of the sternal junction of the rib. The incision is started slightly laterally from the sternal border. The blunt preparation of muscles is recommended. Intercostal nerves and vessels are preserved. Preparation has to be very careful in order not to damage chest wall with pleura. In dicky situation the wound is filled with sterile saline and observed if there occur gas bubbles.Surgeon must be prepared to solve such complication as pleural tear and pneumotorax.

After uncovering the surface, the rib is prepared in its entire thickness. Rib cartilage in its entire thickness or its inferior part in accordance to actual need is resected. Sometimes in young people with enough soft cartilage just the superficial part of the rib can be harvested It is cut by a knife paralell with is longitudinal axis

If a straight graft is needed, only the central part of the cartilage is required. Shortly after dissection, the peripheral layer usually rolls to the outside. In young people the cartilage is soft and can be easily trimmed, creating a graft of the desired shape and size.

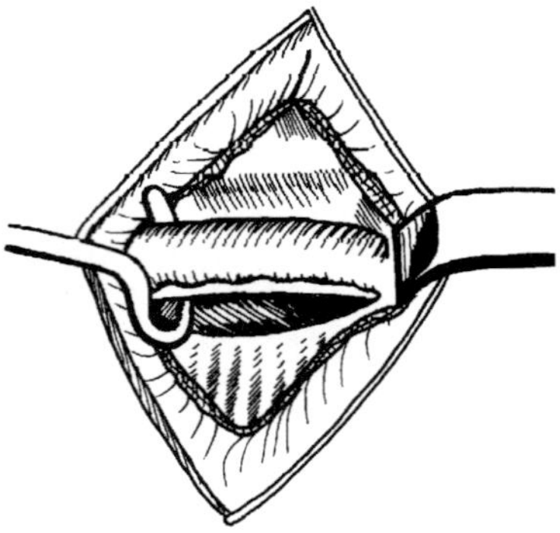

Fig. 26. Rib cartilage prepared for resection

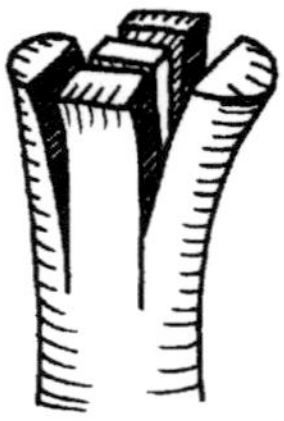

Fig. 27. After dissection the cartilage margins usually roll. The central column is more stable in shape.

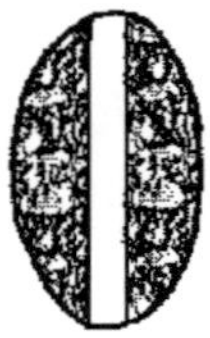

Fig. 28. Middle cartilaginous plate is resected from the rib

If a wider graft is needed, for example for septal cartilage replacement, it can be taken from the central part of a rib. In elderly people this cartilage is usually ossified and modelling is therefore more difficult.

More often in the correction of saddle nose deformity, bony material taken from the periosteum is used. The long edge of the "L"-shaped graft is inserted into the nasal dorsum in order to be in contact with the nasal bones. Thereby its nutrition and proper healing is ensured. The short edge is inserted between the medial crura of the alar cartilages to strut the nasal tip. Both edges are fixed by suture. Other parts of the nasal skeleton are corrected by means of the above-mentioned methods. A cartilaginous graft is rarely used if the patient does not agree to exstirpation of an osseous autograft from the pelvic bone.

Reparation of saddle nose deformity is among the most troublesome procedures in esthetic rhinosurgery. The choice of an optimal reparative method is based mostly on the surgeon´s own experience. Authors dealing with saddle nose deformity correction (4 - 7) consent to use predominantly autogenous materials. Autotransplant is physiologic, it heals easily and is therefore safe. It can be stored for long enough periods using appropriate methods . Homogenous material can be rapidly absorbed or rejected, which was also observed in our patients. Hellmich (8) prefers using homogenous rib cartilage stored in merthiolate. The availability and unlimited amount of well-formed material are the advantages of this method. Using any foreign material (plastic, metal and others) in the nose is risky, because rejection of such a graft may happen even after many years (9). In spite of that, some authors try to find suitable synthetic material shapable and ready for use at any moment (10,11).

Effaced cartilagineous autograft can be used to fill in any drop in the nasal dorsum. One must be gentle when working with this cartilage in order not to crush the whole piece or to destroy its structure. Bujia (12) found that after crushing the cartilage, only 10 to 30% of the chondrocytes survived. Such material can be implanted but tends to be reabsorbed. In cutting the cartilage using a sharp scalpel, the majority of the chondrocytes survive and tend to proliferate. Such cartilage is more suitable as soft tissue support against pressure or traction forces. Haas (13) warns of the possibility of rib cartilage torsion as a cause of secondary nasal deformity even after long periods. It is important to harvest the graft properly and then to trim it until a smooth surface is achieved. In implanting homogenous cartilage, more extensive reabsorption is assumed than in implanting autogenous . The advantages and disadvantages of "L"-shaped cartilage grafts were described by Fomon et al. (14) and Musebeck (15).

Daniel (16) uses an osteocartilaginous segment of a rib as a support in rhinoplasty. The bony part of the rib serves to create a new dorsal nasal contour, whereas the cartilaginous part struts the columella and elevates nasal tip projection. These segments are joined together using microscrews.

An autogenous bony graft is suitable for elevating nasal dorsal projection. It is most frequently harvested from the pelvic bone, rarely from the calva (17, 18). Takato et al. (19) prefer the qualities of an "L"-shaped bony graft. After healing, a narrow nose with elevated tip and columella projection results.

In their work from 1995, Takato and associates explored the survival rate of a bony implant inserted into the nose. The implant was placed subperiostally in order to be in direct contact with the nasal bones. In a group of 14 patients, they found that the graft diminished slightly and its margins became curved during the first 2-3 months in the new enviroment. After six months there were no significant macroscopic changes in the graft. Burian (9) stated that, with the exception of nasal bones and nasal septal bones, every implanted autogenous bone undergoes remodeling of its structure. After some time it is remodeled and replaced by new bony tissue. In correcting saddle nose deformity, the author emphasises direct contact of implanted bone with original nasal bones. If the implanted bone is not in this close contact, it can be completely absorbed later on. The time interval depends on the graft´s structure. Compact bone may be absorbed after several years, spongious usually sooner.

In our first group of 10 patients, with the exception of one case, an autogenous bone or cartilage graft was used in saddle nose deformity correction. The patients were followed up for one to six years post-operation. In all cases, the autogenous material healed and no complications of graft rejection were observed. In one patient, after the implantation of fresh rib cartilage, elevation of the upper margin in the nasal root region became evident. Some patients had marked combined nasal deformity after an injury and therefore the esthetic result following septorhinoplasty was not as perfect as they had anticipated. We are aware that repeated surgical procedure on a previously repaired nose involves some risk because it may endanger the original graft and cause new scar formation. This is why no further correction was performed in these cases.

5.3 Postoperative care

Comprehensive and adequate postoperative care is as important as proper operative technique. This includes external nasal fixation, dressing and internal nasal fixation, and general and local drug therapy during the postoperative period.

6. External nasal fixation

At the end of surgery, after shaping and repositioning the nose into the medial plane, it should be properly fixed. External fixation is achieved with taping, plaster of Paris, metal or plastic splints, stomatologic thermoplastic material, etc. We usually apply modified plaster splints attached to the forehead, which better fix the nose in the middle plane. Nasal skin is first covered using Leukopor (paper tape) by which gives a proportional pressure of skin to subcutis (figure 29). Then a plaster splint accomodated to nasal proportions is applied and held in place by finger pressure until it dries (figure 30,). This part of fixation is very important. If back pressure is not created, the plaster splint will extend and the nasal root will remain wide. Finally, the plaster splint is affixed using Leukoplast (plastic tape) to the cheek and forehead. The splint is changed when postoperative swelling subsides, usually three to five days after surgery. The overall period of external fixation is about ten days. In cases in which an osteotomy was not performed, a smaller plaster splint covering only the external nose is applied. It creates back pressure on the internal dressing and helps to maintain the desired nasal shape in the early postoperative period. Such a splint is left in place for a few days. In patients who for any reason tolerate external splinting badly, a minimum period of 7 days of fixation is recommended.

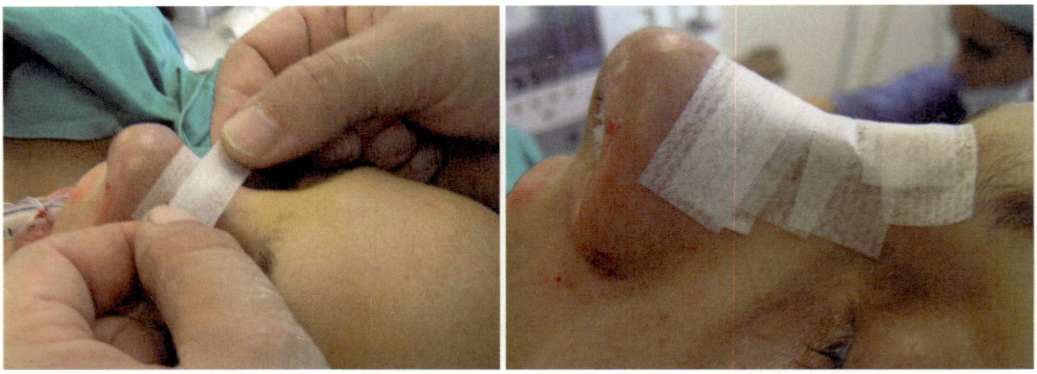

Fig. 29. Nasal dorsum is covered with paper tape

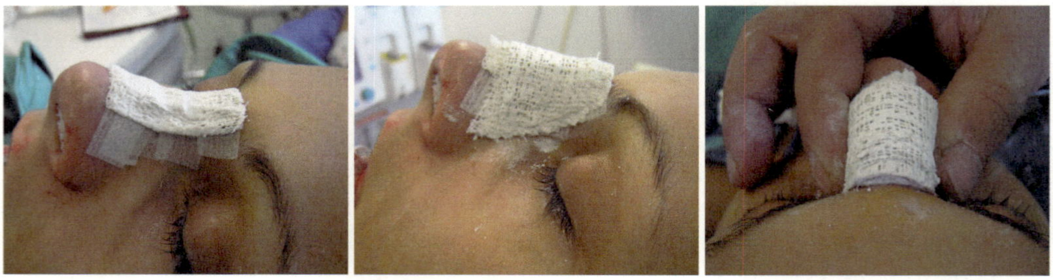

Fig. 30. Modelation of plaster splint

7. Tamponade, internal nasal splints

Nasal cavity packing with vaseline dressing gauze is used after each septorhinoplasty for a postoperative period of 24 hours. Tamponade lessens postoperative bleeding, development of a synechia or hematoma, and fixes and holds together intransal incision margins. The patient tolerates tamponade quite well after surgery using general anesthesia until the next day. After removing the tamponade, the nose is left free.

Internal splints are used after any operation for septal perforation. Original splints from the firm XOMED or thick polyethylene foil is arranged according to the size of the nasal cavity and is placed on both sides of the nasal septum. The splints are fixed by transseptal silon suture. Until the first postoperative day, a light nasal packing is added. Internal splints are removed after 7 days at the earliest. In cases in which bilateral subperichondrial septal tunnels were created, it is not recommended to apply only internal splints without tamponade. An intranasal splint alone does not avoid the formation of a hematoma nor does it improve nasal ventilation in the early postoperative period. Certain improvement of nasal ventilation, and thereby the patient´s comfort, can be achieved by inserting an intranasal plastic splint with a tube for breathing. These splints are expensive but they can be replaced for example by a thin intubation tube.

In our opinion, for proper septal fixation and hemostasis in the early postoperative period, it is necessary to put a vaseline or other type of nasal packing into the nasal cavity. Tamponade must be compact enough in order not to shift into the nasopharynx or to be aspirated. Of course, any foreign body in the nasal cavity causes discomfort. The patient feels pressure in his nose, unpleasant mucosal flow, must breath through his mouth and has a sense of dry mouth, etc.. Serpell and associates (20) examined the influence of nasal packing on blood oxygen saturation during sleep. They discovered that nasal packing does not have a fundamental influence on oxygen saturation in otherwise healthy individuals. Nevertheless, in patients with ventilation nasal tubes better objective and subjective results were observed.

After septoplasty in which a synechia between the nasal septum and the lateral nasal wall is split, a soft polyethylene foil covering the wound surface is inserted. The foil is fixed by septal suture and left in place for 14 days.

8. Local and general therapy in the postoperative period

Standard local therapy after septorhinoplasty includes intranasal antibiotic ointment and paraffin oil. Long lasting swelling mainly at the nasal tip is managed by skin massage with nutritive cream. Local administration of corticosteroids by injection in the case of subcutaneous scarring after surgery is evaluated very carefully. After initial improvement, repeated application may cause subsequent weakening or even atrophy of subcutaneous tissues, with unfavourable consequences.

General antibiotic therapy is indicated in patients after complicated nasal surgery with the open approach and with autotransplant insertion.

9. References

[1] Huizing, E.H., De Groot, J.A.M.: Techniques in functional corrective nasal surgery. Utrecht, Printing Office University Hospital 1995, 33 s.

[2] Orak, F. a spol.: Reversed roof graft for the severely deviated nose. Aesthetic Plast. Surg., 19, 1995, č. 1, s. 31–36.
[3] Mommaerts, M.Y. et al.: Rhinoplasty with nasal bone disarticulation to deepen the nasofrontal groove. Experimental and clinical results. J. Craniomaxilofac. Surg., 23, 1995, č. 2, s. 109–114.
[4] Ortiz-Monasterio, F.: Rhinoplasty. Philadelphia, W.B. Saunders 1994, 291 s.
[5] Candiani, P. a spol.: Anatomical reconstruction versus camouflage of the inferior two thirds of the nasal seotum. Ann. Plast. Surg., 34, 1995, č. 6, s. 625–630.
[6] Johnson, C.M., Toriumi. D.M.: Open structure rhinoplasty, W.B. Saunders Company, Philadelphia, 1990, 516 s.
[7] Nicolle, F.V.: Aesthetic rhinoplasty. London, W.B. Saunders 1996, 126 s.
[8] Hellmich, S.: Der Einfluss unterschiedlicher Konservierungsmethoden auf die biologisme Qalität von Knorpelimplantaten. Larzng Rhinol Otol, 53, 1974,10, p.711-717
[9] Burian, F.: Plastická chirurgie. Praha, Nakladatelství Československé akademie věd 1959, 101 s.
[10] Owsley, T.G., Taylor, C.O.: The use of Gore-Tex for nasal augmentation, a retrospective analysis of 105 patients. Plast. Reconstr. Surg., 94, 1994, č. 2, p. 241–248.
[11] Lindsey, WH., Ogle, RS., Morgan, RF., Cantrell, RW., Sweenyz, TM.: Nasal reconstruction using an osteoconductive collagen matrix. Ach Otolarzngol Head Neck Surg, 122, 1996, 1. p.37-40
[12] Bujia, J.: Determination of the viability of crushed cartilage grafts: clinical implications for wound healing in nasal surgery. Ann. Plast. Surg., 32, 1994, č. 3, s. 261–265.
[13] Haas, E.: Materialbedingte Gefahren bei der Sattelnasenkorektur. Laryngol. Rhinol. Otol., 48, 1969, č. 1, s. 28–34.
[14] Fomon, S. a spol.: Saddle nose and the "L" shaped graft. Arch. Otolaryng., 71, 1960, s. 932–940.
[15] Musebeck, K.: Nachteile der Winkelspäne bei der Sattelnasenkorrektur. Laryngol. Rhinol. Otol., 48, 1969, č. 1, s. 34–37.
[16] Daniel,RK.: Rhinoplasty and rib grafts: evolving a flexible optative technice. Plast Reconstr Surg, 94,1994, 5, p. 597-609
[17] Citardi, MJ., Friedman, CD.: Nonvascularized autogenous bone grafts for craniofacial skeletal augmentationand replacement, Otolaryngol Clin North Am, 27, 1994, p 894–910
[18] Frodel, JL.: Management of the nasal dorsum in central facial injuries. Indications for calvarial bone rafting.Arch Otolaryngol Head Neck Surg., 121, 1995, 3,p 307 - 12
[19] Takato, T., Yonehara, Y, Mori, Y, Susami, T.: Use of cantilever iliac bone grafts fro reconstruction of cleft lip-associated nasal deformities. J Oral Maxilofc Surg, 53, 1995,7, p.757-62
[20] Serpell, MG., Padgham, N., McQeen, F.m, Block, R., Thomson, M.: The influence of nasal obstruction and its reliéf on oxygen saturation during sleep at the early postoperative period. Anesthesia, 49,1994, 6,p.538-540

2

Le Fort I Osteotomy for Maxillary Repositioning and Distraction Techniques

Antonio Cortese
University of Salerno
Italy

1. Introduction

Despite the widespread acceptance of various classifications for midface fractures, the most commonly used for describing these fractures remains the classical one described by the French physician Rene Le Fort in 1901 (Le Fort, 1900, 1901).

The technique for maxillary osteotomy type Le Fort I was performed for the first time by Cheever in 1864 for rinofaringeal tumor resection (Halvorson & Mulliken, 2008).

In 1921 Herman Wassmund performed a Le Fort I osteotomy for dentofacial deformity correction without intraoperative mobilization, which was achieved by orthopedic traction in the post operative time (Wassmund, 1927, 1935).

In 1934 Auxhausen performed a Le Fort I osteotomy mobilization for open bite correction (Axhausen, 1934), but only in 1952, in the USA, Converse described his cases operated by maxillary osteotomy and large vestibular and palatal elevation for Le Fort I osteotomy combined with midpalatal osteotomy (Converse, 1952).

After this report some other surgeons performed maxillary osteotomies for open bite correction, but results were not stable (Steinhausen, 1996). Only in 1974 Stoker and in 1975 Epker, reported encouraging results in dentofacial deformity correction using down fracture technique for complete maxillary mobilization by Le Fort I osteotomy (Stoker, 1974; Epker, 1975).

After encouraging reports by some American surgeons (Converse, 1969) who published several methods for correction of jaw deformities and stressed the importance of close collaboration between surgeon and orthodontist, other surgeons (Obwegeser, Wilmar, Bell) started to widely adopt maxillary osteotomies for dentofacial deformity correction (Obwegeser, 1969; Bell, 1975, Hogeman & Wilmar, 1967).

An important contribution to orthognatic surgery came from Obwegeser's unit in Zurich (Switzerland) and from many excellent textbooks on orthognatic surgery published in the 80s by different American surgeons (Bell, 1980; Bell, 1985, Epker and Fish, 1986; Profitt and White, 1991).

Before 1965 this kind of deformities were commonly treated only by mandibular osteotomies even if skeletal problems were present in maxillary bones, but final results were not aesthetically satisfactory. An important progress in orthognatic surgery was the 'two-jaws surgery' with the simultaneous mobilization of the total maxilla and mandible. Köle introduced bimaxillary alveolar surgery in 1959, but Obwegeser published his experience in 1970 as the first surgeon who had performed total mandibular and maxillary osteotomies (Obwegeser, 1970). Nowadays the Le Fort I osteotomies are widely employed in dentofacial deformities correction in consideration of the new aesthetic concept of facial beauty.

2. Le Fort I osteotomy and facial aesthetic evolution

The first parameter for facial beauty is symmetry, which is probably related to the expression of a correct genetic asset of each individual. In a study by Little (Little et al., 2001), different images (symmetric and asymmetric) of the same subject were shown to a group of young females and the concept of beauty was identified in symmetric images (Perrett et al., 1999). Secondly the concept of beauty has been modifying towards bi-protrusive cephalometric type as shown by most contemporary actors' faces; probably because maxillary bi-protrusion strongly suggests a complete genetic growth expression (Arnett & Gunson, 2010). The third point for a modern concept of beauty of the face is a wide smile without black corridors in the lateral area of the mouth; also a gingival exposure of the upper dental arch is commonly accepted for a durable beauty of the face and young appearance in consideration of the natural drop of the smile height in older age (Arnett & Gunson, 2004).

The fourth point is the association of malar bones and mandibular lower border evidence, resulting in good face skin tension with cheek concavity , without any sub-mental and cheek folds (Naini et al., 2006).

This new concept of beauty largely influences the planning of dentofacial deformity correction with an indication to increase facial skeleton dimension either by Le Fort I osteotomies alone or in association with mandibular surgery.

Because the patient's main request in dentofacial deformity treatment is a new aesthetical balance of the face (see fig.1) involving good occlusion, good masticatory function, aesthetic of the smile, aesthetic of the facial skeleton contour (zygomatic and mandibular border evidence) and high ratio between facial skeleton and skin amount for good skin tension and juvenile looking; a new kind of operation and surgical planning has been developed in maxillofacial surgery (Merli et al., 2007; Triaca et al., 2004, 2009, 2010).

Many of these procedures involve the Le Fort I osteotomies with new variations and techniques like osteodistraction and bone augmentation and a skill team working with intense cooperation between Maxillofacial surgeons, orthodontists, dentists and anesthesiologists (Cortese et al., 2003, 2009, 2010, 2011).

3. Le Fort I type osteotomy: Classic surgical technique

Bleeding control and vascular preservation after complete mobilization of the maxillary segments in order to avoid vascular necrosis were the main problems that maxillofacial surgeons had to face at the beginning of the Le Fort I type osteotomy surgery.

For these reasons vascular studies were performed by Turvey and Fonseca on maxillary artery anatomy (Turvey & Fonseca, 1980) and the importance of accurate surgery technique in the posterior maxilla area to preserve the integrity of the maxillary artery. The importance of soft posterior tissue pedicles for maxillary blood supply was investigated by Bell (Bell, 1973), Justus by a laser Doppler analysis and Jones, who suggested attention to vascular risk, particularly in patients using orthodontic appliances or post-surgical splints (Justus et al., 2001; Jones, 2001). Teeth modification with narrowing of the pulp canals after Le Fort I osteotomy was investigated also by Ellingsen and Artun (Ellingsen & Artun, 1993) but the conclusion over 30 years of Le Fort I osteotomy is that no major problems are usually reported after maxillary osteotomies following recommended techniques (Panula et al., 2001); life-threatening complications are very rare (Van de Perre et al., 1996; Acebal-Bianco et al., 2000).

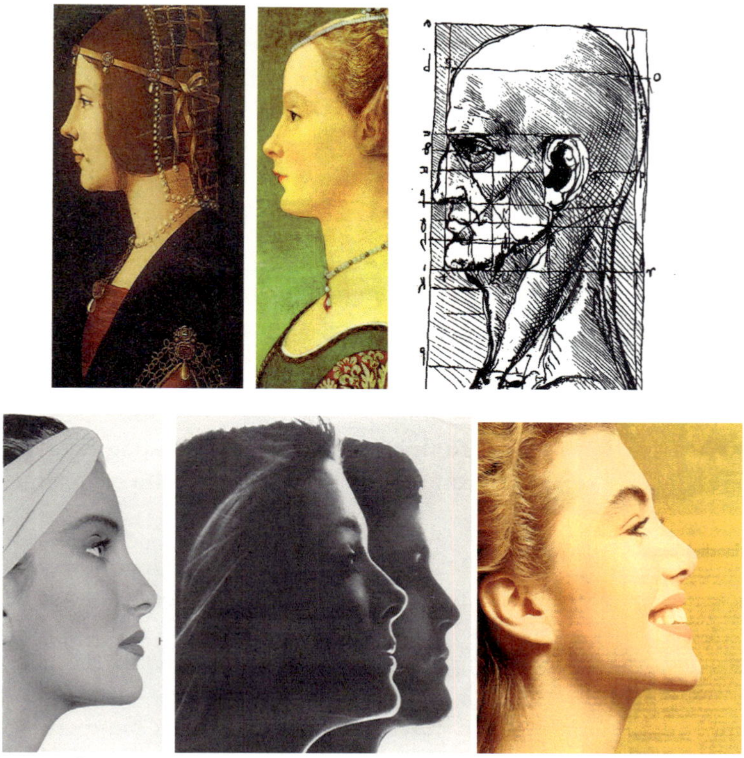

Fig. 1. Classic versus modern concepts of beauty face

Avascular necrosis related to lack in blood supply is one of the main complications after Le Fort I osteotomy and has been reported by some studies (Parnes & Becker, 1972; Lanigan, 1993) with an occurrence fewer than 1% after this kind of surgery.

The main problems related to vascular compromise after maxillary mobilization are rupture of the descending palatal artery, post-operative thrombosis, perforation of the palatal mucosa in segmented maxillary surgery and partial stripping or excessive tension of the palatal fibromucosa in maxillary expansion (Lanigan et al., 1990). Anatomic irregularities such as craniofacial dysplasias, orofacial clefts, or vascular anomalies increase the risks of vascular problems following maxillary osteotomy surgery (Kramer et al., 2004). Expecially in the segmented Le Fort I, palatal fibromucosa preservation is an important factor to avoid partial necrosis and malunion of the maxillary bone fragments particularly in patients with orthodontic appliances or palatal splint causing pressure on the palatal mucosa.

External reference landmarks are established at the nasofrontal area by inserting a pin into bone after a stab incision, in order to record the vertical measurement from the pin to the incisal edge of the maxillary incisors for proper vertical positioning of the maxilla after osteotomies. In the Author experience external reference is more reliable than reference mark on the maxilla, but multiple control references are advised because correct maxillary repositioning is fundamental for postoperative final symmetry of the face. For these reasons, direct control of the bipupillar line and occlusal planes symmetry and the midline alignment of the frontonasal (Nasion), interincisal and Pogonion points must be checked before final fixation of the maxilla.

Also intermediate maxillary splint for maxilla repositioning is not completely reliable because mandibular condyles may be displaced from the glenoid fossae during repositioning and fixation procedures.

3.1 Soft tissue incision

Before proceeding to the surgical incision a solution of local anaesthetic with epinephrine (2% lidocaine with 1:100000 epinephrine) is infiltrated into the buccal mucosa along the entire surface of the maxilla in order to minimize bleeding and increase anaesthesia during surgical procedure. Because palatal soft tissue is an important vascular pedicle for the maxilla after complete LeFort I osteotomy, no injection is performed in the palatal region.

Total blood loss is significantly reduced during surgery also elevating of 15 degrees patient's head and by systolic blood pressure control (about 90 mmHg) with hypotensive anaesthesia (Shepherd, 2004).

Soft tissues incision is performed bilaterally from the midline of the fornix above the central incisors to first molar region, involving mucosa, muscle and periosteum; after the incision, blood supply of the maxilla is guaranteed by a wide pedicle of buccal tissue over the teeth. A subperiosteal dissection made with a periosteal elevator exposes the lateral wall of the maxilla, from the pterygomaxillary junction to the anterior nasal spine. At this point it is important to identify and protect the infraorbital neurovascular bundle; dissection should not be extended to tissues set behind the incision, in order to preserve an optimal perfusion of the maxilla (see fig. 2 and fig. 3).

The dissection continues toward the maxillary tuberosity and pterygoid plate, with an inferior angled fold behind the zygomatic buttress. In this area it is recommended to achieve a mucosal tunnelling under direct vision, to preserve a wide-based, intact part of buccal soft tissues. During this procedure the buccal fat pad can be exposed, covering the surgical field: using a retractor the fat pad can be displaced laterally, after covering it with a moistened gauze.

The piriform aperture is exposed, and the mucoperiosteum is elevated along the piriform rim, the nasal floor and the lateral wall under the inferior turbinate, then reflected with a periostal elevator to expose the anterior floor of the nose. The septopremaxillary ligament is transected as well as the transverse nasalis muscle to completely free the anterior nasal spine. Obviously a careful management of the nasal mucosa, without perforations and cuts, minimizes blood loss and reduces postoperative discomfort.

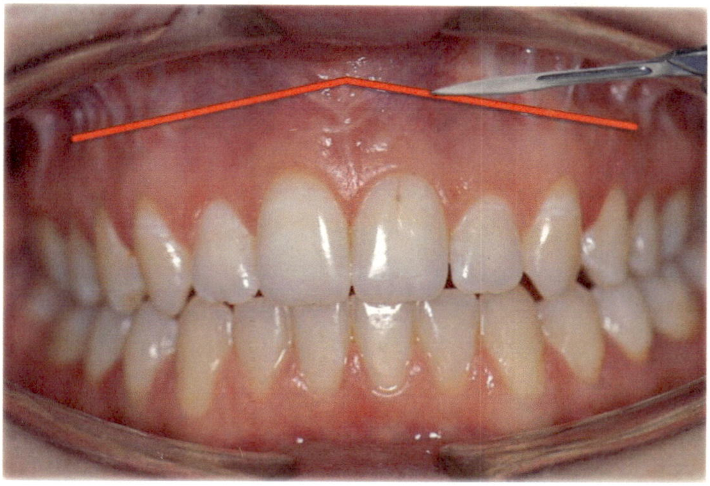

Fig. 2. Buccal mucosa incision starts from the zygomatic buttress 5 mm over the dental roots apices and proceeds across the median region up to the opposite site, from 1.6 to 2.6.

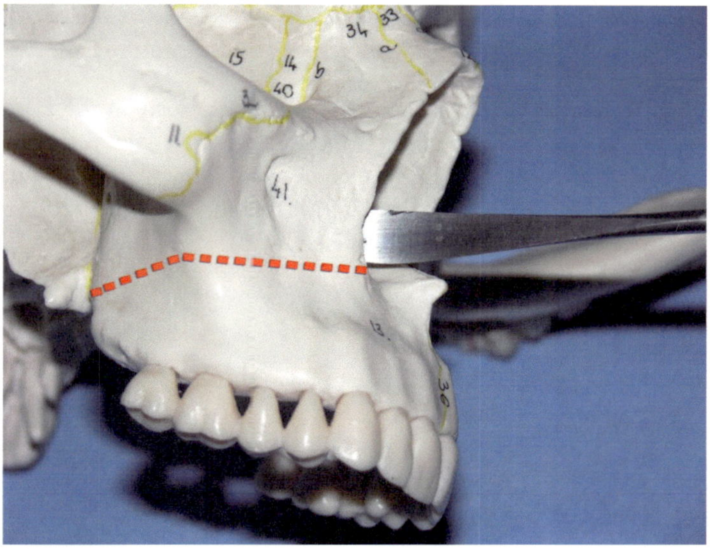

Fig. 3. Periosteum elevation both on buccal and nasal side of the maxilla.

3.2 Osteotomy techniques

Once the dissection is completed, reference points are established before performing osteotomy. Vertical reference landmarks are scratched with a bur at the piriform aperture region and at the zygomatico-maxillary region; the couples of holes in cortical bone stand 5 millimetres above and 5 millimetres beneath the imaginary line of planned osteotomy (see fig. 4); if a maxillary impaction is planned this distance has to be increased, depending on the amount of the impaction. Using the callipers, two holes 4 mm above the apices of the canine and the first molar are marked to help positioning of the first osteotomy line. Together with the external landmarks described before, these intraoral points allow vertical and horizontal positioning of the maxilla after the mobilization is made; also the occlusal splint will help the proper fixation of the maxilla in the sagittal and vertical planes.

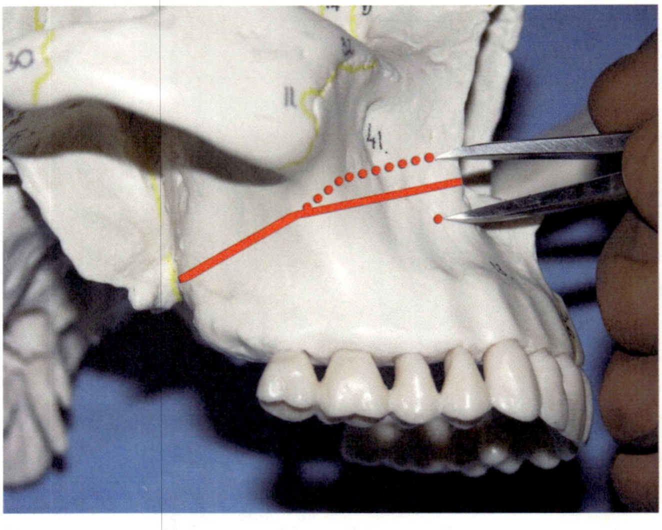

Fig. 4. Amount of bone removal measured by caliper at the osteotomy site.

The osteotomy begins placing a bur or a surgical saw posteriorly at the zygomatic buttress, about 35 mm above the occlusal pane, and advances through lateral maxillary wall to the piriform rim. Before performing the osteotomy of the lateral wall of the nose, a periostal elevator is inserted subperiosteal under the inferior turbinate, at the piriform aperture for 2 cm approximately, to protect the nasal mucosa (see fig. 5).

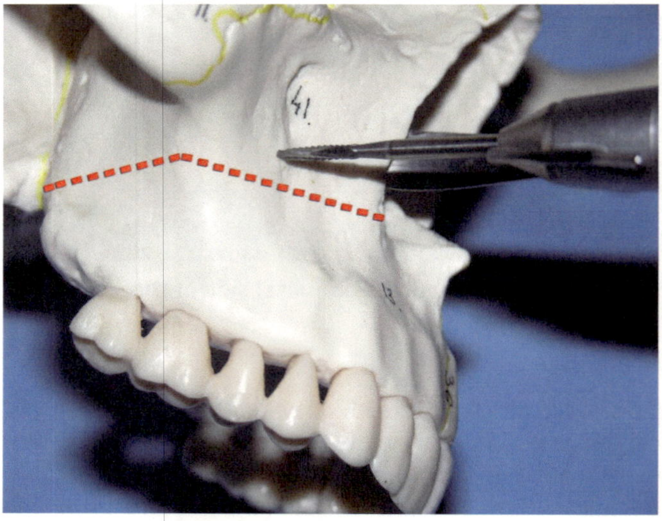

Fig. 5. Maxilla bone cut from the piriform fossae up to the tuber maxillae.

To complete the section of the lateral posterior wall of the maxilla, a flexible retractor must be placed under the periostium at the junction of the maxillary tuberosity with the pterygoid plates, to avoid the risk of damaging the maxillary artery or one of its branches

In this area the osteotomy is directed inferiorly and posteriorly, under direct vision with high carefulness. Once the section of the lateral maxillary wall is completed, the direction of the saw is reversed so that the blade cuts laterally from the sinus to the outside: this shift allows an easy sectioning of the posterior maxillary wall.

Referring to the amount of maxillary impaction planned before surgery, adequate amount of bone will be removed by the saw or bur from the lateral piriform rim to the posterolateral sinus wall. In this posterior aspect, amount of bone removal will be less than planned for impaction, because of the bone thinness and telescopic movements frequently seen in this area.

The osteotomy line should always run at least 5 mm above the second molar roots to reduce the risk of devitalizing teeth. If an impacted molar is placed over the line, the osteotomy design must not be modified: it will be removed at the end of the procedure, after downfracture. The same procedure is repeated on the opposite side and wet gauzes are introduced in the posterior aspect of the wound to minimize blood loss.

At this point osteotomy of the septum and the lateral nasal wall are performed. A septal osteotome is carefully inserted along the septal crest of the maxilla under the intact nasal mucosa, in order to separate the cartilaginous and bony septum from the septal crest of the maxilla (see fig. 6).

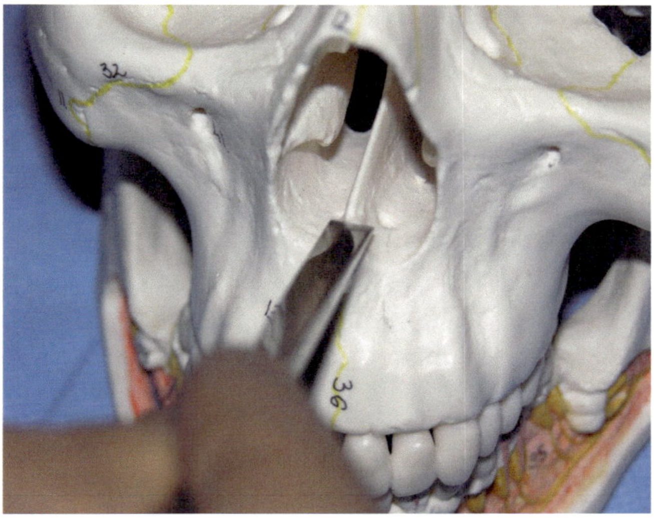

Fig. 6. Nasal septum disarticulation from anterior nasal spine and septal crest of the maxilla.

An elevator protect the nasal mucosa when the nasal lateral wall is sectioned by an osteotome directed posteriorly and inferiorly toward the perpendicular plate of the palatine bone. Particular care must be paid to this step of the procedure: bone of the lateral wall of the nose is thin with few resistance to the chisel; when the vertical pillar of the palatine bone is reached, resistance will increase with detectable change in sound when malleting the chisel (see fig. 7).

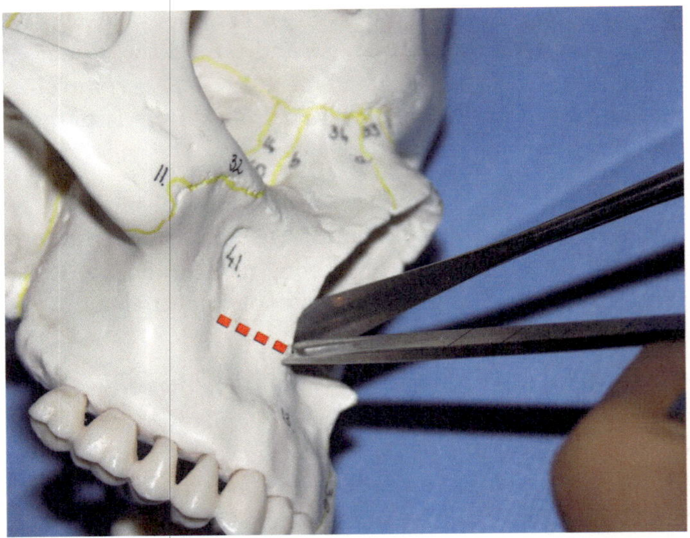

Fig. 7. Nasal wall osteotomy protecting nasal mucosa by elevator (dotted line for osteotomy inside the nasal cavity).

Partial section of the perpendicular plate of the palatine bone must be performed in order to avoid bad-fracture at the downfracture step resulting in an higher fracturing line than the nasal floor plane. This surgical event could lead to disruption of the orbit or even of the cranial base. If the osteotomy is carried out too deeply in the vertical plate of the palatine bone it could result in injury of the descending palatine vessels with a bleeding difficult to control before performing the downfracture. The opposite lateral nasal wall will be sectioned following the same procedure and the osteotomy of the nasal septum will be carried out. If the maxilla remains firmly attached to its bony base posteriorly after complete section of the buccal cortical plane, of the lateral walls of the nasal cavity and septum foot, osteotomy of the pterigomaxillary junction will be performed.

After removing gauze sponges previously placed, a retractor is inserted subperiosteally in order to place a curved osteotome at the junction of the maxilla and pterygoid plate. An index finger is placed on the palate at the amular notch region in order to feel the tip of the osteotome when malleting (see fig. 8). The same procedure will be performed on the other side and downfracture is performed using finger pressure on the anterior aspect of the maxilla or by Rowe forceps. During this procedure nasal mucosa partially attached is carefully elevated from the nasal floor.

Particulary when impaction of the maxilla is planned remaining vomer, septum, septal crest and lateral nasal walls are reduced by rongeur or bur, to accomplish any superior setting. After downfracture, mobilized maxilla freely move in all of the three planes. Usually the neurovascular bundle of the descending palatine vessels are commonly preserved and bone should be removed carefully from the posterior maxilla. If this bundle is injured bleeding can be controlled by packing, cautery or vascular clamps; sensibility in the maxillary area is usually preserved even performing these manoeuvres (Bouloux & Bays, 2000).

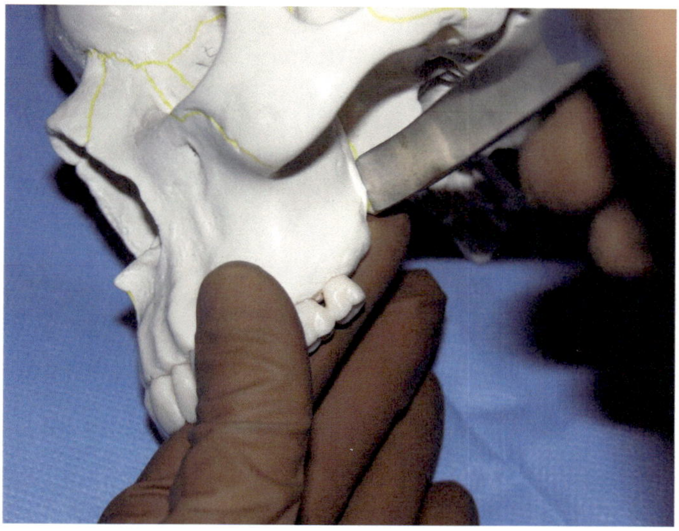

Fig. 8. Section of the pterygo-maxillary junction by curved chisel under finger control on the palatal side.

Also removing bone from the pterygoid plates can cause bleeding from the pterygoid muscles, usually controlled by packing or injecting dilute epinephrine solution. Bone interferences are common in this area and must be carefully eliminated for proper maxillary repositioning even if it's a time-consuming procedure. At this time an occlusal wafer splint is inserted and maxilla and mandible are fixed togheter by 25-Gauge wire for maxillomandibular fixation. Then the maxillomandibular complex with the inserted splint will be turned up to the proper position, detecting bone premature contacts and taking care not to dislocate condyles from glenoid fossae (see fig. 9). Measurement of the distance

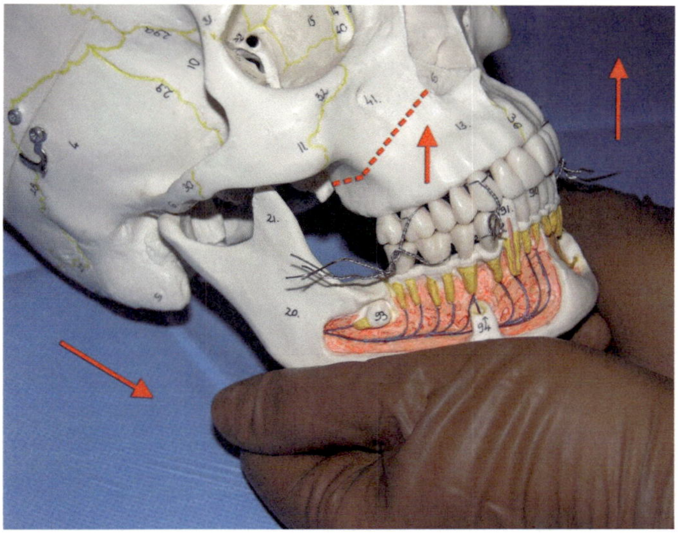

Fig. 9. Maxillary fixation after maxillo-mandibular block checking centric condilar position in the glenoid fossae.

between intraoral and extraoral reference points is performed to ascertain that proper maxilla repositioning has been achieved. Attention must be paid to bone precontacts causing mandibular condyle dislocation and septum deviation with nasal airflow obstruction. If more than 5 millimetres maxillary impaction is planned, also trimming of the inferior turbinates is suggested. Gross tears and nasal mucosa holes must be repaired by 4-0 Vicryl suture to minimize nasal bleeding.

3.3 Maxillary segmentation

If a segmented Le Fort I is planned for maxillary expansion, or for occlusal plane levelling for open or deep bite correction, or for space closure after dental extraction in Class II correction, the segmentation should be performed before the downfracture for better handling of the bone fragments. In the two pieces maxillary segmentation interdental osteotomy il performed between the central incisors roots, under finger control by the palatal side (see fig. 10).

For maintaining vascular supply of the maxillary bones, no more than three or at least four pieces segmentation must be performed, because risks of necrosis increase with multiple segmentation. Also the integrity of the palatal mucosa is mandatory to avoid necrosis problems of the anterior maxilla and teeth. For these reasons sagittal segmentation is usually performed in para-median sites, where bone is thin and palatal mucosa is thicker than the midline, avoiding risks of palatal mucosa perforation (see fig. 11). In the three pieces maxillary segmentation, interdental osteotomy sites are usually located between canine and bicuspidate roots, where a 3 millimetres space must be created with orthodontic treatment for parodontal safety (Dorfman & Turvey, 1979) (see fig. 11 and fig. 12). In this three pieces maxilla segmentation is performed placing the osteotomy sites in a bilateral position between the roots of canine and first bicuspids, lateral sites of the palate, and a transversal osteotomy of conjunction (see fig. 13).

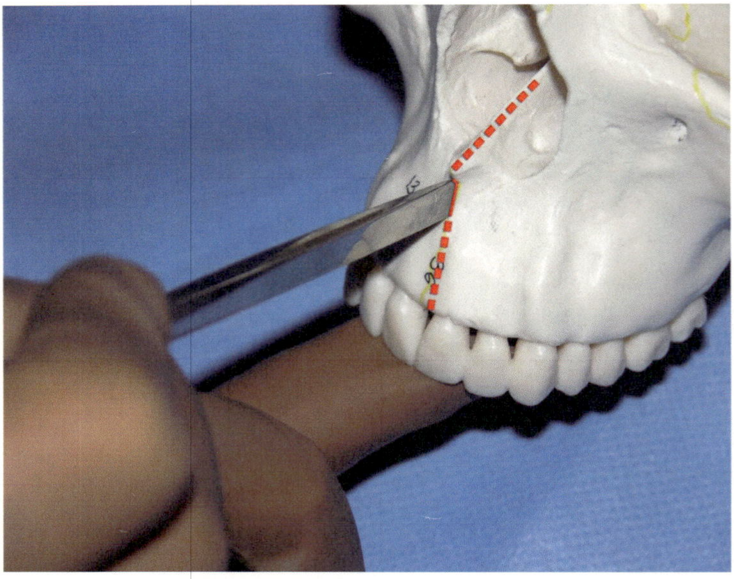

Fig. 10. Interdental midline osteotomy under finger control by the palatal side.

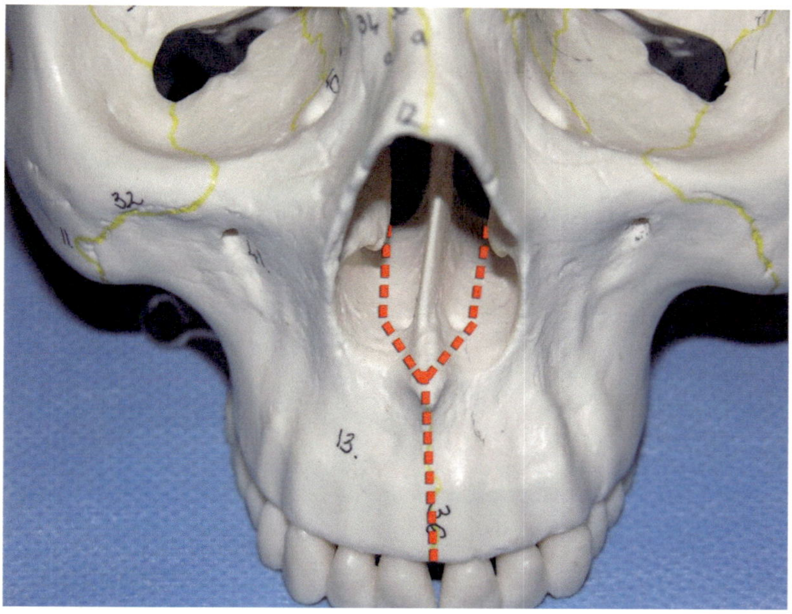

Fig. 11. Midline interdental and palatal para-median osteotomy for the two pieces maxilla segmentation.

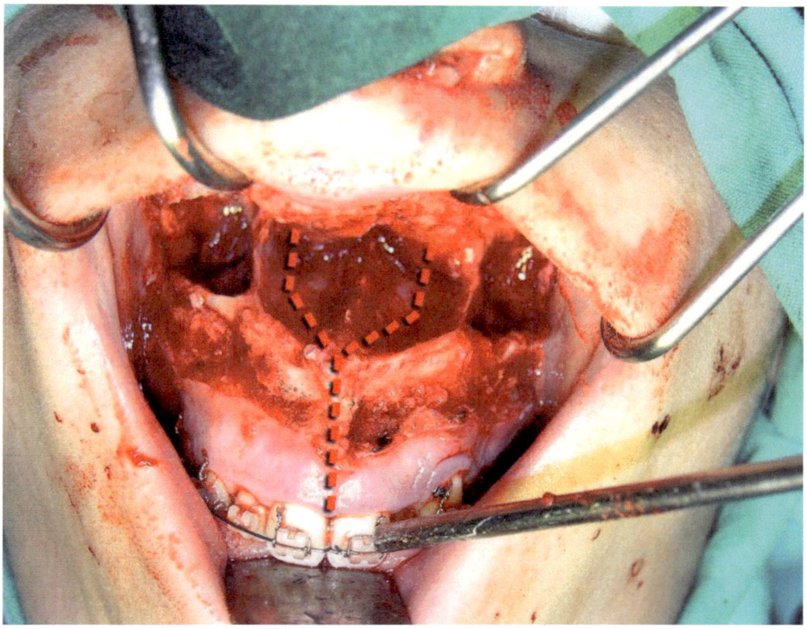

Fig. 12. Down fracture in Le Fort I osteotomy with possibility to perform maxillary segmentation.

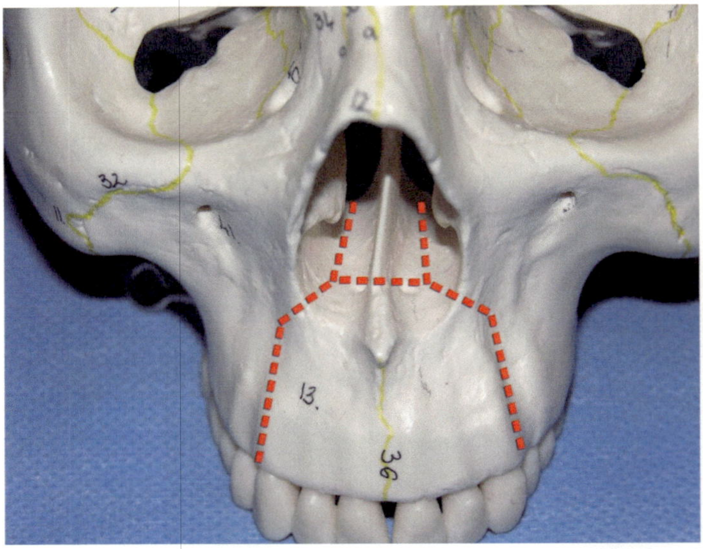

Fig. 13. Interdental and palatal lateral osteotomy plus transversal palatal osteotomy for the three pieces maxilla segmentation.

Even if this kind of segmentation is commonly performed in the Le Fort I osteotomy with down fracture, expansion and three dimensional repositioning (LFI-E), nowadays segmented Le Fort I is frequently associated with other techniques like surgical assisted rapid palatal expansion (SARPE), tooth-borne or bone-borne distraction for specific consideration about related problems, complications and indication:

1. In maxillary two pieces sagittal segmentation for palatal expansion, relapse is a frequent problem, in association with heavy limits to palatal expansion for fibro-mucosa inextensibility and related risks of aseptic necrosis for excessive tension of the fibro-mucosa (Cortese et al., 2010; Haas, 1980; Wertz, 1970.
2. Even if in maxillary three or four pieces segmentation for palatal expansion and occlusal plane levelling, fibro-mucosa tension is distributed in multiple sites, the aforementioned problems and complication occur any way for the extensive dissection need of the palatal fibro-mucosa ; moreover multiple segment management during operation is difficult.
3. About the maxillary segmentation technique for space closure after bicuspidate extraction for Class II correction (Wassmund), it is nowadays frequently avoided in favour of mandibular advancement alone or in combination with maxillary expansion for correct interdental arches relations after mandibular advancement .

For more extensive information about bone-born maxillary expansion techniques, refer to the specific paragraph of this chapter (Palatal expansion: bone born techniques).

3.4 Fixation

Before proceeding with fixation, it is advisable to expose the nasal floor and the posterior maxillary area and wash with saline solution to remove blood clots. Maxillary fixation requires occlusal splint insertion to achieve the correct maxillary position. In the classic technique occlusal splint are taken in place by four transosseous wire sutures (26-Gauge) passing through holes in the piriform area and zygomatic buttress; in this areas the thickness of the bone ensures good retention. To reinforce stability an additional suspension wire (24-Gauge) is placed through a hole in the piriform region, left exposed in the buccal fold with a loop, connected subsequently to the mandibular arch wire to reduce the maxillo-mandibular shift.

In our experience occlusal splint is kept in place by interdental arch wire fixation (26-Gauge), placed on orthodontic arch wire or on dental brackets; maxillomandibular complex is turned upward in position, checking for bone interference that have to be accurately eliminated to avoid dislocation of the condiles resulting in final maxillary malpositioning. For this reason also occlusal splint retainment and maxillary positioning by transosseous wire sutures in the piriform area are avoided, preferring manual positioning of the maxillomandibular complex after studying occlusion at this step on articulator, paying attention not to displace condiles from the centric position in the glenoid fossae. For this purpose maxillomandibular complex must be positioned applying manual pressure on the inferior border of the mandible, particularly in the Gonion area, avoiding excessive pressure on the symphysis.

Nowadays the most common way to achieve maxillary fixation is by rigid osteosintesis with four miniplates and screws; in this procedure maxilla is placed in the new position, then two bone plates (usually small, semirigide, metal or biodegradable) for each side are set to the piriform rim and to zygomatic buttress. The shape of the plates should be similar to the edge of the maxillary walls, to avoid displacement of the bone and unexpected malocclusion. Although stabilization could be reached with one screw holding any repositioned segment, it is recommended to place two screws on each side of the osteotomy line (four screws for each plate). Three or four maxillary segments could not require additional plates, because the fragments are held in the occlusal splint.

After rigid fixation, maxillomandibular stabilization devices are removed and the occlusion must be checked into the splint. With a gentle movement of the fingers posed on the inferior border, the mandible is rotated to the final position with teeth firmly locked into the splint. In case of interferences (deviations or open-bite) maxillary position is evaluated and eventually corrected in order to obtain proper maxillary position with mandibular condiles in centric position in the glenoid fossae. Usually the bone interference is placed posteriorly and medially: once removed, wires on one of the sides of osteotomy are replaced and re-established the maxillomandibular fixation, the entire bony complex is rotated into correct position and the occlusion checked again as before. This procedure is repeated until the surgeon can achieve the expected occlusion, with the mandible placed passively into the splint. If an early jaw function will follow the surgery, all interferences should be removed from the surface of the splint.

4. Bone grafts

After osteotomy and repositioning of the maxilla, an incomplete contact between the lateral bony walls can occur because of their thinness. The bone in the premolar zone can heal with development of fibrous tissue, but this event does not injure maxillary stability or the sinus health. Crucial regions for a good healing are the piriform rim and the zygomatic buttress:

when these areas are in contact a proper osseous union is expected. Otherwise, significant vertical defects (>3 mm) must be filled with bone grafts. Bone grafting helps the stabilization of the new maxillary position and allows faster healing of the bone; sometimes these grafts come from bone removed during surgery and saved sequentially.

Bone scraps can be forced and locked between bone segments, or supported with fixation devices.

Particularly in cases of vertical dimension increase of the maxillary bones with gaps > 3-4 mm rigid fixation by miniplates alone cannot support bone healing, resulting in final compromising of the maxilla stability. In these cases bone grafts are recommended from iliac crests (first choice) or from mandible or calvaria.

The bone grafts can be fixed in the proper position to fit the bone gaps by wire or screw fixation, or by the bone plates used for maxillary fixation across the defects. Additional bone can be placed over the remaining defects of the lateral maxillary walls, but they have to be stabilized primarily by fitting into the defects or by rigid membranes, because displaced bone grafts in the sinus cavities can result in bony sequestration with complain of nasal bad smelling secretions. In these cases if symptomatology doesn't resolve within 15 days, the bone sequestration has to be removed by lateral sinus wall approach; if the infection will interfere with osteotomy bone healing, the final stability might be compromised.

Allogeneic bone grafts from bank bone have also been employed with similar results to autogenous bone grafts and the advantage of avoiding the necessity of a donor surgical site, but the vascularization and healing are delayed when allogenic bone is used.

Also alloplastic material like hydroxyhapatite have also been used into maxillary osteotomy defects, with good properties for stabilizing the bone defects, but the material is not replaced by bone; for this considerations, autogenic bone grafts is still the first choice for maxillary grafting.

5. Soft tissue closure

Maxillary advancement is classically associated with lip shortening; some Authors suggest that this problem is related to excessive tissue compression when suturing with large amount of tissue capturing when stitching. Others suggest that scar retraction or failure to suture the transacted mimic facial muscles are the reason for lip shortening and alar base widening; but probably the main factor is the increase of soft tissue tension after maxillary advancement.

To avoid this problem, two different techniques, alar cinching and double V-Y suture, are commonly performed in soft tissue closure (Howley et al., 2011).

The alar chinching technique is usually performed by a 3-0 Vicryl suture passed through the alar bases of the nose, from lateral to medial on one side, and from medial to lateral on the opposite site; the median region is included in the stitch passing the suture in a little hole of the bone at the anterior nasal spine site. The stitch is tightened until the alar base width will be identical to that dimension measured by a calliper before the surgery.

The muscle suturing technique is performed with four mucoperiosteal stitches, two for each side, passed for the nose alar base and the inferior mucosa at the paramedian region with an anterior direction, in order to pull the lip and the alar base medially when tightened. The posterior suture begins at the first molar region on the superior border of the wound and is passed in a more medial direction at the canine or premolar region of the lower side of the wound. In this way the wound includes periosteum and muscle layer when the needle is inserted. When tightening this sutures, pressure on cheek skin has to be performed in order to allow skin repositioning in a more anterior fashion.

The V-Y mucosal closure with 4-0 Vicryl is performed in a double lateral position in order to avoid excessive bulging in the midline of the upper lip. Placing the V-Y suture in the canine region upper lip advancement and vermillion exposition is uniformly placed on the entire upper lip, minimizing any vermillion surface deficiency on the anterior aspect. Also the bulk from the advancement technique is not concentrated in the midline area.

At the end of the operation a nasogastric tube is placed in order to prevent blood collecting in the gastrointestinal tract, from nasal or paranasal mucosal bleeding immediately after surgery.

6. Problems and complications

Nasal airway obstruction frequently happens in the immediate post operative period; for this reason good care must be taken to keep nasal airways clean from blood crusting and secretions by suction and by wet gauze cleaning , particularly in cases of intermaxillary fixation.

Conspicuous facial oedema frequently may appear immediately after surgery, maximum degree is reached in two or three days and it progressively decrease in two weeks; useful method to decrease the oedema are corticosteroid therapy one day before and two or three days after surgery, upward head position during day and night and cold package by ice for one day after surgery

Also residual bleeding is one of the most common problems in the immediate post operative phase; lack of sensibility for infra orbital or alveolar nerve are the most common complications that usually resolves in at least 6-12 months.

With rigid fixation with miniplates and screws, intermaxillary fixation is not anymore necessary; in case of inter-maxillary fixation necessity for multiple days, extrusion of the frontal teeth frequently happens, for these reason intermaxillary fixation by bone anchorage is recommended.

The most dangerous problem in immediate post operative time after maxillary surgery is partial or total maxillary bone necrosis for vascular supply failure.

Maxillary aseptic necrosis is usually related to the degree of vascular compromise and is a very rare complication occurring in less than 1% of cases after complete Le Fort I osteotomy(Lanigan et al., 1990, 1997; Kramer et al., 2004; Parnes & Becker, 1972).

Failure of the blood supply to the maxilla after the down fracture is usually related to lesion of the descending palatine artery during the osteotomy, perforation of the palatal mucosa when cutting the maxilla in two segments particularly in the median aspect where the palatal fibromucosa is thinner, and excessive tension or stripping of the palatal mucosa when expending the transversal dimension of the maxillary arch. Palatal devices may also cause vascular defeat by pressure on the soft tissue of the palate, particularly in segmented Le Fort I osteotomy. Problems related to a vascular necrosis of the maxillary bones may include loss of tooth vitality, periodontal defects, tooth loss and a major or minor part loss of the alveolar bone up to necrosis of the entire maxilla (Bell et al., 1995).

Risks and complications related to aseptic necrosis of the maxilla after mayor maxillary surgery is also related with vascular anomalies, craniofacial dysplasia and orofacial clefts probably related to scar fibrosis after prior surgery. Aseptic necrosis of the maxilla should be treated by careful hygiene of the mouth with curettage and cleansing of the necrotic tissue, antibiotic therapy, heparinization and hyperbaric therapy (Nilsson et al., 1987; Singh et al., 2008).

Important complications during major maxillary surgery are bad fracture of the maxillary bones particularly at the down fracture surgical time. At this surgical step much attention must be paid to avoid pterygoid plate fracture, usually at a low level of the plates; in a few cases pterigoid plate fracture can cause trauma to the base of the skull with vascular and ophthalmic complications (Kumar et al., 2007; Silverstein, 1992).

Complications in the immediate post operative time are related to malpositions of the nasal septum in relation with nasal floor and mandibular condyle dislocation in the glenoid fossae. In case of major dislocations reoperation is recommended.

Late complications may include major periodontal defects or loss of the vascular supply to the teeth adjacent to the sectorial osteotomy site in segmented Le Fort I operations.

7. Consideration on nasal airway and sinus cavities

Superior repositioning of the maxilla is a procedure commonly used for the correction of vertical maxillary excess: concern for the effect of this procedure on nasal respiration may be appropriate, since superior repositioning of the maxilla may decrease the volume of the nasal cavity, particularly if the septum is not shortened and out of the proper mid-position.

Following results may apparently be in contradiction with the assumption that nasal air flow space is decreased when the palate is impacted in maxillary surgery; but an explanation can be found in the support gain for nostrils when the maxilla is advanced or superiorly repositioned. Scientific studies have been performed evaluating pre- and postoperative nasal-resistance in patients who underwent superior repositioning of the maxilla by the Le Fort I down-fracture procedure. In case of superior repositioning of the maxilla nasal respiratory function was not usually reduced; these findings indicate that superior repositioning of the maxilla, with or without involvement of the nasal floor by osteotomies, usually results in decreased nasal resistance (Turvey et al., 1984; Walker et al., 1998).

Support gain will determinate nostril angle and nasal valve widening resulting in final decrease for nasal airflow resistances.

When analyzing patients who underwent a one-piece Le Fort I-osteotomy with anterior and superior repositioning of the maxilla, using cephalograms, rhinological inspection, anterior rhinomanometry and acoustic rhinometry, results show a significant increase in interalar width and in cross-sectional diameter at the nasal valve too. The mean total nasal airflow is unchanged, indicating no increase in resistance despite decreased intranasal dimensions (Erbe et al., 2001).

These findings show that surgical maxillary impaction rarely compromise nasal breathing; conversely, an increase in nasal patency is usually observed in most of the patients undergoing orthognatic surgery with maxillary expansion or advancement: a deformation of the nasal valve from a teardrop-shape to a postoperatively more rounded fashion was claimed to be responsible for this change (De Mol Van Otterloo et al., 1990).

Maxillary advancement also involves the aesthetic of face and profile, with significant increasing of the nasolabial angle, nasal tip angle, nasal tip inclination, alar base width and columellar angle; also the columellar length and nostril axis angle usually decrease, while the nostril area doesn't show any significant change. In a recent study analyzing nasal tip and alar base width changes using Cone-Beam Computer Tomography (CBCT) in adults with skeletal class III deformities who underwent Le Fort I advancement and impaction osteotomy associated with mandibular setback, an anteriosuperior shift of the nasal tip and widen of the alar base width and nostril was reported (Park et al., 2011). CBCT analysis can be an available tool for measurement of both skeletal and soft-tissue changes enabling, moreover, 3D assessment of nasal morphologic changes.

Also in other studies, an increase in nasal airflow and a decrease in nasal resistance are usually observed in the maxillary impaction and advancement.). After bimaxillary surgery consisting of a 1-piece Le Fort I osteotomy advancement combined with a bilateral sagittal split osteotomy, active anterior rhinomanometry show an increase of mean and median total nasal airflow and of nasal resistance (Ghoreishian & Gheisari, 2009).

Bimaxillary surgery (maxillary advancement and mandibular setback) for treatment of Class III malocclusion, appears to be more effective than mandibular setback alone into keeping patency of the upper airway space. A computed tomography study was performed to evaluate the morphologic changes at the level of soft palate and base of tongue in patients treated with these two different types of surgery. Results show a significantly less reduction in anteroposterior dimensions of the airway in cases treated with bimaxillary surgery, at least not statistically significant; while in the mandibular setback surgery group, the cross-sectional area of the airway decreased significantly (Degerliyurt et al., 2008).

Even if nasal breathing actually increase after maxillary advancement and impaction, in cases where a considerable amount of superior repositioning is planned, much attention must be paid in septum repositioning without deviations or bulking by proper remodeling or reductions of the osteo-cartilaginous portions, septal crest of the maxilla and lower turbinate (Haarmann et al., 2009; Posnick et al., 2007).

Because aesthetic is the main motivation for most of the patients who undergo this kind of surgery and alar flaring of the nasal base is often an unaesthetic modification, the resuturing of the transverse nasals muscle or the alar base cinch suture must be performed to avoid excessive widening of the alar base. Techniques are described in the related paragraph (Soft tissue closure) of this chapter.

8. Classic maxillary segmentation techniques: Anterior sub-apical osteotomies

Segmented maxillary osteotomy surgery was usually performed in the decade of the sixty years to achieve correction of class II malocclusions by frontal teeth set back following the techniques of Wassmund and Wunderer. With the evolution of the Le Fort I osteotomy techniques this anterior subapical osteotomy for pre-maxilla set back was relegated for few particular cases because new concepts about beauty of the face and cephalometric and photometric analysis suggest that maxillary and upper frontal teeth are usually in good position for most of the patients with class II malocclusions. (Arnett & Gunson, 2010)

Also in that few cases where upper frontal teeth are in a protruded position these condition is frequently associated with a narrowed palate : by transversal palatal expansion a consequent set back of the upper teeth is achieved by an orthodontic dentoalveolar movement related to basal bone and dentoalveolar enlargement in the transversal dimension.

For these reasons isolated anterior subapical osteotomy of the maxilla following the classic Wassmund technique is nowadays rarely performed, relegated to particular indications: cases of anteriorly positioned maxilla with normal transversal palatal dimension.

8.1 Surgical technique

The classic Wassmund technique with ostectomy of the palatal premolar segment after extractions is performed on a subperiosteal plane leaving extensive palatal and buccal soft tissue pedicles in order to preserve premaxilla blood supply.

Under general anaesthesia, after infiltrating the buccal mucosa in the canine-bicuspid region, a vertical incision is performed bilaterally between canine and bicuspid (see fig. 14); no solution injection should be performed in the palatal site in order to preserve palatal vascular supply.

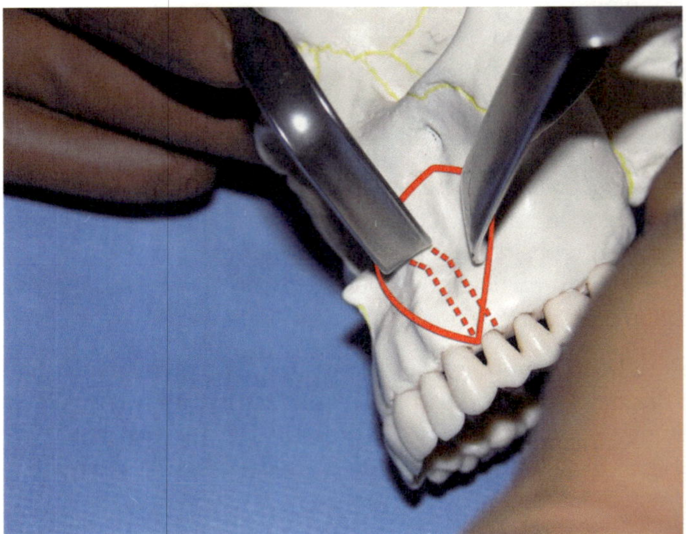

Fig. 14. Buccal mucosa incision at the premolar site with mucoperiosteal flap elevation (continuous line) and osteotomy (dotted line).

Leaving the canine distal papilla intact and in bone contact, a mucoperiosteal flap is elevated from the premolar and tunnellized up to the piriforme aperture. Also nasal mucosa should be carefully elevated from nasal floor together with the palatal mucosa in order to consent palatal bone segment ostectomy (see fig. 15).

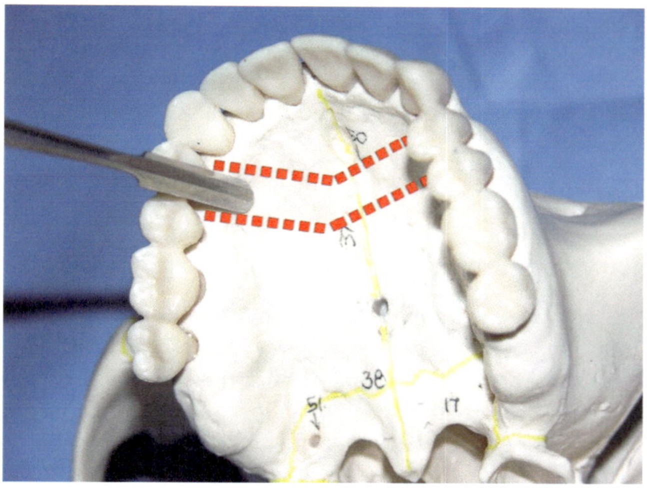

Fig. 15. Palatal mucosa elevation for bone removal.

Before this time, first bicuspids must be extracted if planned, otherwise sufficient space between cuspid and first bicuspid roots should be orthodontically created for planned bone segment removal.

Ostectomy may be performed by bur or in combination with oscillating saw and chisel, starting from the lateral aspect of the maxilla and extending the bone cuts to the lateral wall of the nose and the palate. Amount of bone removal must be carefully evaluated and no more than the planned amount must be performed leaving 2 mm of bone over the adiacent teeth roots (see fig. 16). Then the nasal septum will be disarticulated from the nasal floor by an osteotome and the mobilized premaxilla will be properly repositioned by an occlusal splint.

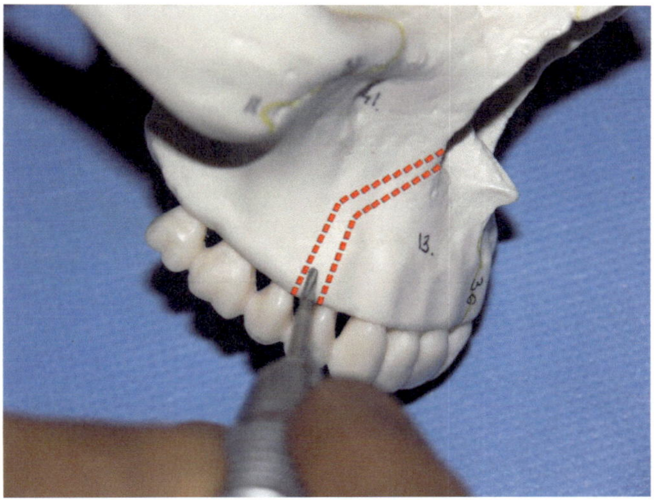

Fig. 16. Buccal bone removal at the inter-bicuspid site or after bicuspids removal.

The anterior fragment can still be splinted in the midline after mucosa incision in the interincisive site; fixation will be performed by miniplates and screws on the facial aspect of the osteotomy at the piriform rim and on auxiliary orthodontic arch wire previously prepared after maxillomandibular fixation on the occlusal splint.

Wound closure will be performed by continuous suture in the buccal aspects and single suture in case of palatal wound to preserve palatal vascular supply.

In most of the cases fixation stability is firm and no additional maxillomandibular fixation is required in the post-operative time.

9. Classic maxillary segmentation technique: Lateral sub-apical osteotomy

Isolated posterior subapical osteotomy is a segmental technique that can be performed in particular cases; following Schuchardt techniques lateral sub apical osteotomies can be performed in case of anterior open bite,unilateral cross-bite or in case of molar intrusion planning, particularly in pre-prosthetic surgery for dentoalveolar segment repositioning when upper molar extrusion occur after lower molar extraction (Ermel et al., 1999).

9.1 Surgical technique

This technique can be performed under general anaesthesia or lower anaesthesia or conscious sedation; surgical treatment must be planned in conjunction with orthodontist to align teeth and create sufficient space between the teeth roots (3mm) for bone osteotomy. Also in preprostetic surgery osteotomy must be planned in cooperation with the prosthodontist to facilitate replacement of the teeth.

After infiltrating with an anaesthetic-vasoconstrictor solution (2% lidocaine 1.100000 epinephrine) in the buccal mucosa a mucoperiostal incision in made from the upper canine to the tuberosity; a mucoperiosteum flap is elevated superiorly living the mucoperiosteum inferior to the incision attached to the bone to preserve proper vascular nutrition to the posterior maxilla bone fragment. Also in the area of the bone vertical cut distal to canine periosteum is carefully elevated tunnelling the mucosa; in the palatal region usually no incision are necessary for bone cut, only in cases of medial repositioning necessity, bone removal is required and a paramedian palatal mucosa cut is necessary. No vasoconstrictor infiltration is performed in the palatal mucosa to preserve vascular supply. Bone cuts are performed by bur in the buccal aspect and by a curved chisel for the palatal cuts through the sinus cavity. Only in cases where bone removal is required from the palatal bone, chilindric bur is used through the palatal mucosa incision. At this time the maxillary tuberosity is separated from the pterigoid plates using a curved osteotomy. Performing bone cuts particular attention must be paid to preserve vascular supply of the bone fragment from facial and palatal mucosa pedicles. After appropriate bone removal the posterior dento-alveolar segment of the maxilla is repositioned by a previously prepared occlusal splint.

Fixation of the fragment is performed combining rigid fixation by mini plates and screws in the buccal aspect with auxiliary orthodontics arch wire and occlusal splint.

When lateral repositioning of the dento alveolar fragment is required amount of palatal mucosa may be insufficient for closure; and incision on the controlateral palate mucosa may be required to mobilize a flap over the palatal osteotomy to allow bone closure without tension. Usually maxillomandibular fixation is not required for the post operative days; occlusion splint fixation for the maxilla can keep dento-alveolar fragment fixed for clinical healing.

9.2 Problems and complications

Facial oedema after sectorial maxillary surgery may be conspicuous and not be strictly correlated to the trauma of the procedure; maximum degree is reached in two or three days and progressively decrease in two weeks.

Useful method to decrease the oedema are corticosteroid therapy one day before and two or three days after surgery, upward head position during day and night and cold package by ice for one day after surgery.

Sensory supply to the mucosa and teeth may be altered for four months to one year; in some cases teeth may maintain vascular supply even if the response to the cold is negative. Also upper lip and paranasal area sensibility may be altered in an immediate short time after surgery.

Forty day after surgery are usually sufficient to remove splint and auxiliary arch wire when the dento-alveolar segment is clinically firm.

Complication in segmental maxillary osteotomy are quite rare and are usually related to periodontal defect in osteotomy sites and failure of the vascular supply to the adjacent teeth: to avoid this complications attention must be paid in leaving 3 mm of bone coverage on adjacent teeth to the osteotomy site.

Also failure to entire dento-alveolar bone segment may happen particularly when the bone segment is not totally firm: in this case the entire dento-alveolar segment can be lost and the repair may be attempted by prosthetic technique or reconstructive surgery.

10. Palatal expansion: Bone born distraction techniques

Transversal maxillary hypoplasia in adolescents and adults is a frequently seen pathology with substantial effects on occlusion with cross-bite malocclusions and dental crowding, on breathing with nasal airflow limitations, on smile aesthetic with buccal corridors evidence when smiling and on TMJ dysfunctions.

Treatment of these dysmorphisms is maxillary expansion which is commonly performed during the growing age by orthodontic appliances (Hyrax and Haas), promoting growth at the suture through the deposition of new bone at the sutural margin by the adjacent cellular layer (Gautam et al., 2009). After maxillary skeletal maturity has been reached, orthodontic treatment can't provide a stable widening of the constricted maxilla. Even if the available literature is inconclusive and in conflict regarding time of closure of the palatal suture ranging from the possibility to easily separate the intermaxillary and palatine sutures at as late an age as 35 years to data expressed (Koudstaal et al., 2008), in clinical practice skeletal correction via orthopaedics appliances is considered successful until the age of skeletal maturation (14-15 years). After this age a combination of surgery and orthodontic treatment is suggested for widening of the maxilla in skeletally matured patients.

Up to two years ago there were three kinds of different techniques for maxillary correction in adult patients after maturation of the facial skeleton has occurred:

1. the segmental Le Fort I osteotomy (LFI-E) (Charezinski et al., 2009; Bailey et al., 1997; Morgan & Kirk, 2001; Phillips et al., 1992; Reinkingh & Rosenberg, 1996);
2. the surgically assisted rapid maxillary expansion (SARME-dental) by a tooth borne devices (Hyrax),
3. the surgically assisted rapid maxillary expansion by bone borne devices (SARME-bone) (Mommaerts, 1999; Pinto et al., 2001; Ramieri et al., 2005);

The first technique allows a simultaneous correction in the three planes of the space in one surgical operation, but it is considered one of the least stable orthognatic procedure (Phillips et al., 1992; Pinto, 2009).

Other negative aspects of this technique are the difficulties found in obtaining large amount of expansion because of the palatal fibromucosa traction, bone fragment tipping, root damage risks in the three peaces segmentation, vascular risks of bone necrosis for premaxilla fragment after wide deperiostation of the palatal bone for allowing segmental movements and difficulties in bone fragment managing at the fixation time during surgery (Pinto, 2009; Quejada et al., 1986; Lanigan et al., 1990).

Other unfavourable occurrences associated with the LFI-E are severe intra and post operative haemorrhage after transsectioning of the descending palatine or other large blood vessels, oroantral or oronasal fistulas, permanent mobility the maxillary fragments and loss of gingival papillae after large immediate widening of the bone fragments (Pinto, 2009).

The second technique SARME-dental requires a two steps surgery with second operation for maxillary advancement, rotation or occlusal plane variation accomplished by a complete Le Fort I osteotomy.

Advantages in this technique consist of new bone formation achieved by osteodistraction and new soft tissue gain achieved by distraction histogenesis particularly useful at the palatal fibromucosa site for avoiding resistance in the expansion movement.

Disadvantages of this technique are related to the tooth borne forces (cortical fenestration with parodontal defects, dental root reabsorption, dental tipping and relapse (Koudstaal, 2009).

Also the third technique SARME-bone requires a two steps surgery for expansion and tridimentional maxillary position correction. This technique avoids teeth related disadvantages of the aforementioned SARME-dental related to the use of a tooth borne appliance because of the employment of the bone borne devices (Cortese et al., 2004, 2010; Matteini & Mommaerts, 2001; Marchetti et al., 2009).

Several bone borne distractor devices have been projected and used in this kind of surgery in the last few years; the most widely used are the TPD device by Mommaerts and the Rotterdam Distractor.

The transpalatal distractor (TPD) (CE 9001, Surgi-tec, Bruges, Belgium) was developed in 1999. The module consists of a two-cylinder screw attached to abutment plates fixed to the palate with screws. The Rotterdam palatal distractor (CE-0297, KLS Martin, Postfach 60, D-78501 Tuttlingen, Germany) is a bone-borne distractor made of titanium grade II based on the mechanical design of a car jack. The two abutment plates (5 x 12 mm) contain 6 nails, each 2 mm long. The activation part consists of a small exagonal activation rod, positioned directly behind the maxillary central incisors. By activating the distractor, the nails of the two abutment plates penetrate the bone and the device is stabilized automatically and no screws are necessary to fix the distractor to the bone.

Major advantages of the bone borne devices are that the forces are directly applied to the bone nearly to the centre of resistance of the maxillary bone avoiding dental tipping and maintaining segmental bone tipping to a minimum level. Relapse of maxillary expansion after distraction or segmented Le Fort I is a widely recognised risk (Chamberland & Proffit, 2008).

Problems concerning the use of the aforementioned two types of palatal distractors are related to the poor stability of the appliances concerning the poor retention on the palatal site and the poor rigidity of the devices. In the authors' experiences with these appliances, problems are related to the absence of fixation screws on the palatal vault and to the possibility of movement of the expansion module with the plates connected to the palatal vault.

According to the Paley classification, these can cause two kinds of complications: detachment of the appliances from the palatal vault with swallowing risks; loose of control of the distraction vector during the expansion phase with asymmetric expansion (Koudstaal, 2009) and three-dimensional malposition of the two maxillary fragments at the end of the distraction. To overtake these limits a new device was developed and used by the Author (Cortese, 2003, 2010) named Palatal Distractor Device (PDD) (see fig. 17).

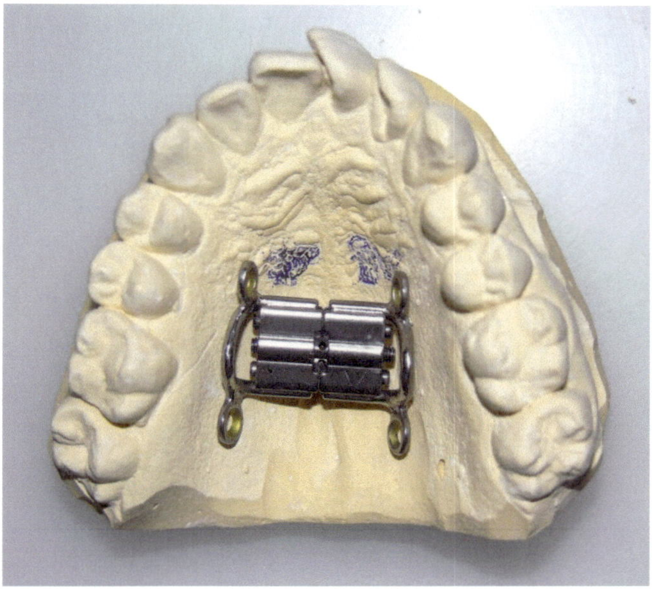

Fig. 17. Rigid bone borne palatal distractor device.

10.1 Appliance design

The functional components of the PDD are a Rematitan titanium expansion jackscrew (Dentarum, Pforzheim, Germany) welded with 2 titanium miniplates (Stryker Leibinger,

Leibinger, Germany). These components are intended to combine a simple expansion system (titanium expansion screw) with a well-tested fixation system (miniplates and screws). A triangular bar is welded to the miniplates to allow proper expansion of the alveolar bone. The PDD is cast on patient models, and activation is performed transorally at its medial part, using a common key for the expansion screw. One full turn is equivalent to an expansion of 0.8 mm; the full expansion is 10 mm. The rationale for using a jackscrew for the activation system is to obtain a transversal activation system on a horizontal stable plane, to avoid inclination of the 2 maxillary bones during activation. With the PDD, it is possible to ensure stability of the 2 maxillary bones in the sagittal and horizontal planes during activation, with palatal distraction in association with an incomplete Le Fort I osteotomy. Advantages of this distractor in comparison to the 2 other palatal distractors (TPD by Mommaerts and Rotterdam palatal distractor) and other most common palatal distractors consists in its intrinsic stability in the three plane of the space because of the jack screw expansion system and the three points of anchorage for each maxillary halves (two screws and one triangular bar for each side).

Because of this characteristics a segmental bodily movement is obtained with full control in the three planes of the space in the cases treated by Le Fort I osteotomy, midline segmentation and maxillary distraction by PDD (See fig. 18). On the other hand the other types of palatal distractors can't assure this stability because they haven't any intrinsic rigidity and have only one point of force application.

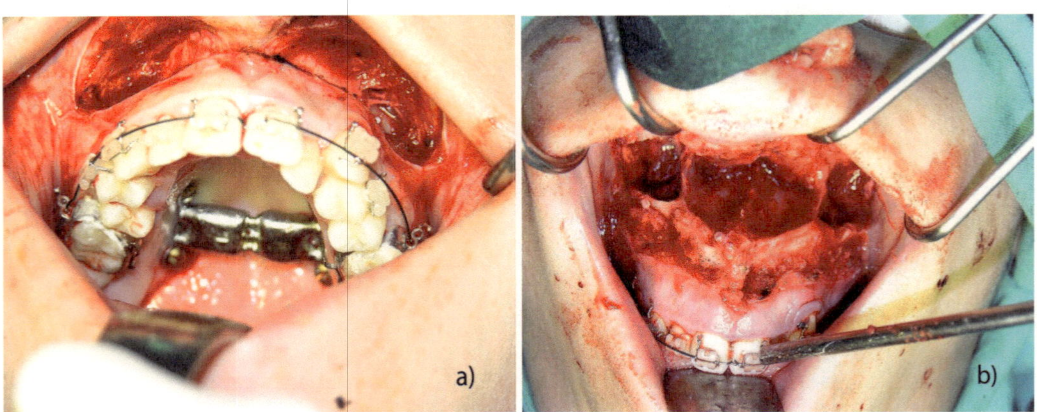

Fig. 18. (A). Palatal distractor fixation by four screws. (B). Downfracture after two pieces Le Fort I osteotomy and palatal distractor fixation by four screws.

This is particularly important in surgically assisted rapid maxillary expansion (SARME) when no fixations systems are applied on the maxilla because only an incomplete Le Fort I is performed (see fig. 19, Case 1).

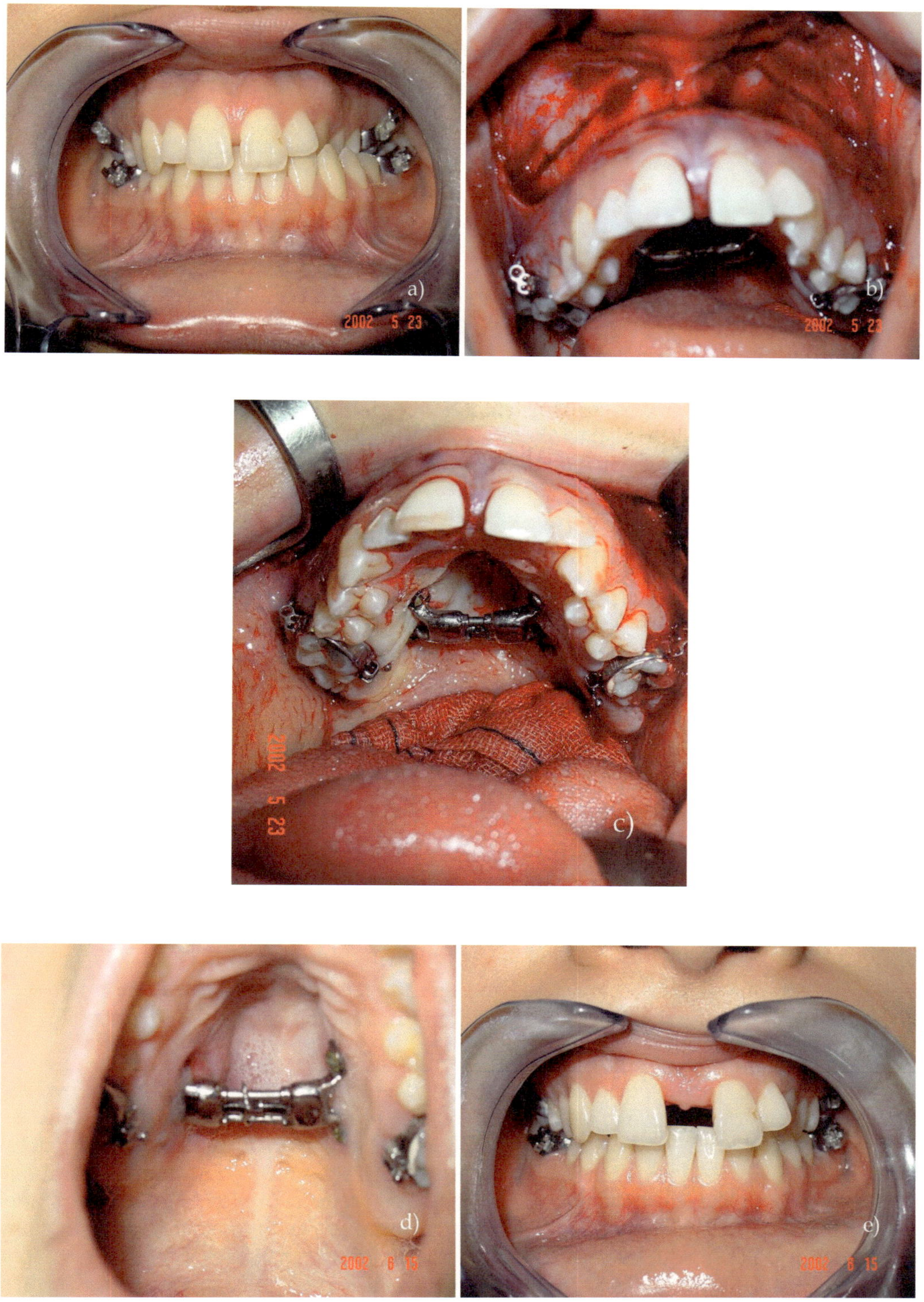
a)
2002 5 23
b)
2002 5 23
c)
2002 5 23
d)
2002 6 15
e)
2002 6 15

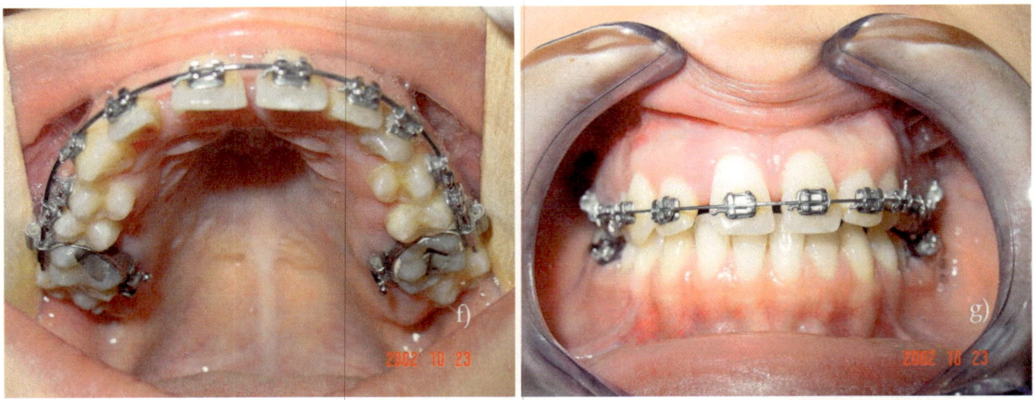

Fig. 19. (Case 1). Patient with maxillary constriction who underwent surgery for maxillary distraction by bone-borne device (SARME-bone). A) Occlusion, pre-operative view. B) Le Fort I and midline osteotomy for maxillary bipartition with palatal distractor in place. C) Palatal distractor fixed at the palatine vault, intra-operative view. D) Post operative palatal mucosa healing after distractor placement. E) Dental occlusion after distraction phase. F) Palatal mucosa healing after palatal distractor removal. G) Dental occlusion after palatal distractor removal.

11. Palatal distraction and maxillary tridimensional repositioning in one stage

One disadvantage of the two techniques for maxillary repositioning (SARME-d with tooth borne device and SARME-b with bone borne device) is the necessity of a second surgery step for three-dimensional maxillary repositioning by a complete Le Fort I osteotomy.

To overtake this problems and combine the best features of the two techniques (stability for osteodistraction osteogenesis and histogenesis in the maxillary distraction by bone borne appliance and one stage expansion and maxillary repositioning by a the LFI-E) a new technique was developed by the Author: a Le Fort I Osteotomy for Maxillary Advancement and Palatal Distraction in 1 Stage (Pinto, 2009; Cortese et al., 2009).

The goal of this technique (LFI-do-bone) was to obtain a good stability in the three-dimensional planes without limiting transversal distraction by PDD.

11.1 Surgical techniques

Under general anaesthesia administered through nasoendotracheal intubation, a Le Fort I osteotomy with down-fracture was performed in combination with a midpalatal osteotomy and palatal distractor setting (LFI-do-bone) (see fig. 20 Case 2).

For this operation, the Le Fort I osteotomy was conducted in the usual manner; however, before the down-fracture was performed, a midline osteotomy was created between the 2 central incisors root up to the posterior nasal spine using a small osteotome. The PDD is typically applied with an epimucosal fixation by four 8-mm screws after predrilling through the holes of the plates and the palatal mucosa. (We prefer using four 8-mm screws after drilling the bone with a bur angled in a vertical direction to avoid the dental roots and any risk of screw release and swallowing). The proper screw position is over the root apex between the first and second bicuspids and between the first and second molars (see fig. 21).

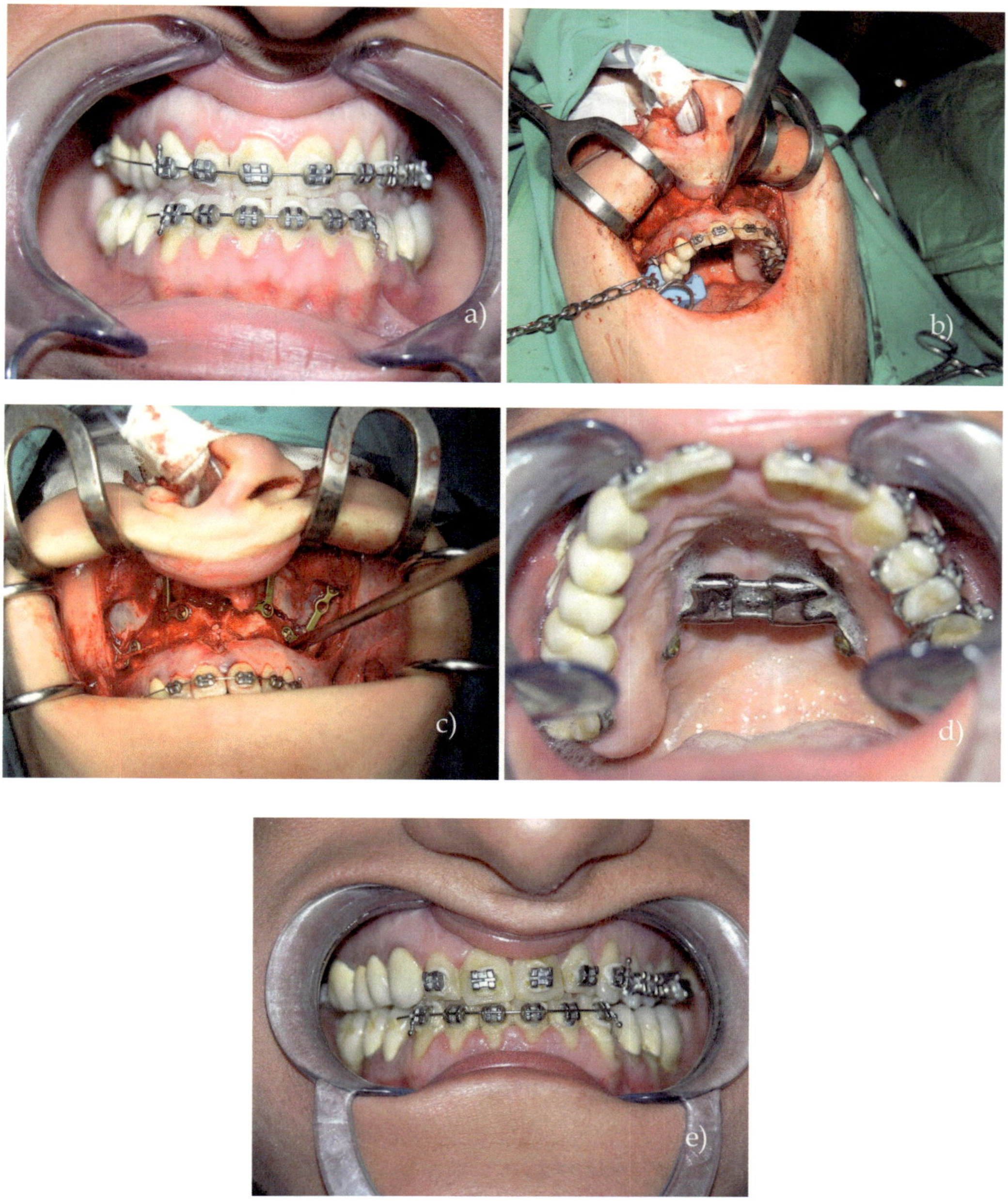

Fig. 20. (Case 2). Patient with class III malocclusion and maxillary constriction who underwent surgery for Le Fort I osteotomy with down fracture, three dimensional maxillary repositioning and distraction with rigid bone borne device in one surgical step (LFI-DO-bone-borne) A) Occlusion, pre-operative view. B) Le Fort I and midline osteotomy for maxillary bipartition with palatal distractor in place. C) Maxillary fixation after down-fracture and maxillary three-dimensional repositioning by four mini-plates and only two screw for each plate to allow maxillary distraction. D) Palatal distractor fixed at the palatine vault, post- distraction view. E) Dental occlusion after palatal distractor removal.

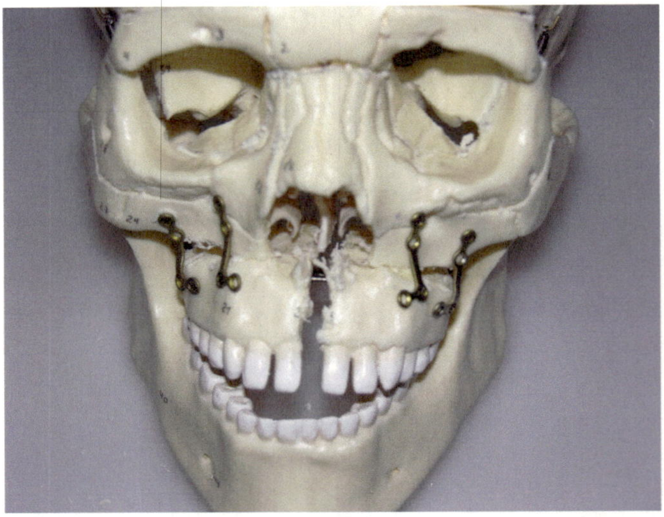

Fig. 21. Complete Le Fort I osteotomy for palatal distraction and maxilla repositioning and semi-rigid fixation by four mini-plate and only 8 screws.

The PDD gives good stability on the horizontal plane, allowing easy management of the 2 fragments of the maxillary bones during the down-fracture procedure. It also facilitates fixation of the maxillary bones in a more advanced position to correct Class III malocclusion or maxillary malposition after down fracture. To allow maxillary expansion when activating the PDD, we perform fixation with 4 miniplates and only 8 or 12 screws (2 or 3 screws for each miniplate) leaving one hole free of the upper part of the miniplate. The miniplates are torqued in the vestibular direction to allow maxillary expansion. The screws are inserted in a very high position in the upper part of the maxillary sinus walls. The goal of this technique is to achieve good stability in the vertical and anteroposterior directions without limiting transversal distraction.

After 7 days of healing, the device is activated in 0.20-mm increments 4 times a day until adequate expansion is achieved. Overexpansion is avoided, because we expect an almost pure skeletal movement without dental share.

Once proper maxillary expansion is obtained, the expansion screw of the device is blocked for 4 months, after which the device is removed under local anaesthesia.

Also when a complete Le Fort I osteotomy is performed in association with a mid palatal distraction, the intrinsic stability of the system is important because in this way it is possible to put 4 mini plates for maxillary fixation taking under proper control the occlusal plane stability particularly in the posterior aspect of the maxilla.

During the post operative time, an inferior molar vestibular torque frequently occurs for decompensation of the lingual inclination of the lower molars. This movement frequently happens because of the new pattern of the bite forces on buccal cuspids of lower molars after crossbite resolution and for the orthodontic appliances effects.

When this situation occurs a little widening of the inferior arch appears with the consequent necessity of further maxillary expansion: in the cases treated with a segmented LFI-e, a new operation is necessary to obtain further maxillary expansion; also in cases treated with SARME-d technique in association with Hyrax or other tooth borne appliances a restart of the expansion system is at risk for tooth borne problems, in relation to the application of the expansion forces on teeth against an increased resistance because of the initial consolidation of the osteotomies.

On the contrary in the cases treated with the PDD, tooth borne risks are avoided and resistance forces may be easily over passed because of the bone borne and rigidity device characteristics which also assure a bodily bone fragment movement with full control in the three planes of the space.

11.2 Considerations about different (tooth born and bone born) palatal expansion techniques

Transverse maxillary deficiency is a common pathology among adults in treatment by orthodontic therapies; this deficiency can be treated with several different surgical therapies but relapse is one of the main problem in maxillary expansion technique.

There is no consensus in the literature regarding the cause and amount of relapse and whether or not over-correction during the distraction phase is necessary.

A consolidation period of 3 months is generally accepted to be sufficient to avoid most of the relapse due to bone incomplete consolidation. A factor to consider in relapse is the mode of distraction.

It is suggested that relapse increases when a tooth-borne rather than a bone-borne distractor is used. An explanation for this might be the tipping of the elements due to the tooth-borne fixation of the expander. Another factor might be the tipping of the maxillary segments instead of parallel expansion due to the different position of the tooth-borne and bone-borne distractors relative to the 'centre of resistance' (Matteini & Mommaerts, 2001).

This 'centre of resistance' is a combination of the area where the maxillary halves are still connected to the skull after the maxillary corticotomy: they are the pterygoid region (in case of SARME without pterygo-maxillary disjunction), the resistance of the surrounding soft tissues and , above of all, the vertical plates of the palatine bones. This latter strong bone structure acts like a pivot during the maxillary expansion: evidence of this is the commonly accepted concept that the resistance centre of the maxillary bones during expansion is located upward and backward, exactly in the position of the vertical plates of the palatine bones (see fig. 22). For this reason maxillary expansion commonly happens with a v-shaped movement, which is of major amount at the frontal teeth level and minor at the molar area. To avoid this v-shaped movement and related orthodontic problems with difficulties in space closure of the frontal teeth and relapse of cross-bite for molar teeth, it's important to adopt a palatal distractor device with intrinsic rigidity and four anchorage point on the horizontal plane.

Also in surgical assisted expansion with three-dimensional maxillary repositioning after down-fracture, a v-shaped expansion may occur probably for bone contacts at the fractured palatine vertical plates,: for this reason a rigid palatal distractor device is recommended.

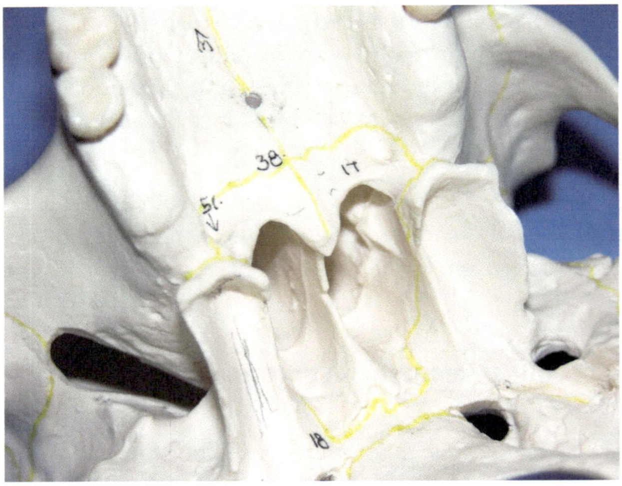

Fig. 22. Horizontal and vertical plates of the palatine bone (n. 17).

Surgical maxillary expansion can be accomplished by several different techniques which can be classified in:

- Segmented Le Fort I with down fracture with expansion and three-dimensional maxillary repositioning (LFI-E)
- Surgical Assisted Rapid Maxillary Expansion by incomplete Le Fort I osteotomy with dental borne devices Hyrax (SARME-dental)
- Surgical Assisted Rapid Maxillary Expansion by incomplete Le Fort I osteotomy with bone borne devices (SARME-bone)
- Le Fort I osteotomy with down fracture, three-dimensional maxillary repositioning and distraction osteogenesis with dental borne device (LFI-DO-dental)
- Le Fort I osteotomy with down fracture, three-dimensional maxillary repositioning and distraction osteogenesis with bone borne devices (LFI-DO-bone)
- Le Fort I osteotomy with down fracture, three-dimensional maxillary repositioning and distraction osteogenesis with rigid bone borne devices (LFI-DO-bone-rigid) (Charezinsky et al., 2009; Cortese, 2009, 2010, 2011; Pinto et al., 2009).

Because of frequent association between maxillary anterior-posterior and vertical deformities with transversal discrepancies, a subsequent orthognatic surgery is necessary in all SARME procedures with consequent costs and risks of an additional procedure under general anaesthesia. In contrast with LFI-E it's possible to obtain palatal expansion and desidered three-dimensional movements, but it's considered one of the less stable orthognatic procedure. With the LFI-DO it's possible to combine the advantages of the aforementioned techniques limiting the relative disadvantages. Also in surgical assisted expansion with three-dimensional maxillary repositioning after down-fracture, a v-shaped expansion occur probably because of bone contacts at the fractured palatine vertical plates: for this reason a rigid palatal distractor device is recommended (Pinto et al., 2009).

11.3 Problems and complications

Even if surgical complications are infrequent, in LFI-E severe intra or postoperative haemorrhage, difficulties in positioning and stabilizing the bone segments, oro-antral or oronasal fistulas, permanent mobility of maxillary segments, and loss of gingival papillae for underling periodontal defects have been reported (Quejada et al., 1986; Lanigan et al., 1990).

With SARME-dental most of the aforementioned problems related with LFI-E are avoided but teeth borne related problems (periodontal defects bone and root reabsorption) may occur and a double stage surgery is necessary when a three-dimensional maxillary repositioning is required.

With SARME-bone related tooth borne problems are avoided but a double stage surgery is necessary if required for a three-dimensional maxillary malposition correction.

With a complete Le Fort I osteotomy wit down fracture, associated with distraction osteogenesis by tooth borne devices (LFI-DO dental), it's possible to associate the advantages of the one step surgery by LFI-E with the advantages of the SARME-dental, avoiding the surgical related problems of LFI-E.

By a LFI-DO-bone, using a bone-borne distractor device it's possible to avoid the teeth related problems of a tooth borne device of the aforementioned technique.

By LFI-DO-bone rigid PDD, using a bone-borne distractor devices, it's possible to avoid the problems related to the use of a non-rigid device like asymmetric maxillary expansion (Koudstaal, 2009, 2010, 2011), device components detachment with swallowing risks (Neyt et al., 2002).

As the rigid palatal distractor device (PDD) held the maxillary segments rigidly like a single unit, advantages of using a rigid tooth borne device are the related facilities in positioning and stabilizing the bone segments at the maxillary fixation time during surgery and possibility to start again with palatal expansion when required if occlusal changes in the lower dental arch occurs.

In the Le Fort I with down fracture and maxillary repositioning associated with the technique of palatal distraction by the use of a rigid tooth borne palatal distractor and semi-rigid contention system (four mini-plates with only two or three screws for each miniplate) it's possible to obtain a variation of the occlusal plane particularly useful when an improvement of the posterior maxillary height is required.

With this technique stability of the maxillary bones is good and to perform osteotomy for mandibular repositioning in the same surgical stage is suitable.

In all of the aforementioned surgical procedures close cooperation between orthodontist, dental prosthetist and maxillofacial surgeon is fundamental: to succeed in creating this kind of cooperation partial overlapping of competence between the different disciplines involved in the treatment of this patients is needed.

12. References

Acebal-Bianco, F. Vuylsteke, PL. Mommaerts, MY. et al. (2000). Perioperative complications in corrective facial orthopedic surgery: A 5-year retrospective study. *J Oral Maxillofac Surg* Vol. 58, No. 7, (Jul 2000), pp. 754-60.

Arnett, GW. Gunson, MJ. (2004). Facial planning for orthodontists and oral surgeons. *Am J Orthod Dentofacial Orthop*, Vol. 126, No. 3, (Sep 2004), pp. 290-295.

Arnett, GW. Gunson, MJ. (2010) Esthetic treatment planning for orthognathic surgery. *J Clin Orthod,* Vol. 44, No. 3, (Mar 2010), pp. 196-200.

Axhausen, G. (1934). Zur Behandlung veralteter disloziert geheilter Oberkieferbrache. *Dtsch Zahn-Mund-Kieferheilk* 6 (1934) 582

Bailey, LJ. White, RP. Proffit, WR. Turvey, TA. (1997). Segmental LeFort I osteotomy for management of transverse maxillary deficiency. *J Oral Maxillofac Surg,* Vol. 55, No.7, (Jul 1997), pp. 728-731.

Bell, WH. (1973). Biologic basis for maxillary osteotomies. *Am J Phys Anthropol* Vol. 38, No. 2, (Mar 1973), pp. 279-89.

Bell, WH. (1975). Le Fort I osteotomy for correction of maxillary deformities. *J Oral Surg.* Vol. 33, No. 6, (Jun 1975), pp. 412-26.

Bell, WH. (1980-1985). *Surgical correction of Dentofacial Deformities.* W.B. Saunders, Philadelphia, USA.

Bell, WH. You, ZH. Finn, RA, et al. (1995). Wound healing after multi- segmental Le Fort I osteotomy and transection of the descending palatine vessels. *J Oral Maxillofac Surg.* Vol. 53, No. 12, (Dec 1995), pp. 1425-33; discussion 1433-4.

Bouloux, GF. Bays, RA. (2000). Neurosensory recovery after ligation of the descending palatine neurovascular bundle during Le Fort I osteotomy. *J Oral Maxillofac Surg.* Vol. 58, No. 8, (Aug 2000), pp. 841-5; discussion 846.

Chamberland, S. Proffit, WR. (2008). Closer look at the stability of surgically assisted rapid palatal expansion. *J Oral Maxillofac Surg,* Vol. 66, No.9, (Sep 2008), pp. 1895-900.

Charezinski, M. Balon-Perin, A. Deroux, E. De Maertelaer, V. Glineur, R. (2009). Transverse maxillary stability assisted by a transpalatal device: a retrospective pilot study of 9 cases. *Int J Oral Maxillofac Surg,* Vol. 38, No.9, (Sep 2009), pp. 937-41.

Converse, JM. Shapiro, HH. (1952). Treatment of developmental malformations of the jaws. *Plast. Surg.* Vol. 10, No. 473, (1952).

Converse, JM. Horowitz, SL. (1969): The surgical orthodontic approach to the treatment of dentofacial deformities. *Am. J. Orthodont.* Vol. 55, (1969), p. 217

Cortese, A. Savastano, G. Saturno, G. & Albano, F. (2003). Tridimensional Intraoral Distractor Device in Adult Severe Mandibular Retrognathia: Management Consideration. *From 7th European Craniofacial Congress,* Bologna (Italy), November 20-22, 2003. Medimond International Proceedings. Volume ISBN 88-7587-031-4 pp. 69-74

Cortese, A. De Cristofaro, M. Papa, F. Savastano, G. (2004). A new transpalatal distractor device. Report of 3 cases with surgical and occlusal evaluations. *Rivista Italiana di Chirurgia Maxillo-Facciale,* Vol. 14, No.1, (Apr 2004), pp. 23-29.

Cortese, A. Savastano, G. Savastano, M. Spagnuolo, G. Papa, F. (2009). New technique: Le Fort I osteotomy for maxillary advancement and palatal distraction in 1 stage. *J Oral Maxillofac Surg,* Vol. 67, No. 1, (Jan 2009), pp. 223-8.

Cortese, A. Savastano, M. Savastano, G. Papa, F. Howard, CM & Claudio, PP. (2010). Maxillary constriction treated by a new palatal distractor device: surgical and occlusal evaluations of 10 patients. *J Craniofac Surg,* Vol. 21, No. 2, (Mar 2010), pp. 339-43.

Cortese, A. Savastano, M. Savastano, G. Claudio, PP. (2011). One-Step Transversal Palatal Distraction and Maxillary Repositioning: Technical Considerations, Advantages, and Long-Term Stability. *The Journal of Craniofacial Surgery*. Vol. 22, No. 5, (Sept 2011), pp. 1714-9.

de Mol van Otterloo, JJ. Leezenberg, JA. Tuinzing, DB. van der Kwast, WA. (1990). The influence of the Le Fort I osteotomy on nasal airway resistance. *Rhinology* Vol. 28, No. 2, (Jun 1990), pp. 107-12.

Degerliyurt, K. Ueki, K. Hashiba, Y. Marukawa, K. Nakagawa, K. Yamamoto, E. (2008). A comparative CT evaluation of pharyngeal airway changes in class III patients receiving bimaxillary surgery or mandibular setback surgery. *Oral Surg Oral Med Oral Pathol Oral Radiol Endod* Vol. 105, No. 4, (Apr 2008), pp. 495-502.

Dorfman, HS. Turvey, TA. (1979). Alterations in osseous crestal height following interdental osteotomies. *Oral Surg Oral Med Oral Pathol.* Vol. 48, No. 2, (Aug 1979), pp. 120-5.

Ellingsen, RH. Artun, J. (1993). Pulpal response to orthognathic surgery: a long-term radiographic study. *Am J Orthod Dentofacial Orthop* Vol. 103, No. 4, (Apr 1993), pp. 338-43.

Epker, BN. Wolford, LM. (1975). Middle third face osteotomies; their use in the correction of acquired and developmental dentofacial and craniofacial deformities. *J. Oral Surg.* Vol. 3, (1975), pp. 491–514.

Epker, BN. Fish, LC. (1986). *Dentofacial Deformities*. Mosby, St. Louis, USA.

Erbe, M. Lehotay, M. Göde, U. Wigand, ME. Neukam, FW. (2001). Nasal airway changes after Le Fort I--impaction and advancement: anatomical and functional findings. *Int J Oral Maxillofac Surg*. Vol. 30, No. 2, (Apr 2011), pp. 123-9.

Ermel, T. Hoffmann, J. Alfter, G. Göz, G. (1999). Long-term stability of treatment results after upper jaw segmented osteotomy according to Schuchardt for correction of anterior open bite. *J Orofac Orthop*. Vol. 60, No. 4, (1999), pp. 236-45.

Gautam, P. Valiathan, A. Adhikari, R. (2009). Maxillary protraction with and without maxillary expansion: a finite element analysis of sutural stresses. *Am J Orthod entofacial Orthop*. Vol. 136, No.3, (Sep 2009), pp. 361-6.

Ghoreishian, M. Gheisari, R. (2009). The effect of maxillary multidirectional movement on nasal respiration. *J Oral Maxillofac Surg* Vol. 67, No. 10, (Oct 2009), pp. 2283-6.

Haarmann, A. Budihardja, AS. Wolff, KD. Wangerin, K. (2009). Changes in acoustic airway profiles and nasal airway resistance after Le Fort I osteotomy and functional rhinosurgery: a prospective study. *Int J Oral Maxillofac Surg* Vol. 38, No. 4, (Feb 2009), pp. 321-25.

Haas, AJ. (1980). Long-term posttreatment evaluation of rapid palatal expansion. *Angle Orthod*, Vol. 50, (Jul 1980), No. 3, pp. 189-217.

Halvorson, EG. Mulliken, JB. (2008). Cheever's double operation: the first Le Fort I osteotomy. *Plast Reconstr Surg* Vol. 121, No. 4, (Apr 2008), pp. 1375-81.

Hogeman, KE. Wilmar K. (1967). Die Vorverlagernng des Oberkiefers zur Korrektur von Gebiganomalien. Fortschr. Kiefer Gesichtschir. Bd 12, Stuttgart; Thieme, 1967

Howley, C. Ali, N. Lee, R. Cox, S. (2011). Use of the alar base cinch suture in Le Fort I osteotomy: is it effective? *Br J Oral Maxillofac Surg*. Vol. 49, No. 2, (Mar 2011), pp. 127-30.

Jones, M. (2001) Human gingival and pulpal blood flow during healing after Le Fort I osteotomy. *J Oral Maxillofac Surg*. Vol. 59, No. 1, (Jan 2001), pp. 2-7, discussion 7-8.

Justus, T. Chang, BL. Bloomquist, D. Ramsay, DS. (2001) Human gingival and pulpal blood flow during healing after Le Fort I osteotomy. *J Oral Maxillofac Surg.* Vol. 59, No. 1, (Jan 2001), pp. 2-7, discussion 7-8.

Köle, H. (1959). Surgical operations on the alveolar ridge to correct occlusal abnormalities. *Oral Surg. Oral Med. Oral Path,* Vol. 12, (1959), p. 277.

Koudstaal, MJ. Wolvius, EB. Ongkosuwito, EM. van der Wal, KG. (2008). Surgically assisted rapid maxillary expansion in two cases of osteopathia striata with cranial sclerosis.. *Cleft Palate Craniofac, J* Vol. 45, No.3, (May 2008), pp. 337-42.

Koudstaal, MJ. Wolvius, EB. Schulten, AJ. Hop, WC. van der Wal, KG. (2009). Stability, tipping and relapse of bone-born versus tooth-borne surgically assisted rapid maxillary expansion; a prospective randomized patient trial. *Int J Oral Maxillofac Surgery,* Vol. 38, No.4, (Apr 2009), pp. 308-15.

Kramer, FJ. Baethge, C. Swennen, G. Teltzrow, T. Schulze, A. Berten, J. Brachvogel, P. (2004). Intra- and perioperative complications of the LeFort I osteotomy: a prospective evaluation of 1000 patients. *J Craniofac Surg* Vol. 15, No. 6, (Nov 2004), pp. 971-7; discussion 978-9.

Kumar, V. Pass, B. Guttenberg, SA. et al. (2007). Bisphosphonate-related osteonecrosis of the jaws: A report of three cases demonstrating variability in outcomes and morbidity. *J Am Dent Assoc* Vol. 138, No. 5, (May 2007), pp. 602-9.

Lanigan, DT. Hey, JH. West, RA. (1990). Aseptic necrosis following maxillary osteotomies: Report of 36 cases. *J Oral Maxillofac Surg* Vol. 48, No. 2, (Feb 1990), pp. 142-56.

Lanigan, DT. (1997). Ligation of the descending palatine artery: Pro and con. *J Oral Maxillofac Surg* Vol. 55, No. 12, (Dec 1997), pp. 1502-4.

Le Fort, R. (1900). Fractures de la machoire supérieure. *Cong intenat. De mèd C-r, Sect. de chir. Gèr.* pp. 275-278.

Le Fort, R. (1901). Etude experimentale sur les fractures de la machoire superieure. *Rev Chir,* Vol. 23, pp. 479-507.

Little, AC. Burt, DM. Penton-Voak, IS. Perrett, DI. (2001). Self-perceived attractiveness influences human female preferences for sexual dimorphism and symmetry in male faces. *Proc Biol Sci,* Vol. 268, No. 1462, (Jan 2001), pp. 39-44.

Marchetti, C. Pironi, M. Bianchi, A. Musci, A. (2009). Surgically assisted rapid palatal expansion vs. segmental Le Fort I osteotomy: transverse stability over a 2-year period. *J Craniomaxillofac Surg,* Vol. 37, No.2, (Mar 2009), pp. 74-78.

Matteini, C. Mommaerts, MY. (2001). Posterior transpalatal distraction with pterygoid disjunction: a short-term model study. *Am J Orthod Dentofacial Orthop,* Vol. 120, No.5, (Nov 2001), pp. 498-502

Merli, M. Merli, M. Triaca, A. Esposito, M. (2007). Segmental distraction osteogenesis of the anterior mandible for improving facial esthetics. Preliminary results. *World J Orthod,* Vol. 8, No. 1, (Spring 2007), pp. 19-29.

Mommaerts, MY. (1999). Transpalatal distraction as a method of maxillary expansion. *Br J Oral maxillofac Surg,* Vol. 37, No.4, (Aug 1999), pp. 268-72.

Morgan, TA. Kirk, LF. (2001). Effects of the multiple-piece maxillary osteotomy on the periodontium. *Int I Adult Orthod Orthognath Surg,* Vol. 16, No.4, (Winter 2001), pp. 255-265.

Naini, FB. Moss, JP. Gill, DS. (2006). The enigma of facial beauty: esthetics, proportions, deformity, and controversy. *Am J Orthod Dentofacial Orthop,* Vol. 130, No. 3, (Sep 2006), pp. 277-82.

Neyt, NM. Mommaerts, MY. Abeloos, JV. De Clercq, CA. Neyt, LF. (2002). Problems, obstacles and complications with transpalatal distraction in non-congenital deformities. *J Craniomaxillofac Surg,* Vol. 30, No.3, (Jun 2002), pp. 139-43.

Nilsson, LP. Granström, G. Röckert, HOE. (1987). Effects of dextrans, heparin and hyperbaric oxygen on mandibular tissue damage after osteotomy in a experimental system. *Int J Oral Maxillofac Surg* Vol. 16, No. 1, (Feb 1987), pp. 77-89.

Obwegeser, H. (1969). Surgical correction of small or retrodisplaced maxillae. *J. Plast. Reconstr. Surg,* Vol. 43, (1969), p. 351

Obwegeser, H. (1970). The one time forward movement of the maxilla and backward movement of the mandible for the correction of extreme prognathism. *SSO Schweiz Monatsschr Zahnheilkd,* Vol. 80, No. 5, (May 1970), pp.547-56.

Panula, K. Finne, K. Oikarinen, K. (2001). Incidence of complications and problems related to orthognathic surgery: A review of 665 patients. *J Oral Maxillofac Surg* Vol. 59, No. 10, (Oct 2001), pp. 1128-1136.

Parnes, EI. Becker, ML. (1972). Necrosis of the anterior maxilla following osteotomy: Report of a case. *J Oral Surg* Vol. 33, No. 3, (Mar 1972), pp. 326-330

Park, SB. Yoon, JK. Kim, YI. Hwang, DS. Cho, BH. Son, WS. (2011). The evaluation of the nasal morphologic changes after bimaxillary surgery in skeletal class III maloccusion by using the superimposition of cone-beam computed tomography (CBCT) volumes. *J Craniomaxillofac Surg.* 2011 Jul 2. (Epub ahead of print).

Perrett, DI. Michael BD. Penton-Voak, IS. Lee, KJ. Rowland, DA. Edwards, R. (1999). Symmetry and Human Facial Attractiveness. *Evolution and Human Behavior,* Vol. 20, No. 5, (Sept 1999), pp. 295-307.

Phillips, C. Medland, WH. Fields, HW. Proffit, WR. White, RP. (1992). Stability of surgical maxillary expansion. *Int J Adult Orthod Orthognath Surg,* Vol. 7, No.3, (1992), pp. 139-46.

Pinto, PX. Mommaerts, MY. Wreakes, G. Jacobs, W. (2001). Immediate post expansion changes following the use of the transpalatal distractor. *J Oral Maxillofac Surg,* Vol. 59, No.9, (Sep 2001), pp. 994-1000, discussion 1001.

Pinto, LP. Bell, WH. Chu, S. Buschang, PH. (2009). Simultaneous 3-dimensional Le Fort I/distraction osteogenesis technique: positional changes. *J Oral Maxillofac Surg,* Vol. 67, No.1, (Jan 2009), pp. 32-9.

Posnick, JC. Fantuzzo, JJ. Troost, T.(2007). Simultaneous intranasal procedures to improve chronic obstructive nasal breathing in patients undergoing maxillary (le fort I) osteotomy. *J Oral Maxillofac Surg* Vol. 65, No. 11, (Nov 2007), pp. 2273-81.

Proffit, WR. White, RP. (1991). Surgical Orthodontic Treatment. Mosby-Year Book, St. Louis, USA.

Quejada, JG. Kawamura, H. Finn, RA. Bell, WH. (1986). Wound healing associated with segmental total maxillary osteotomy. *J Oral Maxillofac Surg,* Vol. 44, No.5, (May 1986), pp. 366-77.

Ramieri, GA. Spada, MC. Austa, M. Bianchi, SD. Berrone, S. (2005). Transverse maxillary distraction with a bone anchored appliance: dento-periodontal effects and clinical and radiological results. *Int J Oral Maxillofac Surg*, Vol. 34, No.4, (Jun 2005), pp. 357-63, discussion 1001.

Reinkingh, MR. Rosenberg, A. (1996). Palatal surgical splint for transverse stability of LeFort I osteotomies: a technical note. *Int J Oral Maxillofac Surg*, Vol. 25, No.2, (Apr 1996), pp. 105-6.

Shepherd, J. (2004). Hypotensive anaesthesia and blood loss in orthognathic surgery. *Evid Based Dent*, Vol. 5, No. 1, (2004), p. 16.

Silverstein, P. (1992). Smoking and wound healing. *Am J Med*, Vol. 15, No. 93, (Jul 1992), pp. 22S-24S..

Singh, J. Doddridge, M. Broughton, A. et al. (2008). Reconstruction of post-orthognathic aseptic necrosis of the maxilla. *Br J Oral Maxillofac Surg*, Vol. 46, No. 5, (Jul 2008), pp. 408-10.

Steinhäuser, EW. (1996). Historical development of orthognathic surgery. *J Craniomaxillofac Surg*, Vol. 24, No. 4, (Aug 1996), pp. (195-204).

Stoker, NG. Epker, BN. (1974). The posterior maxillary ostectomy: a retrospective study of treatment results. *International Journal of Oral Surgery*, Vol. 3, No. 4, (Feb 1974), pp. 153-157.

Triaca, A. Minoretti, R. Merz B. (2004). Treatment of mandibular retrusion by distraction osteogenesis: a new technique. *Br J Oral Maxillofac Surg*, Vol. 42, No. 2, (Apr 2004), pp. 89-95.

Triaca, A. Furrer, T. Minoretti, R. (2009). Chin shield osteotomy - A new genioplasty technique avoiding a deep mento-labial fold in order to increase the labial competence. *Int J Oral Maxillofac Surg*, Vol. 38, No. 11, (Nov 2009), pp. 1201-05.

Triaca, A. Minoretti, R. Saulacic, N. (2010). Mandibula wing osteotomy for correction of the mandibular plane: A case report. *Br J Oral Maxillofac Surg*, Vol. 48, No. 3, (Jul 2010), pp. 182-4.

Turvey, TA. & Fonseca, RJ. (1980). The anatomy of the internal maxillary artery in the pterygopalatine fossa: its relationship to maxillary surgery. *J Oral Surg* Vol. 38, No. 2, (Feb 1980), pp. 92-95.

Turvey, TA. Hall, DJ. Warren, DW. (1984). Alterations in nasal airway resistance following superior repositioning of the maxilla. *Am J Orthod* Vol. 85, No. 2, (Feb 1984), pp. 109-14.

Van de Perre, JP. Stoelinga, PJ. Blijdorp, PA et al. (1996). Perioperative morbidity in maxillofacial orthopaedic surgery: A retrospective study. *J Craniomaxillofac Surg* Vol. 24, No. 5, (Oct 1996), pp. 263-70.

Walker, DA. Turvey, TA. Warren, DW. (1988). Alterations in nasal respiration and nasal airway size following superior repositioning of the maxilla. *J Oral Maxillofac Surg* Vol. 46, No. 4, (Apr 1988), pp. 276-81.

Wassmund, M. (1927). *Frakturen und Luxationen des Gesichtsschgdels*, Meusser, Leipzig, Germany.

Wassmund, M. (1935). *Lehrbuch der praktischen Chirurgie des Mundes und der Kiefer*. Meusser, Bd. I., Leipzig, Germany.

Wertz, RA. (1970). Skeletal and dental changes accompanying rapid midpalatal suture opening. *Am J Orthod*, Vol. 58, (Jul 1970), No. 1, pp. 41-66.

Part 2

Spine

3

Quality Control of Reconstructed Sagittal Balance for Sagittal Imbalance

Kao-Wha Chang
Taiwan Spine Center, Taichung Jen-Ai Hospital, Taiwan, Republic of China

1. Introduction

Sagittal balance is important for biomechanical optimization of forces at segmental interspaces. Sagittal plane malalignment is most often clinically significant when there is loss of normal lordosis of the lumbar spine. Excessive kyphosis across these mobile, unsupported segments increases intradiscal pressures and compromises the mechanical advantage of the erector spinae musculature(White AA, Panjabi MM, 1990). Clinically, the patient with sagittal imbalance presents with intractable pain, early fatigue, and a subjective sense of imbalance and leaning forward, and difficulty with horizontal gaze. Compensation can be gained by extension of the hips and flexion of the knees, although this causes increased fatigue. As patients age, muscular weakness, adjacent disc degeneration, and hip and pelvic disease may decrease compensation and increase disability. Restoration of normal and economical sagittal balance reduces the work of the erector spinae and hamstring muscles to achieve balance during normal activity. During reconstructive surgery, restoration of optimal sagittal balance is crucial for obtaining satisfactory clinical results(Mac-Thiong JM et al., 2009; Glassman SD et al., 2005). However, there is no way to control the quality of the reconstructed sagittal balance before or during surgery.

Many clinicians have investigated regional and global spinal alignment in the normal (asymptomatic) adult population(Schwab F, 2006, 2009; Bernhardt M & Bridwell KH, 1989; Berthonnaud E et al.,2005; During J et al.,1985; Gelb DE et al.,1995; Jackson RP et al.,2000; Vaz G et al.,2002). These data have provided a basic understanding of the normative values of spinal parameters. However, since the work by Vidal and Marnay (Vidal J & Marnay T, 1983, 1984), several authors have enhanced the understanding of global alignment by including the pelvis, which has been described as a regulator of sagittal plane alignment. Numerous studies have been conducted to understand the relationship between pelvic parameters and spinal alignment. This has led to the recognition that pelvic morphology and position are essential components of standing alignment(Schwab F et al.,2006; Duval-Beaupere G et al.,2002; Legaye et al.,1998; Roussouly P et al.,2005; Vialle R et al.,2005) In clinical practice, radiographic reference values help identify regional angulations and linear displacements that can be considered as within the normal alignment range for a given patient. However, because of the large range considered "normal," regional values alone are insufficient in assessing patient-specific harmonious alignment and the optimal values to strive for in realigning a deformity. It is thus important to consider the idea of spinopelvic harmony, which relates to the proportionality of one given regional parameter to another and in practical terms the global spinopelvic alignment of the individual. In a simplified manner, for a given subject, a ground rule of harmonious alignment consist of a lumbar lordosis proportional to pelvic incidence while the thoracic kyphosis is proportional to the lumbar lordosis (to a lesser extent) (Schwab F et al., 2010).

When pathology, such as kyphotic deformity perturbs regional alignment, it leads to a chain of modifications along the standing axis. In severe cases, the consequence is a large sagittal vertical axis and pelvic tilt, lost lumbar lordosis resulting in "spinopelvic mismatch" and sagittal imbalance. Based on the idea of spinopelvic harmony and believing that by a chain of interconnected parameters (Berthonnaud E et al.,2005; Schwab F et al.,2006; Vialle R et al.,2005), spinopelvic harmony can be reconstructed according to and in proportion to pelvic morphology, we developed a method to determine the lumbosacral curve which theoretically would bring sagittal balance to an ideal state by calculation and simulation for each patient preoperatively and made template rods of the curve and a blueprint accordingly for operative procedures to follow. It is a pragmatic approach for optional spinopelvic realignment to a given individual on the basis of their respective pelvic morphology. As a pragmatic tool for clinical application, spinopelvic realignment objectives involve utilizing the key pelvic parameters that are constant for each given patient. (The codes of each patient for optimizing reconstructed sagittal balance).

2. Materials and methods

The medical records of 103 consecutive patients who underwent surgery according to the blueprints and with utilization of the template rods for correction of sagittal imbalance by the same surgeon from 2003-2007 were reviewed. Three patients died of unrelated causes and six were lost to follow-up. The remaining 94 patients (73 women, 21 men; mean age 64.7 years, range 51-81 years) were followed up for 2-6 years.

Diagnoses included degenerative lumbar kyphosis (n=41), degenerative lumbar kyphoscoliosis (n=16), posttraumatic lumbar kyphosis (including osteoporotic compression fracture) (n=27), and iatrogenic lumbar kyphosis resulted from extensive neurological decompression without instrumentation and fusion (n=10). We excluded patients with neuromuscular disease, ankylosing spondylitis, or flatback syndrome with instrumented lumbar fusion, patients with lumbar kyphosis combined with weakness of lumbar extensors proved by inability to lift their trunk from the floor by contraction of the extensor muscles in the prone position with their legs being fixed and patients with major hip pathology (hip osteoarthritis, hip flexion contracture ...) as this affects pelvic position and the ability of compensation for sagittal imbalance through their hip.

The efficacy of a method to correct sagittal imbalance can be assessed by radiographic parameters and absolute correction. Preoperative, 2-month postoperative, and final follow-up radiographs were analyzed. One of the authors, who was independent of the surgical team, made all the radiographic measurements. Sagittal measurements were made on 36-in. standing lateral views of the entire spine and upper femur obtained with the hips and knees fully extended. Thoracic kyphosis was measured from the upper endplate of T1 to the lower endplate of T12, and lumbar lordosis was measured from the upper endplate of L1 to the upper endplate of S1. Positive values were used to denote kyphosis and negative values were used to indicate lordosis. Sagittal global balance was measured as the horizontal distance between vertical lines through the hip axis and sacral promontory and represented as sacrofemoral distance (SFD, positive values for femoral anterior to the promontory). The acceptable range of the reconstructed sagittal global balance was -2 to 2 cm (HA nearly under the promontory). Sagittal spinal balance was measured as the horizontal distance between the C7 sagittal plumb line and the posterior superior corner of S1. Because the posterosuperior aspect of the S1 body was the reference, the normal neutral range for sagittal spinal balance was ≦3 cm from this point (plumb line through or behind the L5-S1 disc). Sacral inclination angle (SIA) was defined as the angle subtended by the sacral endplate and horizontal reference line (positive for anterior inclination). The proximal junctional angle was defined as the angle of the inferior endplate of the upper instrumented vertebrae (UIV) to the superior endplate of one suprajacent vertebra above the UIV. Abnormal proximal junctional kyphosis was defined by the proximal junction sagittal Cobb angle +10° or more and proximal junction sagittal Cobb angle being at least 10° higher than the preoperative measurement. Fracture of the UIV or one suprajacent vertebra above the UIV was noted as a junctional fracture. Segmental lordosis from L1 to S1 was measured by the Cobb method from the superior endplates of adjacent vertebrae and was utilized to distribute segmental lordosis of the determined lumbosacral curve. Closing-opening wedge osteotomy (COWO) angle was the segmental lordosis of the segment with COWO. L4-S1 lordosis was the Cobb angle between the superior endplates between L4 and S1.

Magnetic resonance imaging was used to confirm spinal stenosis and identify neural compression (retropulsed bone or disc). All patients received the standard method of measuring bone density via dura-energy radiographic absorptiometry. Thirty-four patients were osteopenic (T scores between -1.0 and -2.5) and 43 patients were osteoporotic (T scores < -2.5). Seventeen patients had normal bone stock (T scores between 1 and -1).

Paired t tests were used for continuous variables between time points and between estimated and reconstructed values. Statistical significance was set at $p < 0.05$.

2.1 Making template rods and blueprint for surgery

2.1.1 Identify the center of gravity line

The center of gravity (CG) is over the HA and normally directly under the promontory of the sacrum (Takemitsu Y et al.,1988). The CG line is a vertical line through the CG, and it was used as a guideline for the reconstruction of optimal sagittal balance in this study. The ideal sagittal balance to be reconstructed was to have a sagittal global balance with the CG directly under the promontory with SFD = 0 (Figure 1A).

2.1.2 Determine pelvic orientation

Each person has a unique posture and spinopelvic balance with a particular set of sagittal alignment. Pelvic morphology has been shown to affect standing lumbosacral lordosis and pelvic balance significantly around the hips in studies involving both adult volunteers and patients with spinal disorders.(Jackson PR, 1997, 1998, 2000; During J et al.,1985; Kobayashi T, 2004). Measurements of pelvic morphology have been made by determining the approximate centers of the hip joints on lateral radiographs (Jackson RP & Hales C, 2000). Jackson and Hales (Jackson RP & Hales C, 2000) described a specific "pelvic radius technique, which involved locating a midpoint between the hip centers called the pelvic "hip axis" and drew a line from this axis to the posterior superior corner of S1.

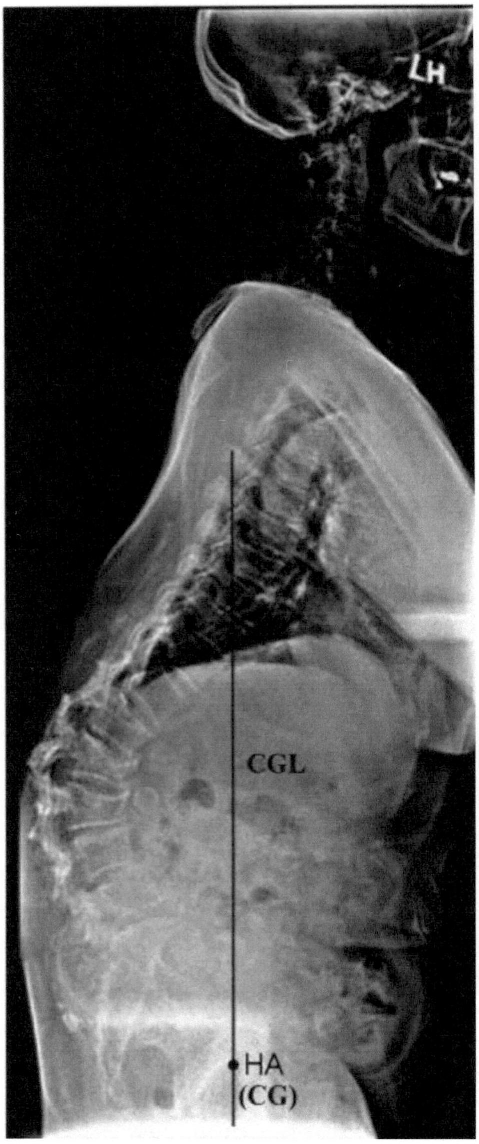

(A) subfigure 1

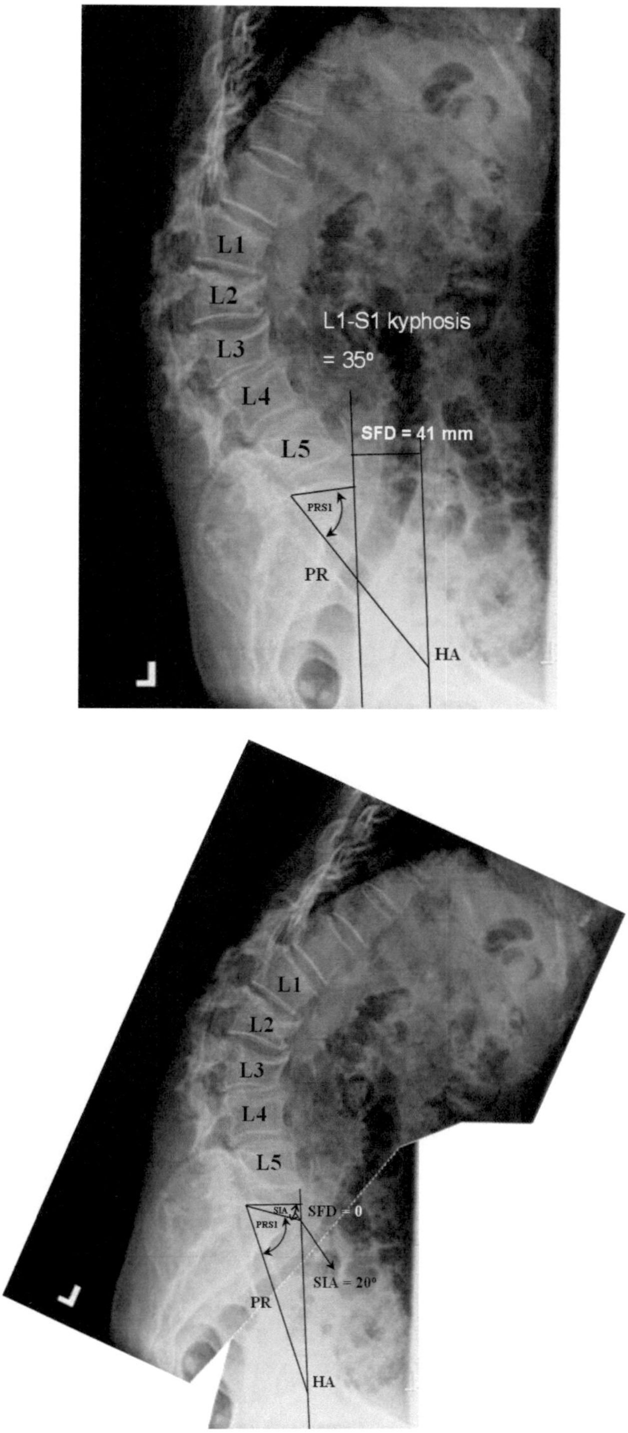

(B) subfigure 1

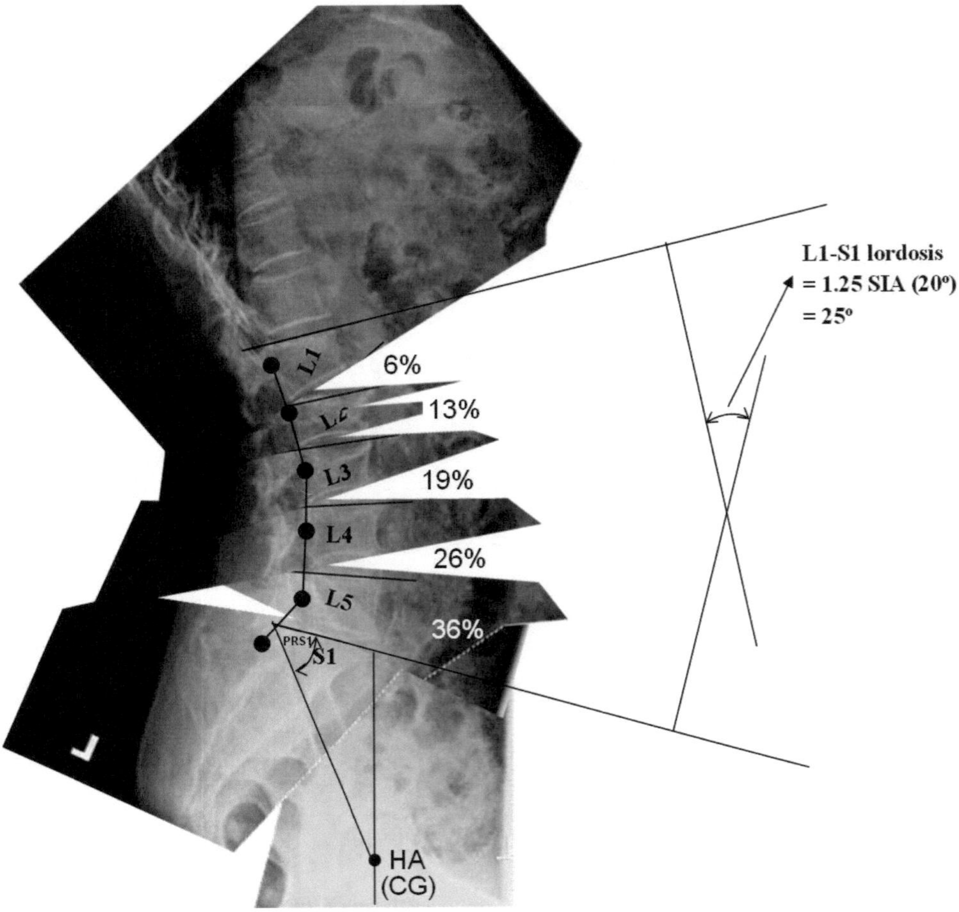

(C) subfigure 1

Fig. 1. A representative example of quality control of reconstructed sagittal balance for sagittal imbalance. A 67-year-old woman with iatrogenic lumbar kyphosis. The preoperative value of L1–S1 lordosis, sacral inclination angle (SIA), sacrofemoral distance (SFD), and sagittal spinal balance were 35°, −9°, 41 mm, and 150 mm, respectively. A, Identify the center of gravity line (CGL). Hip axis (HA) is the midpoint between the hip centers. The center of gravity (CG) is over the HA. The CGL is a vertical line through the CG and is a guideline for reconstruction of optimal sagittal balance. B, Determine pelvic orientation. The lumbopelvic portion of the standing radiograph was magnified to life size and the values of pelvic-radius length and pelvic radius-S1 angle were measured, which are constants for each patient. The lumbopelvic portion was divided into the hips and spinopelvic portion. Given the two anatomic constants and 0-mm SFD, pelvic orientation can be determined by translating and rotating the paper with the spinopelvic portion to a position with the values. C, Determine the lumbosacral curve. The Cobb angle between L1 and S1 is equal to the estimated L1–S1 lordosis. The lumbosacral curve was made approximately according to the reported distribution by simulation of operative procedures and motion behavior of vertebral segments.

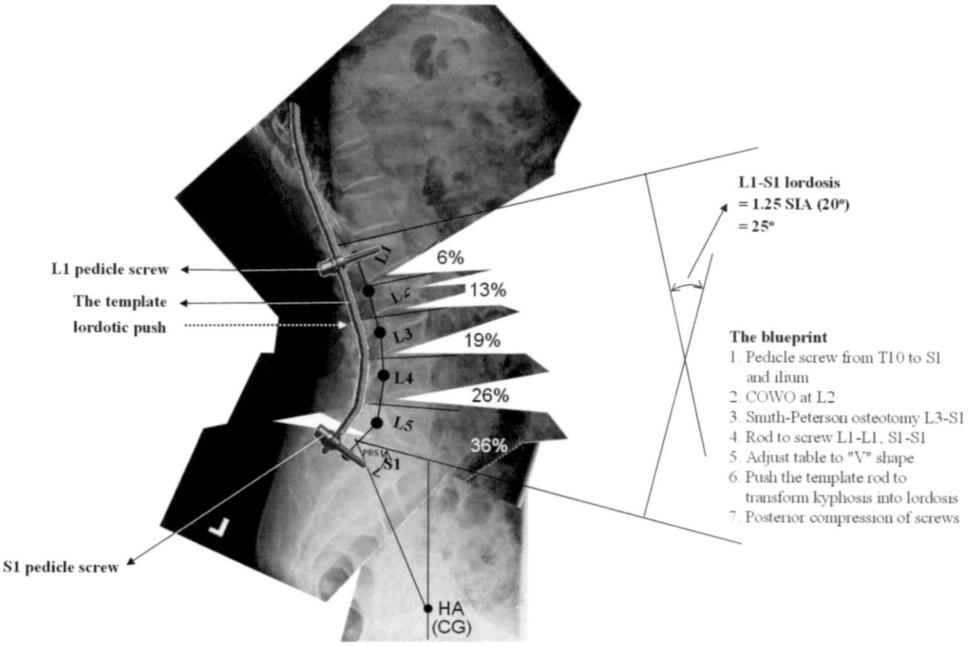

(D) subfigure 1

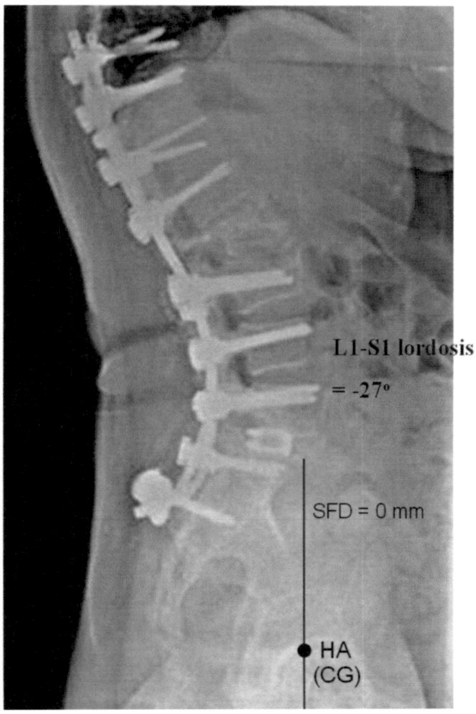

(E) subfigure 1

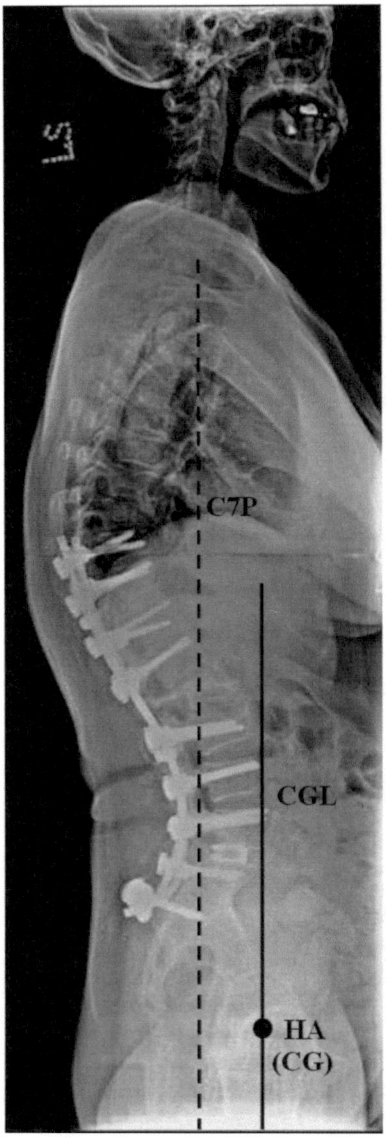

(F) subfigure 1

Fig. 1. D, The template, a rod positioned 15 mm (the average length of the patient's lumbar pedicles) posterior to the curve and contoured to match the lumbosacral curve. The two marks on the rod would be connected to the pedicle screw of L1 and S1. The blueprint is for operative procedures to follow. E, After instrumentation-assisted correction with the template rod. The estimated values of L1–S1 lordosis, SIA, SFD, closing-opening wedge osteotomy angle, and L4–S1 lordosis were −25°, 20°, 0 mm, −3.3°, and −15.5°, respectively, as compared with the reconstructed values −27°, 19°, 0 mm, −11°, and −14°. F, Sagittal spinal and global balance improved from 150 mm and 41 mm before surgery to 0 mm and 0 mm 2 months after surgery.

This line segment was named the "pelvic radius" (PR) because the sacrum rotated around the HA along an arc that can be defined by this radial line. Intraobserver and interobserver assessments for lumbopelvic lordosis and sacropelvic alignment, as well as for pelvic morphology, have been reported as very reliable and reproducible by the PR technique (Jackson RP, 2000a, 2000b).

Individual pelvic anatomy should be constant in the adult and therefore not changing much over time. PR lengths and PRS1 angles are constants for each person (Jackson RP et al., 2000) and should not change with pelvic rotation or sagittal translation. In adult volunteers and in patients with spinal disorders, pelvic morphology and lumbosacral lordosis are strongly correlated and complementary in determining lumbopelvic lordosis (Jackson RP et al., 2000), which are strongly correlated with pelvic balance around the HA. The SFD determines pelvic balance. Therefore, given the two anatomic constants and 0-mm SFD, pelvic orientation can be determined. The lumbopelvic portion of the standing lateral radiograph was magnified to life size and printed on transparent paper, which was divided into the hips and spinopelvic portions. We located the HA and rotated and translated the paper, with the spinopelvic portion to a position with the original PR length and PRS1 angle (constants for each individual) (Jackson RP et al., 2000) and with an SFD value of 0 mm. (The CG line normally is directly under the promontory (Takemitsu Y et al.,1988). Pelvic orientation and the SIA could thus be identified (Figure 1B).

2.1.3 Determine lumbosacral lordosis

Spinal balance is conceived as the result of an optimal lordotic positioning of the vertebrae above a correctly oriented pelvis (Legaye J et al, 1998). Kobayashi et al (Kobayashi T et al.,2004) substantiated their previous results showing that the strongest determinant of lumbar lordosis is sacral alignment. Appropriate lumbar lordosis was estimated to be 80% of sacral inclination by using standing radiographs. The study provides practical data for the assessment of sagittal spinal alignment. For L1-L5 lordosis, 40% are at L4-L5 in the aging spine.(Hammerberg EM & Wood KB, 2003) L5-S1 lordosis/L4 L5 lordosis ave aged 1.4 (Jackson RP & McManus AC, 1994). Total L1-S1 lordosis was estimated accordingly: L1-S1 lordosis = $([\text{SIA} \times 0.8] \times 0.4) \times 1.4 + \text{SIA} \times 0.8 = 1.25\ \text{SIA}$.

2.1.4 Determine the lumbosacral curve that can bring the promontory directly above the center of gravity

COWO (Chang KW et al.,2008) (Figure 2) and Smith-Peterson osteotomy (SPO) (Smith-Peterson MN et al.,1969) were performed in this study to provide adequate release and flexibility for optimal correction. The apex of the lumbar kyphosis was usually between L2 and L4. The site of COWO for three-column release was as close to the apex as possible (usually L2 or L3) and also allowed enough segments below for rigid fixation. The site of COWO was located and marked on the paper of the spinopelvic portion. The spinopelvic portion was divided at the site of COWO and at each disc to simulate release provided by COWO and SPO. Each divided portion of the paper was rotated and translated with correction hinges, either at the pedicular base of the COWO vertebra to simulate closing and opening wedge of COWO or at the posterior border of each divided disc to simulate lordotic correction until the angle between superior end plate of L1 and S1 was equal to the estimated L1-S1 lordosis. For L1-L5 lordosis, the distribution of lordosis had been reported to be approximately 10% at L1–L2, 20% at L2–L3, 30% at L3–L4, and 40% at L4–L5 and L5–S1 lordosis/L4–L5 lordosis averaged 1.4 (Jackson RP & McManus AC, 1994) Therefore, the distribution of L1–S1 lordosis was approximately 6% at L1–L2, 13% at L2–L3, 19% at L3–L4, 26% at L4–L5, and 36% at L5–S1. The estimated distribution of lordosis at the COWO segment of the determined lumbosacral curve would be either 13% if COWO was at L2 or 19% if COWO was at L3. The estimated distribution of lordosis at L4–S1 segments would be 62%. The lumbosacral curve connecting each pedicle base of L1–S1 was approximately made (Figure 1C).

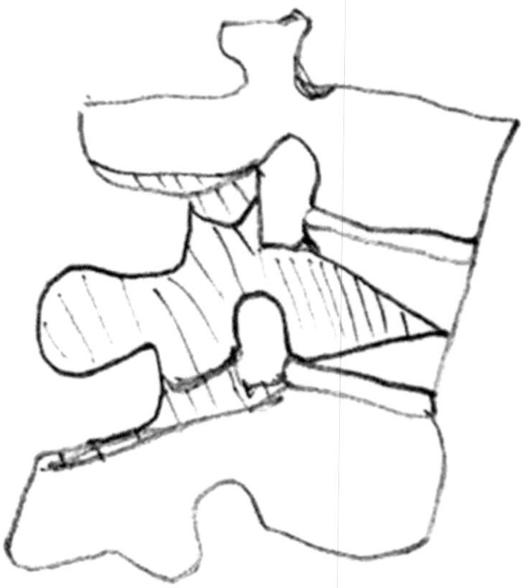

(A) subfigure 2

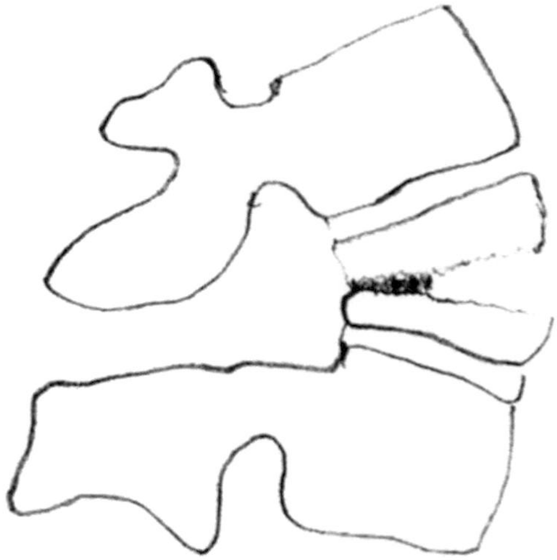

(B) subfigure 2

Fig. 2. Diagram of closing-opening wedge osteotomy. A, Lateral view outlines the bone block to be resected. B, Postoperative view shows that the correction is achieved by hinging on the closed middle column, closing the intravertebral osteotomy and creating an open wedge of the anterior column.

2.1.5 Make template rod and blueprint for reconstruction of optimal sagittal balance

The template, a rod, positioned at the distance of the average length of the patient's lumbar pedicles posterior to the curve and contoured to match the lumbosacral curve, was marked on points L1 and S1, which would be connected with pedicle screws of L1 and S1 (Figure 1D). In theory, the promontory of the sacrum could be brought near to the CG line if the lumbosacral curve could be reconstructed accordingly. Through simulation, the site of osteotomy was noted, and what corrective forces, such as translation, compression, distraction, or rotation, were required during correction was noted on the paper as a blueprint for operative procedures to follow (Figure 1D). The previously mentioned method of template generation can also be done on a computerized model instead of paper cutouts. (Figure 1)

2.2 Surgery

Patients were placed in the prone position with padding at the iliac crests, knees, shoulders, and chest. The abdomen was left free to reduce intraoperative bleeding. The osteotomy site

(L2 or L3) was kept over the hinge in the table so that as the osteotomy was closed and the table could be moved from the neutral to "V" position. A standard posterior midline incision was made (usually from T10 to the sacrum). The spine was bilaterally exposed to the tip of the transverse processes with a strictly subperiosteal approach to reduce bleeding. Pedicle screws were inserted (usually from T10 to the sacrum and ilium except at the COWO level). Intraoperative lateral radiographs were used to adjust the length between the bases of the pedicle and screw head to be the average length of the patient's lumbar pedicles.

Wide posterior decompression and formal lateral-recess decompression and foraminotomy of the involved stenotic levels were usually necessary to treat neurogenic claudication and pain. According to the blueprint, COWO (Chang KW et al., 2008) for three-column release was performed as close to the apical vertebra of the deformity as possible (either L2 or L3). Laminectomy and facetectomy at the level of osteotomy were performed. After both pedicles to be resected were identified, holes were made through them to the vertebral body and curettes were used to enlarge the holes. The transverse processes were excised at their bases. With angled curettes, the cancellous bone was pushed anteriorly into the body to create a cavity. The anterior, posterior, and lateral cortexes of the body were thinned with angled curettes, and both pedicles were enucleated with a small osteotome. The posterior cortex was then pushed down into the body. A rongeur was used to resect the appropriate lateral cortex bilaterally. The anterior cortex was weakened by bilateral penetration with a blunt-end cage trial to facilitate its fracture and opening during corrective procedures for patients with sagittal imbalance requiring large magnitude of correction. Correction was achieved by hinging on the closed middle column, closing the intravertebral osteotomy, and creating an open wedge of the anterior column of the osteotomized vertebra. Before correction, abundant autogenous bones from laminectomy and facetectomy were pushed into the anterior portion of intravertebral osteotomy as bone grafts for the open wedge of the anterior column created by correction. SPO was performed at the other levels for posterior release. These osteotomies provide enough flexibility for optimal correction. A template rod was connected to the pedicle screws with mark S1 connected to the S1 pedicle screw and mark L1 connected to the L1 pedicle screw. The pedicle screws were long-arm pedicle screws. The ample space within the screw head and the flexibility of the rod allow the rod to connect to the screw heads. The operating table was slowly moved to a "V" position to facilitate correction and provide space for sagittal translation and rotation around the site of COWO and the HA. The rod was rotated to correct any scoliosis. The surgeon and assistant pushed the rod against the lumbosacral spine to transform kyphosis into lordosis and compressed the pedicle screws to each other to create lordosis between segments and thus create the lordotic lumbosacral curve (Figure 1E, F). The sacrum of the properly oriented pelvis, which had been brought above the HA, needed to be confirmed by intraoperative lateral radiographs. Wake-up tests were performed. Iliac screws were used for all arthrodeses. Anterior bone grafts were not routinely used for segments added to the arthrodesis. However, interbody fusion with wedge-shaped cages placed posteriorly for anterior-column support and fusion at L5–S1 were performed along with neurologic decompression procedures for 32 patients combined with spinal stenosis at L5–S1 because of the known difficulty of obtaining a long fusion to the sacrum. For patients with T scores less than -1.0, we augmented the UIV and its one suprajacent level with polymethylmethacrylate (PMMA) bone cement to prevent the junctional fracture (Figure 3).

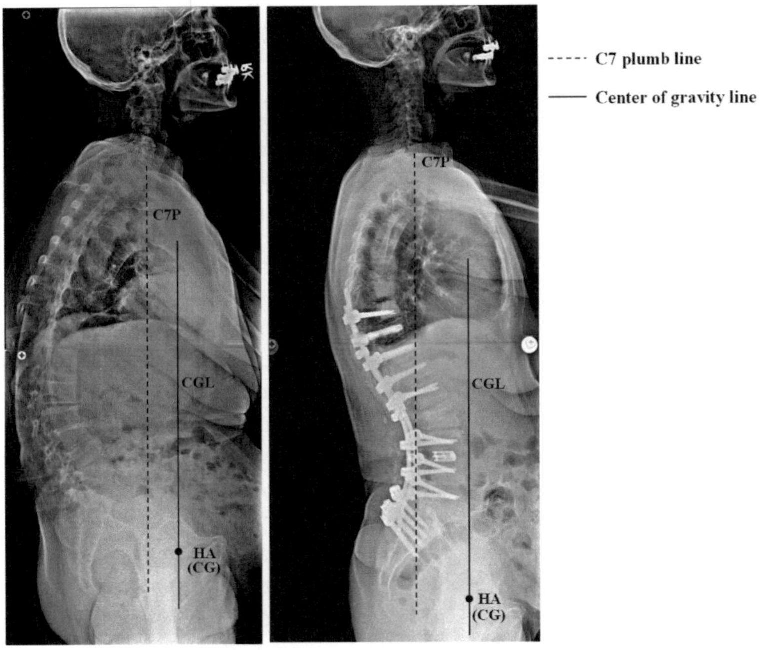

Fig. 3. A 69-year-old woman with degenerative lumbar kyphosis. The preoperative values of L1-S1 lordosis, sacral inclination angle, sacrofemoral distance, and sagittal spinal balance were 17°, −10°, 74 mm, and 75 mm, respectively, compared with postoperative values −48°, 30°, 10 mm, and 0 mm. The upper instrumented vertebrae and its one suprajacent vertebra were augmented with PMMA bone cement to prevent junctional fracture.

Patients ambulated 48 hours later and used custom-made thoracolumbar orthoses for 6 months. Rehabilitation of lumbar extensor musculature by standing straight as much as possible for 15 to 30 minutes every 2 hours during day time began 1 week after the operation.

3. Results

The average preoperative T1-T12 kyphosis was 13°. This increased to 25.2° 2 months after surgery and to 34.5° at the most recent follow-up. The average preoperative L1-S1 lordosis was 19.1°. The curve was corrected to -41.1° 2 months after surgery and to -40.4° at the most recent follow-up. Mean sagittal spinal balance improved from 97.4 mm before surgery to 11 mm 2 months after surgery. Normal sagittal spinal balances (≦3 mm) were reconstructed in 85 of the 94 patients. At the final postoperative visit, the mean sagittal balance increased to 25.4 mm, and there was a significant loss of the reconstructed sagittal spinal balance ($P < 0.01$); however, the normal sagittal spinal balance appeared to be maintained. Mean SFD improved from 61.4 mm before surgery to 3.9 mm 2 months after surgery and to 1.3 mm at the final visit. Acceptable sagittal global balances (SFD = -2 to 2 cm) were reconstructed in all patients. There were no significant differences in the mean value between the 2-month and most recent postoperative visits ($P = 0.3$). Mean SIA improved from -5.4° before surgery to 23.3° 2 months after surgery and to 25.7° at final follow-up. There was no significant change of SIA at the final postoperative visit ($P = 0.4$). (Table 1)

Measurement	Preoperative	Postoperative 2 months	Last Follow-up	Correction	Loss of Correction
T1–T12 kyphosis (°)	13 ± 5.2 (-13 to 22)	25.2 ± 11.1 (11 to 34)	34.5 ± 11.3 (18 to 41)	12.2 ± 3.1 (3 to 14)*	9.3 ± 2.1 (5.1 to 11.1)*
L1–S1 lordosis (°)	19.1 ± 8.3 (-7 to 42)	-41.1 ± 15 (-21 to -51)	-40.4 ± 13 (-20 to -51)	60.2 ± 18.1 (31 to 78)*	0.7 ± 0.4 (0.3 to 2.5)
Sagittal balance (mm)	97.4 ± 24.3 (23 to 193)	11 ± 5.3 (-34 to 43)	25.4 ± 7.3 (-31 to 51.3)	86.4 ± 21.1 (23 to 161)*	14.4 ± 5.3 (7.4 to 37.2) *
SIA (°)	-5.4 ± 3.9 (-12 to 13)	23.3 ± 8.8 (14 to 34)	25.7 ± 7.4 (13 to 34)	28.7 ± 11.3 (19 to 37)*	2.4 ± 0.8 (0.1 to 3.5)
SFD (mm)	61.4 ± 17 (25 to 83)	3.9 ± 2.1 (-13 to 19)	1.3 ± 2.1 (-11 to 24)	57.5 ± 15.8 (25 to 83)*	0.4 ± 0.3 (0 to 5.1)

Table 1. Summary of Radiographic Data. Data are presented as the mean ± standard deviation (range). * means $P < 0.05$. SFD indicates sacrofemoral distance or the distance between the plumb line through the hip axis and the sacral promontory; SIA, sacral inclination angle or the angle between the upper surface of the sacrum and the horizontal line.

COWO was performed at L2 in 46 patients and at L3 in 48 patients. The mean lordosis at the COWO site was -17° and 41% of the reconstructed L1–S1 lordosis 2 months after surgery. The mean estimated lordosis at the COWO site was -5° and 16.1% of the reconstructed L1–S1 lordosis, which was significantly different from the reconstructed value. The mean postoperative L4–S1 lordosis was -19° and 46% of the reconstructed L1–S1 lordosis. The mean estimated lordosis at the L4–S1 segment was -19° and 62% of the reconstructed L1–S1 lordosis. The magnitude was not significantly different from the reconstructed value; however, the percentage of distribution was significantly different from the reconstructed value ($P < 0.01$). The estimated L1–S1 lordosis was –30.8°, which was significantly less than the reconstructed L1–S1 lordosis. The estimated values of SIA and SFD were 24.6° and 0 mm, respectively, which were not significantly different from the reconstructed values (23.3° and 3.9 mm). (Table 2) Only three patients developed junctional kyphosis. No junctional fracture occurred.

Measurements	Estimated value	Postoperative 2 months	Difference
L1-S1 lordosis (°)	-30.8 ± 6.8 (-19 to -43)	-41.1 ± 15 (-21 to -49)	10.5 ± 3.1 (1 to 18.3)*
Dsitribution			
COWO angle (°)	-5 ± 2.6 (-3 to -7)	-17 ± 5.7 (-9 to -20)	12 ± 4.7 (8 to 18)*
% of L1-S1 lordosis	16.1	41 ± 13.1 (33 to 57)	24.9 ± 8 (16.9 to 40.9)*
L4-S1 lordosis (°)	-19 ± 5.8 (-12 to -27)	-19 ± 4.9 (-10 to -23)	0 ± 1.1 (-3 to 5)
% of L1-S1 lordosis	62	46 ± 12.3 (39 to 52)	16 ± 4.3 (10 to 23)*
SIA (°)	24.6 ± 7.4 (15 to 34)	23.3 ± 8.8 (14 to 34)	1.3 ± 0.3 (-2 to 2.5)
SFD (mm)	0	3.9 ± 2.1 (-13 to 19)	3.9 ± 2.1 (-13 to 19)

Table 2. Summary of Estimated and Reconstructed Data. Data are presented as the mean ± standard deviation (range). * means $P < 0.05$. COWO indicates closing-opening wedge osteotomy; SFD, sacrofemoral distance or the distance between the plumb line through the hip axis and the sacral promontory; SIA, sacral inclination angle or the angle between the upper surface of the sacrum and the horizontal line.

4. Discussion

Patients with sagittal imbalance cannot stand erect without compensatory hip extension, knee flexion, and overwork of the erector spinae musculature because reduced moment arm compromises the mechanical advantage. The result is muscle fatigue and activity-related pain. As patients age, muscular weakness, adjacent disc degeneration, and hip and pelvic disease may decrease compensation and increase disability. During reconstructive surgery, restoration of optimal sagittal balance is crucial for obtaining satisfactory clinical results. The spine should be fused in a balanced position that is as close to the normal configuration as possible because insufficient deformity correction involving posterior instrumentation alone may lead to lost correction, pseudarthrosis, increased reoperation rates, or poor clinical results (Grubb SA & Lipscomb HJ, 1992; Bradford DS et al., 1999).

Global sagittal spinal alignment has been historically quantified by measuring a vertical line from the center of the C7 vertebral body with respect to the posterior superior corner of S1 (Gelb DE et al., 1995; Van Royen BJ et al., 1998; Vedantam R et al., 2000). This sagittal vertical axis describes the cumulative balance of the sagittal spinal curves of the trunk but not the entire body, which occurs at the CG. Assessment of the gravity line is gaining interest among spine surgeons in the evaluation of sagittal global balance in normal subjects (Roussouly P et al, 2006; Gangnet N et al., 2003; Legaye J & Duval-Beaupere G, 2008; Schwab F et al., 2006) and in patients with spinal deformity (Allard P et al., 2004; El Fegoun AB et al., 2005; Geiger EV et al.,2007; Nash ML et al., 2002). The CG is near the axis through the hip for pelvic rotation and normally is directly under the promontory (Takemitsu Y et al., 1988). Some patients in this study presented with a lumbar kyphosis and a compensatory thoracic lordosis had a normal sagittal spinal balance and a severely abnormal sagittal global balance (Figure 4). Improved association of the spine, pelvis, and CG or economical sagittal balance reduces the work of the erector spinae and hamstring muscles to achieve balance during normal activity.

According to normal standards (Jackson RP & Hales C, 2000; Takemitsu Y et al., 1988; Kobayashi T et al., 2004), all patients in this study had decreased inclination in the upper sacral surface, or backward rotation, which can be explained by compensated lumbar kyphosis. The line connecting both hip joints was far in front of the promontory, increasing the SFD. Even in natural standing, the lumbar extensors overworked to secure balance against a center of gravity located far in front of the lumbosacral junction. Muscle fatigue, spasm, and pain are clinical symptoms of attempted correction of truncal and whole-body imbalance. Correction of lumbar kyphosis and improvement of sagittal spinal balance without relocating the promontory close to the CG line does not relieve myogenic pain in lumbar kyphosis.

Adult pelvic anatomy is stable, and the pelvic-radius length and pelvic-radius-S1 angle are considered to be constant (Jackson RP et al., 2000) and should not change with pelvic rotation or sagittal translation. In adult volunteers and in patients with spinal disorders, pelvic morphology and lumbosacral lordosis are strongly correlated and complementary in determining lumbopelvic lordosis (Jackson RP et al., 2000), which is strongly correlated with pelvic balance around the hip axis. The SFD determines pelvic balance and sacral inclination, which determines L1-S1 lordosis. Therefore, given the 2 anatomic constants and 0-mm SFD, and simulated motion behavior of the kyphotic lumbar spine which is adequately released by osteotomies during correction, a lumbosacral curve with reported distributions to bring the promontory close to the CG line theoretically could be approximately simulated.

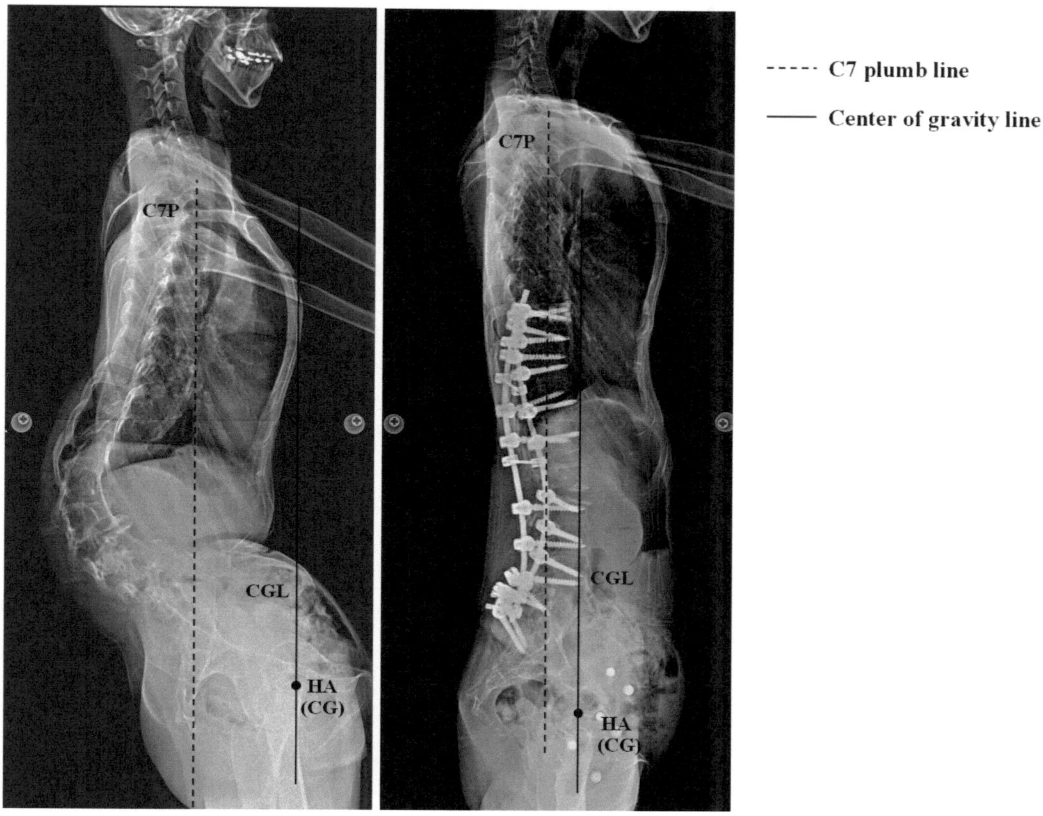

Fig. 4. A 57-year-old woman presented with a lumbar kyphosis and a compensatory thoracic lordosis had a normal sagittal spinal balance and a severely abnormal sagittal global balance. Sagittal global balance was satisfactory reconstructed by the pragmatic approach presented in this study.

Because the caudal end of the construct was sacral and ilial, and because correction of lumbar kyphosis and restoration of lumbosacral lordosis was accomplished by pushing the template rods toward the "V" position of the operating table, the lumbar spine around the apex, which had been three-column released by COWO, translated anteriorly and the lumbopelvic segment caudal to the apex rotated around the hip axis. When the pelvis rotated anteriorly, the distance from the promontory to the CG line decreased and inclination of the upper sacral surface increased. Therefore, the SFD decreased and the SIA increased. All patients obtained significant decrease in SFDs and increase in the SIA.

Because of the rigidity of the deformities, proper release is needed to provide adequate flexibility before posterior instrumentation-augmented correction can be successful. COWO is a three-column release procedure and is responsible for transforming kyphosis into lordosis by lengthening of the anterior column and shortening of the middle and posterior columns. Smith-Peterson osteotomy is a posterior column-only release procedure. The flexibility of a segment with COWO is more than the flexibility of the other segments provided by SPO. It is reasonable that the magnitude of correction obtained at the segment with COWO is the largest (41%) among all segmental lordoses of the reconstructed L1-S1 lordosis. Spinal balance is conceived as the result of an optimal lordotic positioning of the vertebral column above a correctly oriented pelvis (Legaye J et al., 1998). Anatomically, the L4-S1 angle is an important source of lordosis in the lumbosacral spine and about two thirds of an L1-S1 lordosis is distributed below L4 to maintain a "correctly oriented pelvis." Correction by pushing the template rod, with 62% of the estimated L1-S1 lordosis being contoured into the portion of template rod connected to L4-S1 segments, obtained only 46% lordosis of the reconstructed L1-S1 lordosis at L4-S1 segments. This is 16% less than the preoperatively estimated distribution at L4-S1 segments. However, the reconstructed L1-S1 lordosis was 33% larger than the estimated L1-S1 lordosis. We believe this was due to pushing the flexible and deformable template rod during correction. The magnitude of reconstructed L4-S1 lordosis was not significantly different from the estimated value of L4-S1 lordosis (-19° vs -19°). Therefore, a properly oriented pelvis can be reconstructed according to the preoperatively made template and blueprint. We reconstructed a lumbosacral curve with L1-S1 lordosis of -41.1° and proper oriented pelvis with an SIA of 23.3°, which improved sagittal spinal balance from 97.4 mm to 11 mm and improved sagittal global balance by decreasing the SFD from 61.4 to 3.9 mm. We approximated lumbopelvic and sagittal balance to the physiologic state. Although the method were approximate, the results demonstrated it was efficient.

We compared the estimated and reconstructed values of L1–S1 lordosis, L4–S1 lordosis, and the SIA. The reconstructed L1–S1 lordosis was 33% larger than the estimated L1–S1 lordosis, and the reconstructed L4–S1 lordosis was 16% less than the estimated L4–S1 lordosis, so the reconstructed L4–S1lordosis and SIA were not significantly different from the estimated value. Evidently, the lumbar spine was comparatively overlordosed; however, optimal sagittal spinal and global balance were obtained. Sagitta l balance is conceived as the result of an optimal lordotic positioning of the vertebrae above a correctly oriented pelvis (Nash ML et al., 2002). On the basis of this study, a "correctly oriented pelvis" is probably more crucial than "optimal lordotic positioning" for quality control of optimal sagittal balance reconstruction. It is necessary to create enough L1–S1 lordosis with adequate distribution at L4–S1 segments to obtain a "correctly oriented pelvis" and optimal sagittal balance, sometimes at the expense of overcorrection of the lumbar spine. In this study, we excluded patients with ankylosing spondylitis or fl at-back syndrome with instrumented lumbar fusion, because the fused L4–S1 segments, unlike motion behavior at L4–S1 segments in this series, would not accept enough distribution from reconstructed L1–S1 lordosis to obtain a "correctly oriented pelvis" during reconstructive surgery. However, the exclusion does not mean that this study is not helpful for these patients who represent a challenging group of patients that constitute a significant proportion of adult spinal deformity surgeons' practices. Additional release procedures at L4–S1 levels to provide adequate flexibility allow L4–S1 segments to accept enough lordosis for obtaining a correctly oriented pelvis and optimal sagittal balance. Of course, all these additional procedures would increase operation time, blood loss, and complications. Overlordosating the lumbar spine to distribute enough lordosis at L4–S1 segments is another option for these patients. (Chang KW 2005a, 2005b, 2006, 2009). However, more-severe proximal junctional problems and compensatory changes of the thoracic spine above might compromise the reconstructed sagittal balance.

The pelvic incidence (Legaye J et al., 1998) (PI) is defined as the angle between the line perpendicular to the sacral plate at its midpoint and the line connecting this point to the axis of the femoral heads. It is an anatomic parameter, unique to each individual, independent of the spatial orientation of the pelvis. This parameter can be considered as a constant because it is an anatomic one, independent of the position of the pelvis, and independent of the age, once growth is completed. PI is an important component of assessing and reconstructing the sagittal alignment. In fact, it determines it. In this study, we used PRS1 angle (the angle between PR and sacral plate) instead of PI, because PRS1 angle is much easier to be identified and measured than PI. Jackson and Hales (Jackson RP & Hales C, 2000) demonstrated that PRS1 angle was one of the most reliable radiographic measurements of pelvic morphology. PRS1 angle can be utilized in place of PI and is based on the following mathematical calculation (A) and mechanic analysis (B).

A. Mathematical calculation (Figure 5)

1. According to the law of sine: Principle of trigonometry, stating that the lengths of the sides of any triangle are proportional to the sines of the opposite angles. When a, b, and c are the sides and A, B, and C are the opposite angles.

$$\frac{a}{\sin(A)} = \frac{b}{\sin(B)} = \frac{c}{\sin(C)} = \text{constant}$$

2. Refer to Figure 5 and the triangle OAB, ∠OBA+∠BOA+∠OAB =180°, the angle α (ie; pelvic incidence) is a constant , Because(∵)AD is perpendicular to BC so(∴) the angle OAB= α+90°is a constant.

$$\frac{\overline{OB}}{\sin(\angle OAB)} = \frac{\overline{OA}}{\sin(\angle OBA)} = \frac{\overline{AB}}{\sin(\angle BOA)} = \text{constant}$$

$$\Rightarrow \frac{\overline{OB}}{\sin(\alpha + 90^\circ)} = \frac{\overline{OA}}{\sin(\beta)} = \frac{\overline{AB}}{\sin(180^\circ - \alpha - 90^\circ - \beta)} = \text{constant}$$

∵the length of AB=1/2BC is a constant
∴angle BOA is a constant.
∵the angle BOA=180° − ∠OBA − ∠OAB, and the angle OAB is constant.
∴ the angle OBA= β (ie; PRS1 angle) is a constant.

B. Mechanic analysis (Figure 6)

The PI (angle α) is an anatomic parameter. The anatomic components involved in the make-up of this parameter were the first three sacral vertebrae, the sacroiliac joints, and the posterior segment of the iliac bone. HA was considered to be a fixed or stationary reference point as the hinge of motion. The mobility of sacroiliac joint is considered negligible. According to this characteristic property, we can assume that it is a rigid-body; any rigid-body displacement can be considered to be a combination of a rigid-body translation and a rigid-body rotation. The resulting displacements are such that there is no change in the distance between any two points in the body and in any way of moving in rigid-body motion in a fixed axis or plane; all the points maintain the relative distance, and the relative position between points stays the same (Jansson PA & Grahn R, 1995). In this case, the angle α (i.e., PI) and angle β (i.e., PRS1 angle) are constants and the distance between any two arbitrary points of the body is constant and should not change with pelvic rotation or sagittal translation (Figure 6).

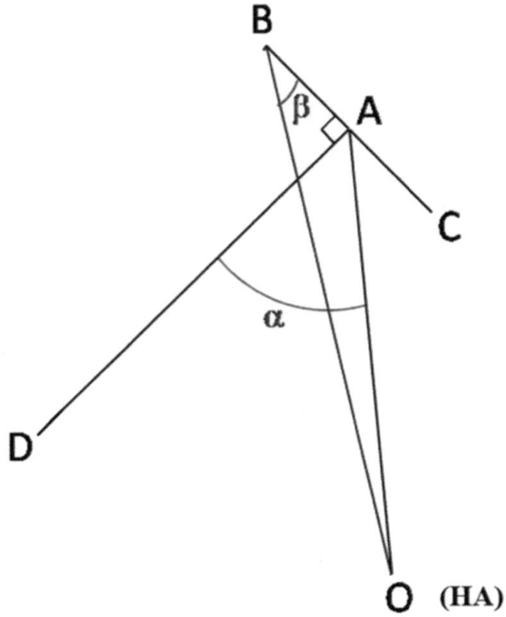

Fig. 5. Mathematical calculation of PI and PRS1 angle. Point O is the hip axis. Point B is the posterosuperior corner of sacrum. Point A is the midpoint of sacral plate. Point C is promontory of sacrum. BC is sacral plate. AD is perpendicular to BC. OB is pelvic radius. Angle α is pelvic incidence. Angle β is PRS1 angle.

On the basis of the above calculation and analysis, both PI and PRS1 are constants and should not change with pelvis rotation or sagittal translation.

The ideal sagittal balance to be reconstructed was to have a sagittal global balance with the CG directly under the promontory, with SFD = 0 (Figure 1A). Given the two anatomic constants (PR and PRS1 angle instead of PI) and 0-mm SFD, pelvic orientation to be reconstructed could be determined before surgery. The results of this study demonstrated that optimal sagittal balance could be reconstructed for sagittal imbalance if the pelvic orientation could be reconstructed accordingly.

There was no significant loss of correction of the reconstructed lumbosacral curve. With the aid of abundant bone grafting the anterior portion of intravertebral osteotomy before correction as bone grafts for the open wedge of the anterior column of the osteomized vertebra created by correction, the union of the anterior open wedge of the anterior column is like the union of a close fracture with rigid fixation, which is fast and definite. During union period, there might be some loss of correction; we believe that it should be minimal.

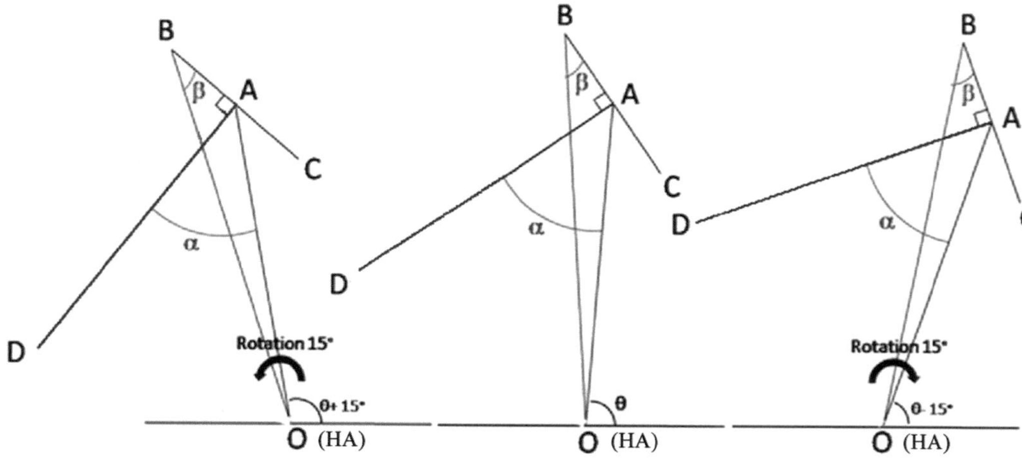

Fig. 6. Mechanical analysis of PI and PRS1 angle. The anatomic construct of pelvic incidence can be considered as a rigid body. Pelvic incidence (angle α) and PRS1 angle (angle β) stay the same, no matter pelvis moves around the hinge (Point O, the hip axis). The illustrations show that angle α and angle β stay the same while the pelvis is rotating 15° and translating posteriorly, staying in neutral position, or rotating 15° and translating anteriorly.

At the level of L5–S1, anterior-column support and anterior bone grafting reduced but did not eliminate the complications such as pseudarthrosis and rods breakage. So, it was not our routine practice to perform structural grafting at L5–S1 through anterior approach. Interbody fusion, with wedge-shaped cages placed posteriorly for anterior-column support, and grafting with high concentrations of autogenous bone and bone morphogenetic protein anteriorly and posteriorly at L5–S1 were performed along with neurologic decompression procedures for patients combined with spinal stenosis at L5–S1 because of the known difficulty of obtaining a long fusion to the sacrum.

For patients with fusion of long segments, and especially for osteoporotic patients, increased motion and stress concentration at a junctional area can induce junctional failure at or above the UIV and adjacent-disc degeneration, leading to junctional kyphosis. Junctional fracture and kyphosis may result in catastrophic neurologic injury, significant loss of sagittal balance, and require reoperation for progressive junctional kyphosis or neurologic deficit. In this study, the lumbar spine was overlordosed; hence, more-severe proximal segmental junctional problems might occur. Preventing the occurrence of junctional problems is crucial for maintaining the reconstructed sagittal balance. DeWald and Stanley (DeWald CJ & Stanley T, 2006) believe that the occurrence of junctional kyphosis is an inevitable consequence of multilevel instrumentation in patients with poor bone stock. They suggested that a potential approach to this problem was to perform limited fusion with the intention of staging proximal extension as the junctional kyphosis progresses. On the basis of our observation of 33 osteoporotic patients who were older than 65 years, had a T score less than −2.5, had a fusion of long segments, and were followed up for an average of 3.7 years, 26%

developed junctional fracture and 29% developed junctional kyphosis, whereas among 46 patients who were older than 65 years, had a T score less than −2.5, had long-segment fusion with PMMA augmentation of UIV and its one suprajacent vertebra to prevent junctional fracture, and were followed up for 4.7 years, none had junctional fracture and nine (20%) developed junctional kyphosis. The cause of junctional kyphosis was suprajacent disc degeneration rather than junctional fracture, so the severity of junctional kyphosis was diminished. We also observed 43 patients older than 65 year who had osteopenia (T score <−0.1) with fusion of long segments and found that 8% developed junctional fracture and 11% developed junctional kyphosis.

In this study, PMMA augmentation of UIV (usually T10) and its one suprajacent vertebra was performed to prevent junctional fracture for osteopenia or osteoporotic patients with a T score less than −1. No junctional failure occurred, and 13 (14%) patients developed junctional kyphosis because of suprajacent disc degeneration. This technique could effectively prevent junctional failure and minimize the severity of junctional kyphosis and the risk of jeopardizing the reconstructed sagittal balance.

The primary cause of lumbar kyphosis might be the following: (1) decline of the anterior elements, multiple disc narrowing, and vertebral wedging or collapse; (2) weakness and loosening of the posterior elements and atrophy of the extensor muscles; (3) combined factors (Takemitsu Y et al.,1988). Spinal alignment can be reconstructed surgically; however, sagittal balance cannot be restored in the presence of weak and atrophic extensor spinal musculature. Therefore, in this study, we excluded patients with neuromuscular disease and those with lumbar kyphosis who could not lift their trunks from the floor by contraction of the extensor muscles in the prone position with legs being fixed. Undoubtedly, the severe reconditioning of the lumbar extensor musculature that occurs as the result of the posterior exposure influences the patient's ability to stand erect. Postoperative rehabilitation of the lumbar extensor muscles is crucial for maintaining the reconstructed sagittal balance and should be started as early as possible and continued.

The average increase of the thoracic sagittal Cobb angle between T1 and T12 at 2 months after surgery was 25.2° and at final follow-up was 34.5°. Although how the thoracic spine would change above was unpredictable and there were significant compensatory changes of the thoracic spine above and significant loss of sagittal spinal balance, the optimal reconstructed sagittal global and spinal balance appeared to be maintained by effective prevention of occurrence of junctional failure and persistent rehabilitation of extensor spinal musculature.

5. Conclusion

Sagittal imbalance can present with a wide range of clinical symptoms and radiographic findings. Recent work has identified key structural parameters to consider in the evaluation and treatment of sagittal imbalance. In addition to the clinical affect of spinal and pelvic parameters, recognition of the interrelationship and necessary harmony between values is critical to optimize individualized treatment. In a simplified manner, for a given subject, a ground rule of harmonious alignment consist of a lumbar lordosis proportional to pelvic incidence while the thoracic kyphosis is proportional to the lumbar lordosis.

When pathology, such as kyphotic deformity perturbs regional alignment, it leads to a chain of modifications along the standing axis. In severe cases, the consequence is a large sagittal vertical axis and pelvic tilt, lost lumbar lordosis resulting in "spinopelvic mismatch" and sagittal imbalance. Based on the idea of spinopelvic harmony and believing that by a chain of interconnected parameters, spinopelvic harmony can be reconstructed according to and in proportion to pelvic morphology. A pragmatic approach for reconstruction of optimal sagittal balance has been presented in this study. Sagittal vertical axis (including C7 plumb line and center of gravity line), and fixed pelvic constants (PR and PRS1 angle) are key parameters and permit a framework to a pragmatic approach for reconstruction of sagittal balance. A correctly oriented pelvis, which can be determined before surgery, reconstructed by restoration of enough L1–S1 lordosis with adequate distribution at L4–S1 segments is a matter of critical importance for optimizing reconstructed sagittal balance. Prevention of junctional fracture and persistent rehabilitation of surgically injured lumbar extensor musculature are crucial for maintaining reconstructed sagittal balance.

The significance of this approach is that quality control of the reconstructed sagittal balance for surgical treatment of sagittal imbalance is possible. It should be noted that the complexity of standing alignment and deformity leaves much work to be done. Surgical planning should strive for ideal alignment while being tempered by risk factors and limitations in the patient's healthcare environment. Ongoing clinical outcome studies are certain to offer useful algorithms in the near future.

6. References

Allard P, Chavet P & Barbier F. (2004). Effect of body morphology on standing balance in adolescent idiopathic scoliosis. *Am J Phys Med Rehabil*, 83:689–97.

Bernhardt M & Bridwell KH. (1989). Segmental analysis of the sagittal plane alignment of the normal thoracic and lumbar spines and thoracolumbar junction. *Spine*, 14:717-21.

Berthonnaud E, Dimner J & Roussouly P. (2005). Analysis of the sagittal balance of the spine and pelvis using shape and orientation parameters. *J Spinal Disord Tech*, 18:40-7.

Bradford DS, Tay BK & Hu SS. (1999). Adult scoliosis: surgical indications, operative management, complications, and outcomes. *Spine*,24:2617–29.

Chang KW, Chen YY & Lin CC. (2005). Closing wedge osteotomy versus opening wedge osteotomy in ankylosing spondylitis with thoracolumbar kyphotic deformity. *Spine*, 30:1584-93.

Chang KW, Chen YY & Lin CC. (2005). Apical lordosating osteotomy and minimal segment fixation for the treatment of thoracic or thoracolumbar osteoporotic kyphosis. *Spine*, 30:1674-81.

Chang KW, Chen HC & Chen YY. (2006). Sagittal translation in opening wedge osteotomy for the correction of thoracolumbar kyphotic deformity in ankylosing spondylitis. *Spine*, 31:1137-42.

Chang KW, Cheng CW & Chen HC. (2008). Closing-opening wedge osteotomy for the treatment of sagittal imbalance. *Spine*, 33:1470–7.

Chang KW, Cheng CW & Chen HC. (2009). Correction hinge in the compromised cord for severe and rigid angular kyphosis with neurologic deficits. *Spine*, 34:1040-45.

DeWald CJ & Stanley T. (2006). Instrumentation-related complications of multilevel fusions for adult spinal deformity patients over age 65. *Spine*, 31:S144–51.

During J, Goudfrooij H & Keessen W. (1985). Toward standards for posture. Postural characteristics of the lower back system in normal and pathologic conditions. *Spine*, 10:83-7.

Duval-Beaupere G, Marty C & Barthel F. (2002). Sagittal profile of the spine prominent part of the pelvis. *Stud Health Technol Inform*, 88:47-64.

El Fegoun AB, Schwab F & Gamez L. (2005). Center of gravity and radiographic posture analysis: a preliminary review of adult volunteers and adult patients affected by scoliosis. *Spine*, 30:1535–40.

Gangnet N, Pornero V & Dumas R. (2003). Variability of the spine and pelvis location with respect to the gravity line: a three-dimensional stereoradiographic study using force platform. *Surg Radiol Anat*, 25:424–33.

Geiger EV, Müller O & Niemeyer T. (2007). Adjustment of pelvispinal parameters preserves the constant gravity line position. *Int Orthop*,31:253–8.

Gelb DE, Lenke LG & Bridwell KH. (1995). An analysis of sagittal spinal alignment in 100 asymptomatic middle and older aged volunteers. *Spine*, 20:1351-8.

Glassman SD, Berven S & Bridwell K. (2005). Correlation of radiographic parameters and clinical symptoms in adult scoliosis. *Spine*, 30:682-8.

Glassman SD, Bridwell K & Dimar JR. (2005). The impact of positive sagittal balance in adult spinal deformity. *Spine*, 30:2024-9.

Grubb SA & Lipscomb HJ. (1992). Diagnostic findings in painful adult scoliosis. *Spine*, 17:518–27.

Hammerberg EM & Wood KB. (2003). Sagittal profile of the elderly. *J Spinal Disord Tech*, 16:44–50.

Jackson RP & McManus AC. (1994). Radiographic analysis of sagittal plane alignment and balance in standing volunteers and patients with low back pain matched for age, sex, and size: a prospective controlled clinical study. *Spine*, 19:1611–8.

Jackson PR. (1997). Spinal balance, lumbopelvic alignments around the "hip axis" and positioning for surgery. *Spine State Art Rev*, 11:33–58.

Jackson PR, Peterson MD & McManus AC. (1998). Compensatory spinopelvic balance over the hip axis and better reliability in measuring lordotic to the pelvic radius on standing lateral radiographs of adult volunteers and patients. *Spine*, 16:1750–67.

Jackson RP & Hales C. (2000). Congruent spinopelvic alignment on standing lateral radiographs of adult volunteers. *Spine*, 25:2808–15.

Jackson RP, Kanemura T & Kawakami N. (2000). Lumbopelvic lordosis and pelvic balance on repeated standing lateral radiographs of adult volunteers and untreated patients with constant low back pain. *Spine*, 25:575-86.

Jansson PA & Grahn R. (1995). Engineering Mechanics: Vol. 2, Dynamics. *Prentice Hall International*, 253–370. Hemel Hempstead, Hertfordshire, United Kingdom

Kobayashi T, Atsuta Y & Matsuno T. (2004). A longitudinal study of congruent sagittal spinal alignment in an adult cohort. *Spine*, 29:671–6.

Legaye J, Duval-Beaupere G & Hecquer J. (1998). Pelvic incidence: a fundamental pelvic parameter for three-dimensional regulation of spinal sagittal curves. *Eur Spine J*, 7:99-103.

Legaye J & Duval-Beaupere G. (2008). Gravitational forces and sagittal shape of the spine. Clinical estimation of their relations. *Int Orthop*, 32:809–16

Mac-Thiong JM, Transfeldt EE & Mehbod AA. (2009). Can C7 plumbline and gravity line predict health related quality of life in adult scoliosis? *Spine*, 34:E519-27.

Nash ML, Allard P & Hinse S. (2002). Relations between standing stability and body posture parameters in adolescent idiopathic scoliosis. *Spine*, 27:1911–7.

Roussouly P, Gollogly S & Berthonnaud E. (2005). Classification of the normal variation in the sagittal alignment of the human lumbar spine and pelvis in the standing position. *Spine*, 30:346-53.

Roussouly P, Gollogly S & Noseda O. (2006). The vertical projection of the sum of the ground reactive forces of a standing patient is not the same as the C7 plumb line: a radiographic study of the sagittal alignment of 153 asymptomatic volunteers. *Spine*, 31:E320–5.

Schwab F, Lafage V & Boyce R. (2006). Gravity line analysis in adult volunteers: age-related correlation with spinal parameters, pelvic parameters, and foot position. *Spine*, 31:E959-67.

Schwab F, Lafage V & Patel A. (2009). Sagittal plane considerations and the pelvis in the adult patient. *Spine*, 34:1828-33.

Schwab F, Patel A & Ungar B. (2010). Adult spinal deformity-postoperative standing imbalance. *Spine*, 35:2224-2231.

Smith-Peterson MN, Larson CB & Aufranc OE. (1969). Osteotomy of the spine for correction of fl exion deformity in rheumatoid arthritis. *Clin Orthop Relat Res*, 66:6–9.

Van Royen BJ, Toussaint HM & Kingma I. (1998). Accuracy of the sagittal vertical axis in a standing lateral radiograph as a measurement of balance in spinal deformities. *Eur Spine J*, 7:408–12.

Vaz G, Roussouly P & Berthonnaud E. (2002). Sagittal morphology and equilibrium of pelvis and spine. *Eur Spine J*, 11:80-7.

Vedantam R, Lenke LG & Bridwell KH. (2000). The effect of variation in arm position on sagittal spinal alignment. *Spine*, 25:2204–9.

Vialle R, Levassor N & Rillardon L. (2005). Radiographic analysis of the sagittal alignment and balance of the spine in asymptomatic subjects. *J Bone Joint Surg Am*, 87:260-7.

Vidal J & Marnay T. (1983). Morphology and anteroposterior body equilibrium in spondylolisthesis L5-S1. *Rev Chir Orthop Reparatrice Appar Mot*, 69:17-28.

Vidal J & Marnay T. (1984). Sagittal deviations of the spine, and trial of classification as a function of the pelvic balance. *Rev Chir Orthop Reparatrice Appar Mot*, 70(suppl 2):124-6.

White AA & Panjabi MM. (1990). Practical biomechanics of scoliosis and kyphosis. In: *Clinical biomechanics of the spine.* White AA, Panjabi MM, eds, 127-68. Philadelphia: Lippincott-Raven.

Part 3

Hip

4

Pelvic and Hip Osteotomies in Children

I. Gavrankapetanovic
Orthopedic and Traumatology Clinic,
Clinical Center University of Sarajevo,
Bosnia and Herzegovina

1. Introduction

In this chapter four tipe of pelvic osteotomy in children will be addressed. We think that is very important to share our 25 years long experience in this field with other colleagues and help with variety of practical advices.

Congenital dysplasia of the hip involves the acetabular roof, which doesn't adequately cover the femoral head. Many pelvic operations are done to achieve better coverage of the femoral head. Among them are various types of pelvic osteotomies.

We have operated many children becouse of poor develope early ultrasound hip screening in past decades in our contry or failure in diagnose on early screening. In this chapter we would like to describe two types of pelvic osteotomies with case presentations for each.

We commenly use following two types of pelvic osteotomies:

1. Innominate Osteotomy of Salter
2. Chiari Medial Displacement Osteotomy of the Pelvis

2. Innominate osteotomy of salter

2.1 Definition

The Salter innominate osteotomy is sort of derotating osteotomy, usually performed in combination with an open reduction for dislocated hip in developmetnal dysplasia of the hip (DDH), and also in treatment of acetabular dysplasia in the child with a concentrically reduced hip.[1]

2.2 Anatomy

The line of osteotomy extends from the sciatic notch to the anterior inferior iliac spine, perpendicular to the sides of the ilium.

The acetabulum is reorientated without changing its size or shape. It is rotated to improve anterior and lateral femoral head coverage.

Bone graft increases anterior and lateral femoral head coverage.[6]

2.3 Indications

1. Age of patient: patient 18 months of age and older till 8 year old
2. Coplete and concentric reduction of the hip
3. Congruous hip joint
4. Absence of contracture

2.4 Pathogenesis

Acetabular dysplasia can have different couses:

- Lack of a reduced, spherical head within the growing acetabulum[1]
- Abnormal interstitial or appositional growth within the acetabular and triradiate cartilage[1]
- Abnormal development of the secondary centers of ossification of the ilium, pubis, and ischium[1]

2.5 Patient history and physical findings

- patient with DDH are usually female and first - born children
- can be breech presentation at birth
- physical examination findings:
  - Hamstring tightness test - implies hip dislocation or flaccid paralysis of the hamstring muscles
  - Gluteus medius lurch - positive test - trunk lean over the stance phase leg
  - Galeazzi sing - positive test is when there are knees at different levels (nonspecifik sing)
  - Limitation of hip abduction - asymmetric abduction signify unilateral hip dislocation, bilateral hip dislocation is shown by bilaterally decreased abduction
  - Trendelenburg sing- the test is positive if the pelvis dips away from the affected leg during single limb stance (nonspecific sign)
  - Inguinal skin fold - asymmetric skin fold (nonspecific sign)

2.6 Imiging and other diagnostic studies

- AP radiography, supine frog - leg lateral pelvis radiography
- to diagnose acetabular dysplasia it is necessary to measure acetabular index on the AP film, also Shenton's line is inspected for discontinuity, which implies hip subluxation
- subtle cases of acetabular dysplasia can be identify by false - profile view of the hip
- in older children for assessing acetabular morphology can be useful 3D CT scanning of the acetabulum, MRI of the hip

2.7 Diferential diagnosis

- Congenital short femur
- Proximal femoral focal deficiency
- Legg - Calve - Pertes disease
- Developmental coxa vara

2.8 Nonoperative management

- Observation of acetabular index after successful closed reduction during the period of 12 - 18 month
- Salter innominate osteotomy can be perfomed if residual acetabular dysplasia exist[9]
- Open reduction of dislocated hip can be performed if a child less than 18 months old fails closed reduction
- If acetabular development is deficient after observation for improvement in the acetabular index Salter innominate osteotomy should be performed

2.9 Surgical management

2.9.1 Preoperative planing

- In cases of hip dysplasia before patient positioning confirmation of concentric reduction is done by hip arthrogram
- If concentric reduction is not achieve before performing a Salter innominate osteotomy than other procedures like open reduction, proximal femoral osteotomy sould be perfomed to achieve it
- Salter innominate osteotomy can be performed including intramuscular psoas lengthening without open hip reduction if patient is older than 18 monts and if a gentle concentric closed reduction is achieved
- To decide whether a concurrent femoral derotational osteotomy is necessary it is used fluoroscopy for estimation of femoral anteversion
- If femoral anteversion is greater than 45 degrees femoral derotational osteotomy is performed

2.10 Positioning

- We placed patient on the operating table with a gel roll under the thoracolumbar spine on the affected side.
- The area of sterile preparation is from the midline anterior and posterior, to the inferior rib cage proximaly, and entire leg distally

2.11 Approach

- It is used an anterior Smith - Peterson approach to the hip

Surgical incision is placed over the anterior aspect of the hip, centered about 2 cm below the anterior superior iliac spine. Proximaly it goes following the contour of the iliac crest but distal to it. Distally, incision curves between the sartorius and tensor fascia lata muscles.

2.12 Surgical techniques

- anterior surgical approach to the hip;
- release of adductor and iliopsoas muscles;
- Gigli saw is used for osteotomizing innominate bone from the sciatic notch to the anterior inferior iliac spine;
- acetabulum together with pubis and ischium is rotated anteriorly and laterally with symphysis acting as a hinge;

- the osteotomy is opened anteriorly by external rotation of the femur;
- osteotomy is held open anterolaterally by bone graft, and thus roof of acetabulum is shifted more anteriorly and laterally;
- bone graft is secured with Steinmann pins;
- it is necessary to take intraoperative radiograph with the pins in place to ensure they do not enter the triradiate cartilage

2.13 Pearls and pitfalls

- the osteotomy should be considered only for anterior and lateral acetabular deficiency in the concentrically reduced hip;
- the osteotomy should be avoided in conditions with known posterior hip displasia, such as myelomeningocele or cerebral palsy;
- it is essential strict subperiosteal exposure of the sciatic notch;
- Gigli saw passage is facilitated by twisting the retractors in opposite directions;
- to determine the proper osteotomy exit postition the anterior inferior iliac spine needs to be fully exposed;
- pulling the distal fragment anterior and keeping the posterior cortex of the osteotomy opposed will hinge open osteotomy;
- estimation of proper pin length;
- obtain an intraoperative radiograph;
- extra - articular pin placement shuld be ruled out by direct palpation or by placing the hip through a full range of motion and feeling and listening for crepitus;
- proper medial pin placement is achieved by pins aimed deep to the medial cortex in the proximal and distal fragments and the graft;
- proper posterior pin placement is achieved by pins aimed in the posterior half of the graft

2.14 Postoperative care

- patient is immobilized in cast for about 6 weeks

2.15 Outcomes

- good to excellent functional outcomes scores at over 30 years are expected after Salter innominate osteotomy, in the abscence of avascular necrosis

2.16 Complications

- during surgical exposure it can be injured: neurovascular structures in the sciatic notch, lateral femoral cutaneous nerve;
- consequence of inadquate patient selection preoperatively or inadequate acetabular rotation intraoperatively is inadequate correction of acetabular dysplasia;[7]
- injury of the femoral nerve can appear due to prolonged retraction of the psoas muscle or incorrect identification of the psoas tendon during intramuscular tenotomy;
- pin penetaration into the hip joint or triradiate cartilage ;
- nonunion at the osteotomy site,
- migration of the graft,[7]

- avascular necrosis of the femoral epiphysis[7]
- growth arrest of the triradiate cartilage

2.17 Case presentation

A boy born august 2008

x – ray took before surgery

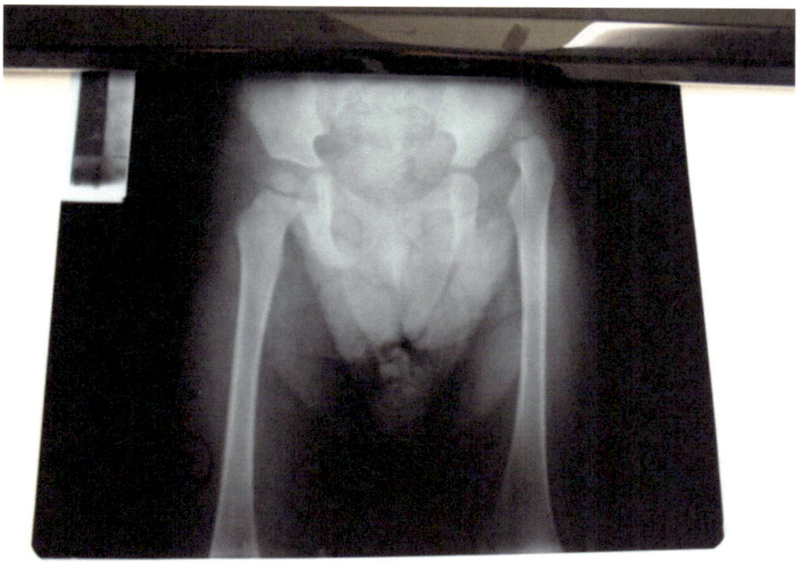

x – ray took 30.12.2010.

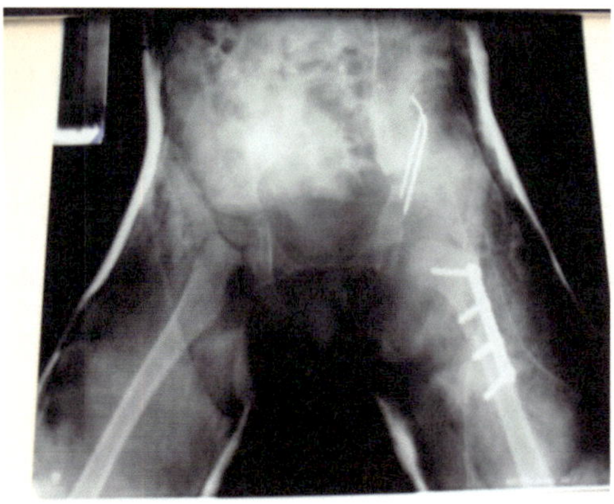

x – ray took 17.05.2011.

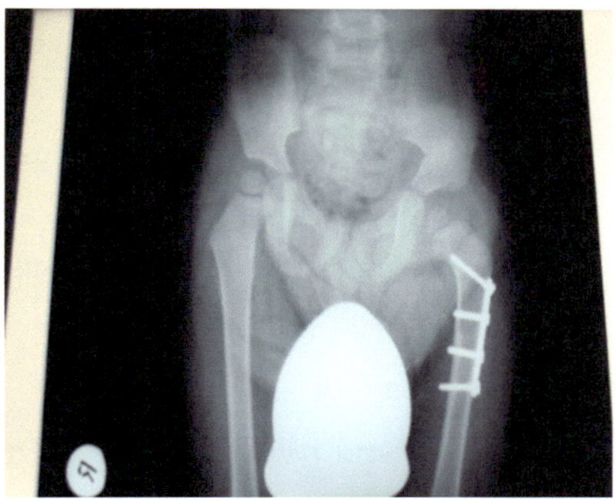

3. Chiari medial displacement osteotomy of the pelvis

3.1 Definition

Chiari osteotomy is a acetabular osteotomy salvage procedure which is indicated in patients without concentrically reducible hip;

- goes through the iliac bone of the pelvis; [1]
- medial deplacement of acetabulum and hip joint;
- improving posterior and lateral coverage;
- shelf over the dysplastic, subluxated hip is formed by ilium;
- goal is create a stable, pain – free hip

3.2 Indications

1. Age of patient: patient over 8 year old, adolescents, young adult
2. An irreducible lateral subluxation of the hip with moderate incongruity of the joint

3.3 Contraindications

- severe arthrosis;
- age over 45;
- greater proximal migration of the femoral head

3.4 Anatomy

- **DDH** – deficiency of the anterior and anterolateral acetabulum;
- **Spastic hip dysplasia** – deficiency of lateral and posterolateral acetabulum;
- When planning the shape and orientation of the osteotomy and positioning of the iliac shelf over the hip joint it is necessary to consider location of acetabular deficiency;
- Femoral head deformity usually involves coxa breva, coxa magna, or coxa plana;
- Abductor mechanicd may be improved by simultaneous advancement of the greater trochanter;
- In cases of high dislocation of the hip and in the pelvis in patients with advanced neurologic conditions Chiari osteotomy may not provide adequate coverage;
- Additonal bone graft to supplement posterior, lateral and anterior coverage is usually necessary;
- Contcentric reduction of the femoral head into the acetabulum is not required;
- Increasing the surfice area of coverage provides decreasing the force across the hip joint;
- Obligatory shortening of the gluteal muscle length and abductor moment arm is caused by lateralizing the ilium to form a shelf that weakness the muscle and contribustes to postoperative Trendelenburg limp;
- Resting length of the gluteus medius can be restored by advancing the greater trochanter

3.5 Pathogenesis

Advanced hip disease requiring salvage surgery may be caused by following:

- late diagnosis of developmental dysplasia of the hip;
- spastic or neuromuscular hip dysplasia;
- failed prior hip procedures;
- acetabular trauma

Incomplete or incongruous femoral head coverage can be caused by following femoral head conditions:

- primary malformation,
- secondary avascular necrosis,
- slipped capital femoral epiphysis,
- epiphyseal - metaphyseal dysplasia,
- secondary malformation from longstanding subluxation or impingement

3.6 Patient history and physical findings

3.6.1 Main parts include

- family or personal history of DDH,
- other hip disorder,
- trauma,
- skeletal dysplasias
- cerebral palsy
- birth order and weight

3.7 The phyisical examination

- limb length,
- gait,
- strength,
- assistive devices

3.8 Specific hip tests

- Trendelenburg test: weakness in abductors
- Anterior apprehension test: patient's subjective feeling of fear or instability
- Strength of gluteus medius and maximus
- Anterior impingement test
- Bicycle test
- Range of motion: testing internal and external rotation at multiple degrees of flexion because of variation of femoral head and acetabular deformities that can help in location of pathologic articulation
- Galeazzi sign: shows hip subluxation or dislocation
- Preoperative requirements: flexion to 90 degrees, full extension, at least 10 to 20 degrees of abduction
- Preoperative gait assessement: discern of limp antalgia what can be improve by Chiari osteotomy

3.9 Imaging and other diagnostic studies

- Radiography includes: weight - bearing AP views of bilateral hips,false profile of hips, AP of hips in maximal abduction and internal rotation what can provide assessment of lateral and anterior coverage of the femoral head as well as congruency of the hip joint.
- 3D CT can be used in preoperatively assessing the amount and direction of acetabular deficiency

- MRI can help in preoperative assessment of articular and labral cartilage

3.10 Diferential diagnosis

- DDH
- Spastic hip dysplasia
- Legg - Calve - Perthes diseas, avascular necrosis
- Posttraumatic hip or femoral dysplasia
- Multiple or spondyloepiphysealdysplasia

3.11 Nonoperative management

- The patient who is candidate for Chiari oteotomy usually have pain and arthrosis;
- The onset of arthritic symptoms can be delayed by activity, job modification, weight loss
- Physical therapy can be useful in increasing of range of motion and strength but can not stop the onset of arthritis in the dysplastic hip

3.12 Surgical management

- Onset of spastic hip dysplasia can be delayed by hip adductor tenotomy, lengthening or Botox if performed before age 4 to 6 and if hip abduction is less than 45 degrees with hip flexed and extended;[4]
- Surgical correction is necessary in painful, unstable, moderate to severe dysplasia with incongruent articualtion with or without femoral head deformity;
- Arthrodesis, shelf procedures and arthroplasty are additional options to Chiari

3.13 Preoperative planning

- A complete physical examination and radiographs
- If there is marked proximal migration, preoperative traction for 2 to 3 weeks can be used to improve the position of the femoral head relative to the acetabulum

3.14 Positioning

- The position of the patient is supine ;
- Antibiotic profilaxis and placement of catheter;
- General anesthesia is one that we prefer

3.15 Approach

There are two approaches:

- ilioinguinal approach - begins from the iliac crest and continues medially for about 10 cm
- iliofemoral approach provides better visualisation in larger patients and combined pelvic and femoral procedures to be done through one incision

3.16 Surgical tehnique

- iliac osteotomy is angled from the sciatic notch to the ASIS - anterolateral distally to posteromedial proximally;

- placing iliac buttress into horizontal position should be avoided since this will cause persistently unstable joint laterally;
- following osteotomy, a triangular osseous defect anteriorly which is stabilized with curved plate of bone graft from iliac wing;
- consequence of inadequate stabilization of anterior defect is anterior instability;
- acetabulum is displaced medially;
- acetabulum is abducted into a more vertical and medial position and replaces it with joint capsule supported by osseous buttress of the iliac wing;
- distal acetabular fragment is displaced medially and adducted;
- proximal iliac fragment sould not be move laterally;
- inferior surface of proximal fragment forms roof over femoral head;
- the osteotomy is fixed in place with cortical screws either along the iliac crest or along the outer table of the ilium

3.17 Pearls and pitfalls

- adequate patient selection;
- Chiari osteotomy may incompletely manage severe arthrosis or proximal migration;
- we pay special attention when considering Chiari osteotomy in young patients or in patients with neuromuscular disease as they may have insufficient thickness of ilium to provide adequate coverage;
- the contents of the sciatic notch must be carefully protected by subperiosteal placement of retractors;
- screws are placed at the iliac crest for fixation or along the outer table of the ilium in increased displacement;
- for augmenting deficient coverage we use a corticocancellous segment of the inner table of the ilium;
- after displacement our recommendation is palpation of the posterior edge of the osteotomy to confirm there is no soft tissue entrapment

3.18 Postoperative care

- Patients are placed in long – leg casts held in abduction by a connector bar

3.19 Outcomes

- Good to exellent outcomes for pain relief;[2,3,5,7]
- We have better outcomes in younger patients with mobile hips and adequate corrected coverage

3.20 Complications

- Infection;
- Heterotropic ossification;
- Incomplete correction and resubluxation;
- Neuropraxia of sciatic and of the lateral femoral cutaneous nerve obtained by sciatic nerve entrapment or injury during osteotomy

3.21 Case presentation

A boy born in february 1998. Operatively treated out of our Institution, when he was one year old

x - ray took 19.10.2010. x - ray took 01.11.2010.

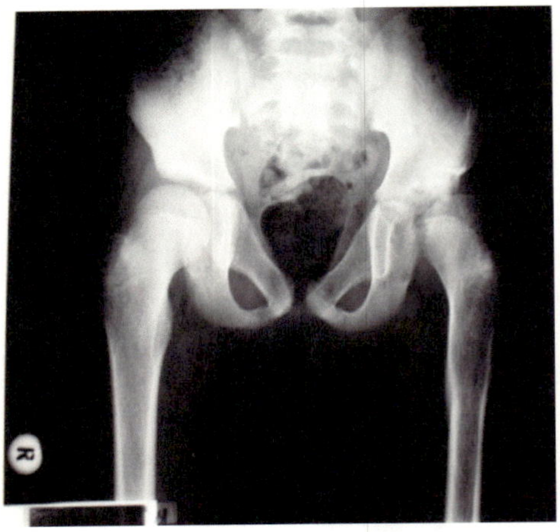

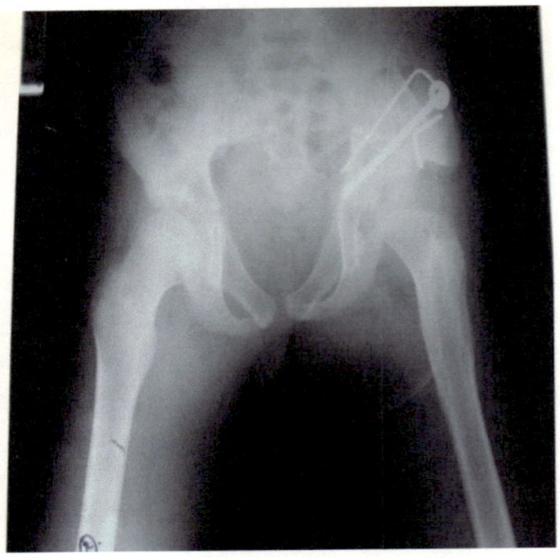

x - ray took 14.12.2010.

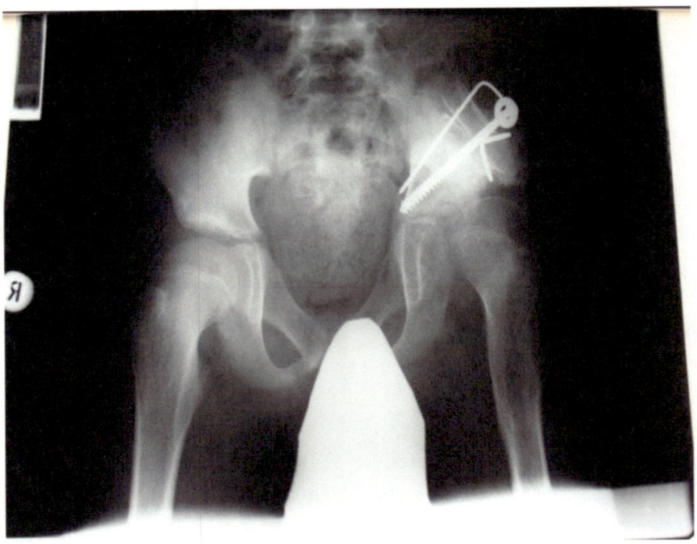

4. References

4.1 References part 1

[1] Flynn JM, Wiesel SW. Operative tchniques in pediatric orthopaedics (Lippincott Williams &Wikins, 2011).

[2] Tukenmez M, Tezeren G. Salter innominate osteotomy for treatment of developmental dysplasia of the hip. Journal of Orthopedic Surgery 2007;15(3):286-90.

[3] Barrett WP, Staheli LT, Chew DE. The effectiveness of the Salter innominate osteotomy in the treatment of congenital dislocation of the hip. J Bone Joint Surg Am 1984;68A:79-87.

[4] Macnicol MF, Bertol P. The Salter innominate osteotomy: should it be combined with concurrent open reduction? J Pediatr Orthop B 2005;14:415-421.

[5] Böhm P, Brzuske A. Salter Innominate Osteotomy for the Treatment of Development Dysplasia of the Hip in Children: Results of Seventy - three Consecutive Osteotomies After Twenty - sixt to Thirty five years of follow - up. JBJS 2002;84:178-186.

[6] Rab GT. Biomechanical aspects of Salter osteotomy. Clin Orthop Relat Res 1978;132:82-87.

[7] Gur E, Sarlak O. The complications of Salter innominate osteotomy in the treatment of congenital dislocation of the hip. Acta Orthop B 2005;14:415-421.

[8] Sarban S, Ozturk A, Tabur H, et al. Anteversion of the acetabulum and femoral neck in early walking age patients with developmental dysplasia of the hip. J Pediatr Orthop B 2005;14:410-414.

[9] Gillingham BL, Sanche AA, Wenger DR. Pelvic osteotomies for the treatment of hip dysplasia in children and young adults. J Am Acad Orthop Surg 1999;7:325 - 337

4.2 References part 2

[1] Flynn JM, Wiesel SW. Operative tchniques in pediatric orthopaedics (Lippincott Williams &Wikins, 2011).

[2] Yanagimoto S, Hotta H, Izumida R, Sakamaki T. Long - term results of the Chiari pelvic osteotomy in patients with developmental dysplasia of the hip: indications for the Chiari pelvic osteotomy according to disease stage and femoral head shape. J Orthop Sci. 2005; 10(6):557-63.

[3] Ito H, Matsuno T, Minami A. Chiari pelvic osteotomy for advanced osteoarthritis in patient with hip dysplasia. J Bone Joint Surg Am 2004; 86A: 1439 - 1445.

[4] Debnath UK, Guha AR, Karlakki S, et al. Combined femoral and Chiari osteotomies for reconstruction of the painful subluxation or dislocation of the hip in cerebral palsy: a long - term outcome study. J Bone Joint Surg Br 2006;88B:1373 - 1378.

[5] Bailey TE, Hall JE. Chiari medial displacement osteotomy. J Pediatr Orthop 1985;5:635 - 641.

[6] Windager R, Pongracz N, Schonecker W, et al. Chiari osteotomy for congenital dislocation and subluxation of the hip: results after 20 to 34 years follow - up. J Bone Joint Surg Br 1991;73B:890 - 895.

[7] Gagala J, Blacha J, Bednarek A. Chiari pelvic osteotomy in the treatment of hip dysplasia in adults. Chir Narzadow Ruchu Ortop. Pol. 2006;71(3):183-5

5

Acetabular Augmentation by Residual Hip Dysplasia

Borut Pompe and Vane Antolič

Department of Orthopaedic Surgery, University Medical Centre Ljubljana, Slovenia

1. Introduction

Residual hip dysplasia is one of the most common causes of secondary osteoarthritis of the hip joint. It is suggested that excessive hip joint contact stress due to small weight-bearing area is an important precipitating factor for the development of hip arthrosis (Hadley et al., 1990; Hipp et al., 1999; Maxian et al., 1995). Dysplasia of the hip refers to mechanical deformations and deviations in the size and shape or mutual proportions between the upper part of the femur and acetabulum (Durnin et al., 1991). The dysplastic hips are diagnosed according to anatomical changes in the hip that are visible in the radiographs (Durnin et al., 1991; Legal 1987; Pauwels, 1976). Usually, the center-edge angle of Wiberg (ϑ_{CE}) is used as the main radiographic parameter for the assessment of the hip dysplasia (Legal 1987; Pauwels, 1976). The range of ϑ_{CE} from 20–25° is considered as the lower limit for normal hips, while the value of ϑ_{CE} below 20° is pathognomonic for the hip dysplasia (Legal 1987). The size of the angle ϑ_{CE} correlates with the size of the weight bearing area and may therefore serve as an indirect measure of the hip joint contact stress (Brinckmann et al., 1981; Hipp, 1999; Iglic et al., 1993; Kummer 1988; Malvitz & Weinstein, 1994). However, it was suggested that besides ϑ_{CE} other geometrical parameters such as the radius of the femoral head (Brinckmann et al., 1981; Legal 1987) or the pelvic shape (Iglic et al., 1993, 2001; Kersnic et al., 1997) should be taken into account in assessment of the contact stress distribution. Therefore, the direct calculation of the contact stress in the hip joint has been introduced in the assessment of the biomechanical status of the hip (Brinckmann et al., 1981; Kummer, 1991;Legal 1987; Vengust, 2001) (Fig.1).

Dysplastic hips in adults are treated by redirectional (Ganz et al. 1988; Salter et al. 1984; Steel, 1973; Sutherland & Greenfield 1977) and periarticular osteothomies of the acetabulum (Pemberton, 1965), as well as by Chiari osteotomy (Chiari, 1953) and by extraarticular augmentation of the acetabular roof (Staheli, 1981), consisting of interposition of the joint capsule between the femoral head and the reconstructed acetabular roof. The aim of these procedures is to relive pain and to postpone the development of hip arthrosis.

The slotted acetabular augmentation (SAA), described by Staheli, is designed to treat mildly or severely dysplastic hips (Staheli, 1981). SAA seems to be a safer technique than complex redirectional and periarticular acetabular osteotomies (Staheli, 1991). In SAA, the acetabular roof is extended laterally, posteriorly and anteriorly by the grafts harvested from the ilium and placed into the slot above the acetabulum in the radial and tangential directions. Grafts are held in place by an elongated reflected tendon of the rectus femoris muscle. No pin fixation is required. After the operation, patients are immobilised in a single hip spica cast for six weeks (Staheli, 1981). SAA is a well-established technique fort the treatment of children and adolescents with hip dysplasia. It has not been widely accepted for treating hip dysplasia in adults altought good outcomes have been reported with other augmentation techniques in adults.

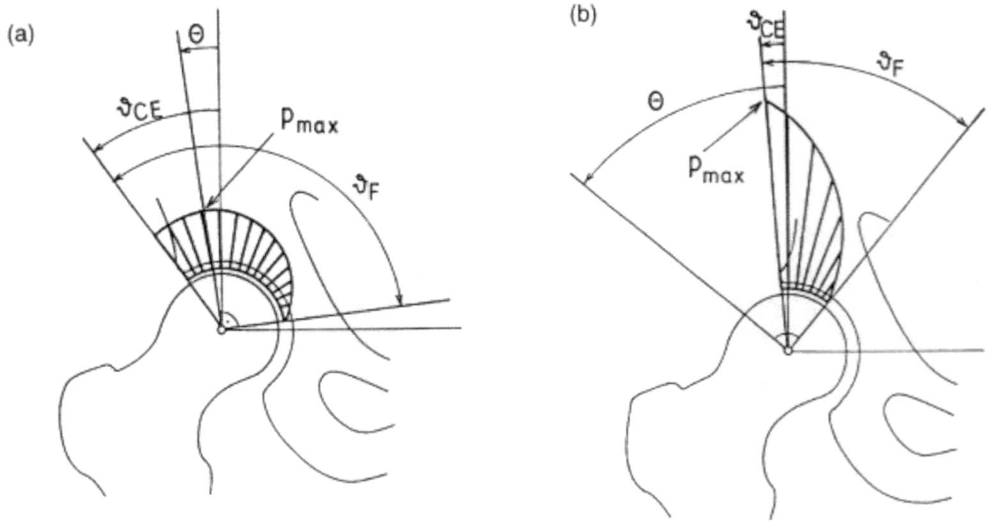

Fig. 1. Schematic presentation of the contact stress distribution in the normal (a) and dysplastic hip joint (b). The center-edge angle (ϑ_{CE}), the coordinate of the pole of stress distribution (θ), the functional angle of the weight bearing area (ϑ_F) and the location of the peak contact stress (p_{max}) are shown.

The purpose of this article was to review our early results of SAA done for residual hip dysplasia in adults. Preoperative values of the centre-edge angle of Wiberg, peak stress on the weight-bearing area of the hip and clinical Harris Hip Score were compared with the values determined at the latest follow-up. The joint-space width was used as an indicator of cartilage degeneration. The level of patient satisfaction was determined.

2. Patients and methods

Between 1997 and 2005, 14 consecutive patients underwent SAA for hip dysplasia. The study included 12 patients undergoing 14 SAAs for residual hip dysplasia; two patients were lost to follow-up and were excluded from the study. All our patients were women, who had a median age of 38.5 (17–42) years at the time of operation. Two of them were operated on bilaterally. All the operated hips showed spherical congruency and had been painful for an average of 4 years before the procedure. Based on the classification system of the Commission for the study of hip dysplasia of the German Society for Orthopaedics and Thraumatology (Tönnis et al., 1985) hips are classified according to the age of the patient and the ϑ_{CE} into the following four grades: grade 1—normal hips with the ϑ_{CE} equal to or greater than 30°; grade 2—mildly pathological hips with the angle equal to or greater than 20° and less than 30°; grade 3—moderately pathological hips with the ϑ_{CE} equal to or greater than 5° and less than 20°; and grade 4—extremely pathological hips with the ϑ_{CE} of less than 5°. All hips evaluated in our study had a ϑ_{CE} of less than 30°, thereby meeting the criteria for hip dysplasia. Preoperatively, two hips were grade 2, eight hips grade 3 and four hips grade 4. None of the hip was subluxated or dislocated before the surgery. The median follow-up period was 4 (1–8) years after surgery.

2.1 Preoperative planning

Previous studies found that in dysplastic conditions where ϑ_{CE} is small or negative, hip joint contact stress is higher than in hips with a larger ϑ_{CE}; however, stress can also be higher due to a higher or a too vertical resultant hip joint force (Iglič et al.,1993a; Ipavec et al.,1999; Genda et al.,2001). The direction and magnitude of the resultant hip joint force **R** depends, among other factors, on the femoral and pelvic geometry (Brand , 1997; Iglič et al.,1993b). It has been suggested that a computer model could be useful for guiding clinical decision-making to determine optimal treatment (Genda et al.,2001;Hsin et al., 1996; Michaeli et al., 1997) The influence of both the ϑ_{CE} and **R** are expressed by the contact stress distribution. Some recent studies indicate that the distribution of the contact stress is the most important biomechanical parameter for predicting successful hip development (Pompe et al., 2003).

Peak contact stress in the weight bearing area of the hip (p_{max}) was calculated using a computer program, HIPSTRESS (Iglič & Kralj-Iglič, 1999; Iglič et al., 2002). The program consists of two procedures. First, the hip joint resultant force **R** transmitted from the acetabulum to the femur is determined by a threedimensional biomechanical model of the human hip (Iglič et al., 2002). This model is based on solving of the static equilibrium equations for the forces and torques acting on the pelvis and the loaded leg in the one-legged stance (Iglič et al., 1993b, 2002). In the one-legged stance the activity of the hip abductor muscles is necessary to maintain the balance of the pelvis. In our model, nine effective muscles are included (Iglič et al., 1993b, 2002). It is assumed that the force of the individual muscle acts in the straight line connecting the attachment point of the muscle on the pelvis to the attachment point on the femur. The individual variations in the femoral and pelvic geometry influence the directions of the muscle forces as well as the radius vectors of the application points of the muscle forces on the pelvis and femur. Therefore the geometry of the hip should be adapted for each patient individually according to the data determined from standard anteroposterior radiographs (Daniel et al., 2001; Iglič et al., 2001, Vengust et al., 2001; Zupanc et al., 2001). The input geometrical parameters of the model for determination of **R** are shown in the Fig. 2.

It was shown that the resultant hip joint force **R** determined in one-legged stance lies nearly in the frontal plane of the body (Iglič et al., 1993b, 2002). Therefore in the second mathematical model for determination of the contact stress distribution (Daniel et al., 2001; Iglič et al., 2002) the force **R** is assumed to lie in the frontal plane. The hip joint reaction force in the frontal plane can be expressed by its magnitude (R) and by its inclination in the frontal plane with respect to the vertical plane ϑ_R (Fig. 2). The angle ϑ_R is taken to be positive in the medial direction from the vertical axis and negativ in the lateral direction from the vertical axis (Daniel et al., 2001; Iglič et al., 1993a).

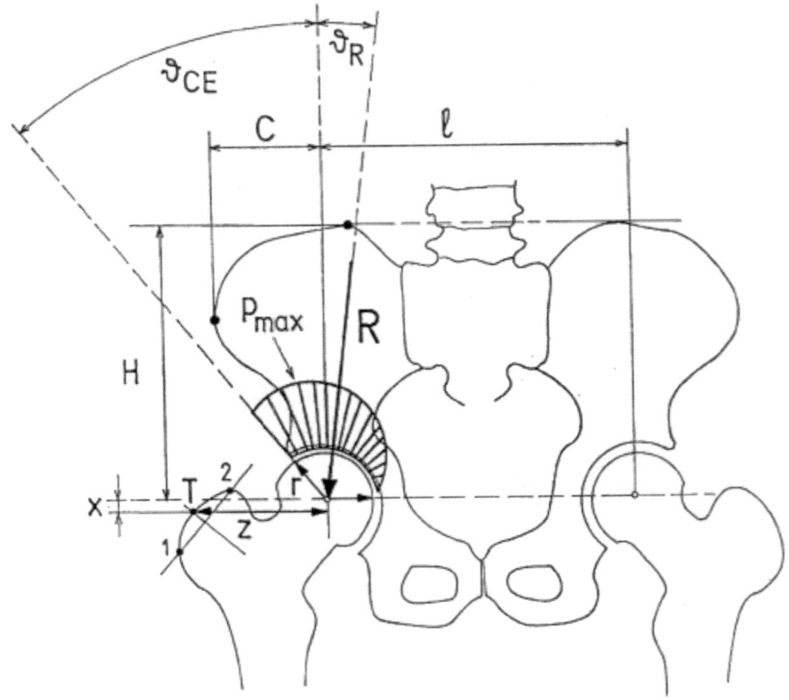

Fig. 2. The geometrical parameters used for determining the resultant hip force (R) include: interhip distance (l), pelvic height (H), pelvic width (C) and coordinates of the muscle attachment point (T), on the greater trochanter (z and x) and the centre-edge angle of Wiberg (ϑ_{CE})

In the second step the mathematical model for calculation of the stress distribution in the hip joint (Daniel et al., 2001; Iglič et al., 2002; Ipavec et al., 1999) is used. The model assumes the non-uniform distribution of the contact stress (Ipavec et al., 1999). Area of the hip where stress differs from zero is called the weight-bearing area. The size of the weight-bearing area and distribution of the contact stress are not fixed but depend on the load and geometry of the hip (Ipavec et al., 1999). The basic idea of the model is described below.

Besides the magnitude of the resultant hip force **R** and inclination of the resultant hip force ϑ_R the input parameters of the mathematical model for calculation of the hip joint contact stress are also the center-edge ϑ_{CE} and the radius of the femoral head r (Fig.2). The ϑ_{CE} is taken to be positive in the lateral direction from the vertical axis and negative in the medial direction from the vertical axis (Fig. 2).

Within the model of stress distribution the contact stress at any point of the weight-bearing area (p) is taken to be proportional to strain in the cartilage layer. The cartilage fills in the cleft between the femoral head and the acetabulum. It is assumed that the femoral head has spherical shape and acetabulum is the portion of the sphere, symmetric with respect to the frontal plane.

After loading there is one point where the spherical surfaces of the acetabulum and the femoral head are the closest. Due to symmetry of the articular surfaces with respect to the frontal plane and due to position of the hip joint reaction force in the frontal plane this point lies in the frontal plane and is called the stress pole (Ipavec et al., 1999). Position of the stress pole can be determined by the spherical coordinate θ (Brinckmann et al., 1981; Ipavec et al., 1999) which is angular displacement of the pole from the vertical axis in the frontal plane. θ is positive in the lateral direction and negative in the medial direction from the vertical axis as well as ϑ_{CE}. The above assumptions lead to the cosine dependency of the contact stress distribution in the hip joint (Brinckmann et al., 1981). The lateral border of the weight-bearing area is determined by the acetabular geometry while the medial border is determined as the curve where stress vanishes.

In the case of dysplastic hips (usually with small ϑ_{CE}) the stress pole lies outside the weight bearing area, therefore the peak contact stress is located at the point of the weight bearing surface which is closest to the pole, i.e. at the lateral acetabular rim. For small ϑ_{CE} the contact stress distribution is highly nonuniform all over the weight bearing area.

The peak stress on the weight-bearing area of the hip was determined before the operation and at the latest follow-up. The Harris Hip Score was calculated preoperatively and at the latest follow-up. The joint-space width was measured in line with the centre of the femoral head. Patient satisfaction with the results of SAA was graded as very satisfied, satisfied and not satisfied. The paired Student's *t*-test was used to detect difeerences between preoperative and followup values. The level of significance was set at 5%.

2.2 Surgical technique

All patients were treated by the same operative technique (Staheli, 1991) performed by the second author (V.A.). The median surgical time was 120 min (90-180). The patients were operated on lying supine on a standard operating table. A Smith- Petersen approach was used to expose the hip joint. The sartorius attachment was detached. It was important to avoid lateral famoral cutaneous nerve damage. A tendon of the reflected head of the rectus femoris was divided as posteriorly as possible, and prepared for a Z-shaped elongation. A slot in the subchondral bone at the acetabular margin was made by drilling 1-cm holes into the acetabular margin. It was important to drill the holes as close to the joit capsule as posible. The holes were joined with a narrow rongeur (Fig 3).

Autologous bone grafts harvested from the ipsilateral pelvic wing were used for additional coverage of the femoral head. The grafts were rectangular in shape, approximately 1 cm wide, 2 to 5 cm long and up to 1 cm thick, with cortical bone on one side and cancellous bone on the other (Fig. 4).

In the layer above the femoral head, the grafts were placed in the acetabular slot with the cortical side down. The graft should be placed in the acetabular slot as press fit as possible. A part of the graft which is not in the acetabular slot should lie on the joint capsule and form a new acetabular roof. The size of the graft should be measured precisely by planning the operation to avoid the acetabular roof overcorrection. The next layer of grafts is perpendicular to the firs leyed and it lies in the tangential direction to the acetabul (Fig. 5).

The two layers of the graft were secured by suturing the tendon back in its original position. The uppermost layer consisted of irregular bone chips which were "hammered" in place. When viewed from the side, the uppermost layer was triangular in shape, with the base on the tangential layer providing additional mechanical support to the first two layers (Fig. 6).

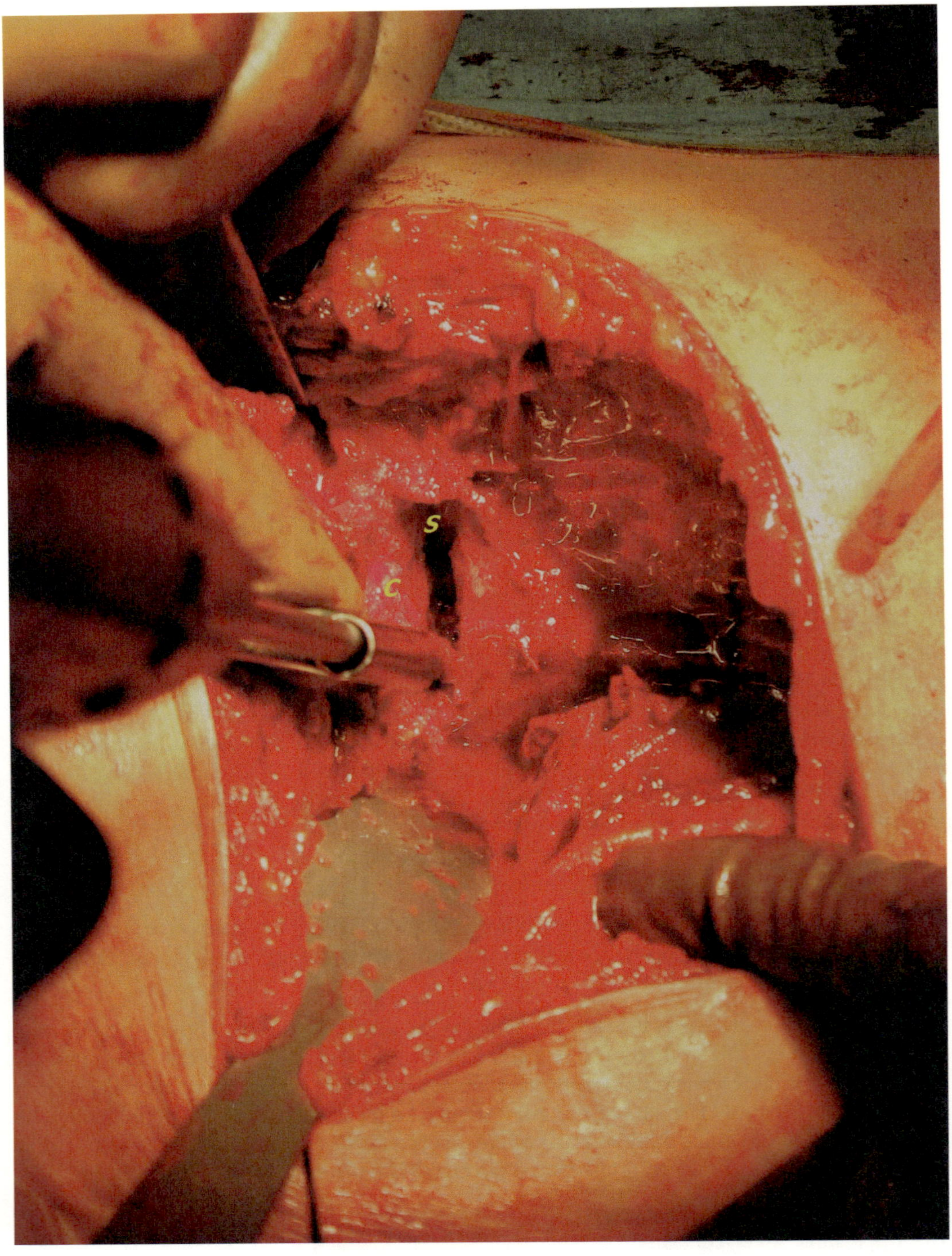

Fig. 3. Drilling the slot into acetabular margin (*S*) as close to the joit capsule (*C*) as posible

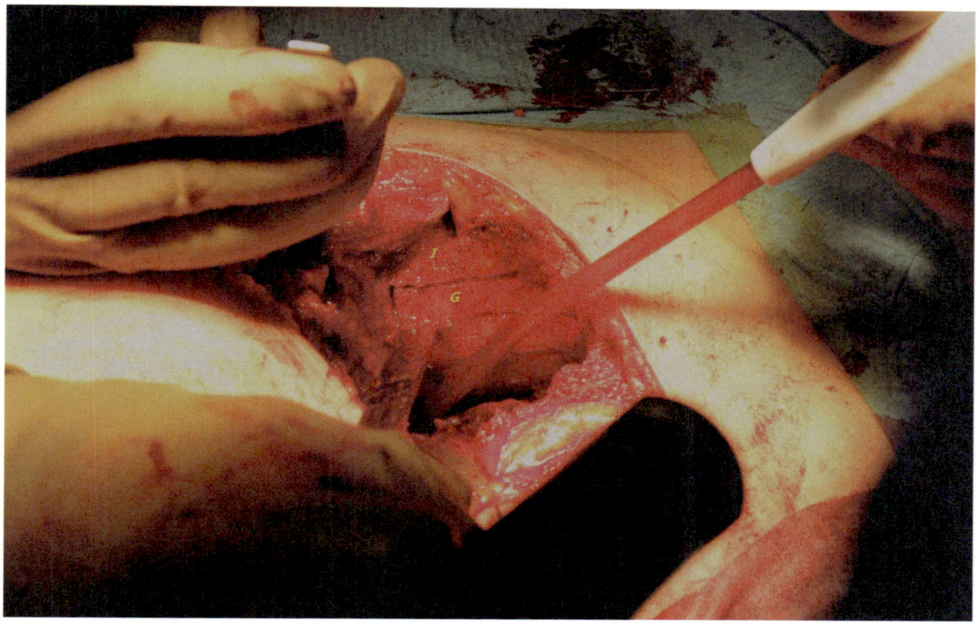

Fig. 4. The preparation of grafts (*G*) from the os ileum (*I*)

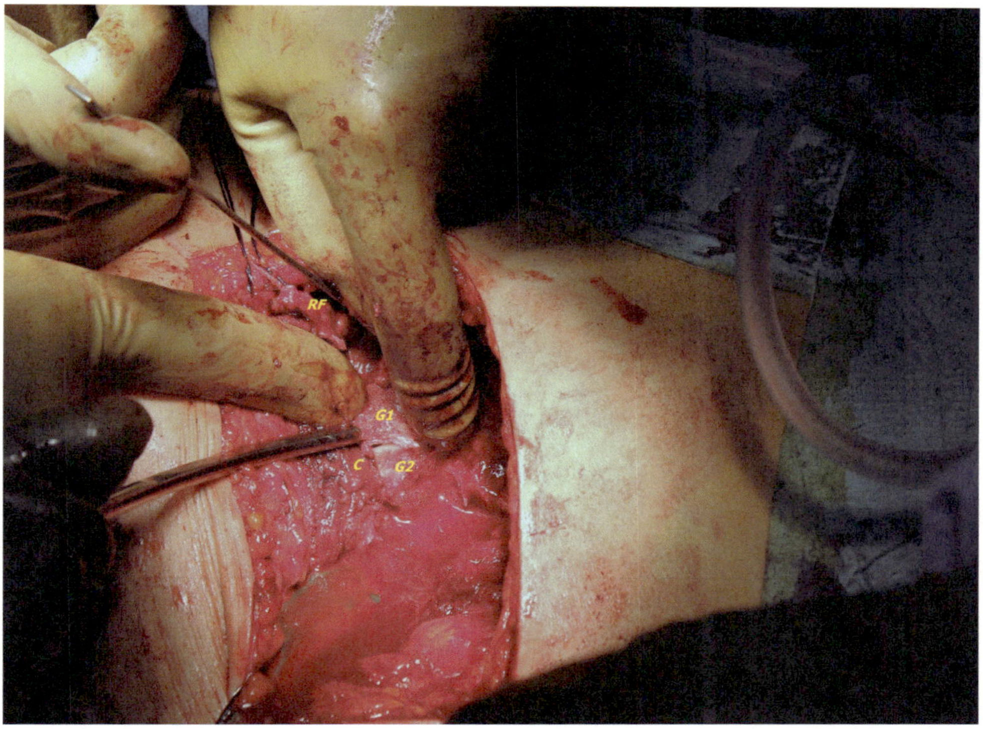

Fig. 5. Inserting the grafts into the slot. *RF:* Anterior part of the reflected head of the rectus femoris prepared for a Z-shaped elongation, *G1:* Insertio of the graft, *G2:* Inserted graft, *C:* Joint capsula

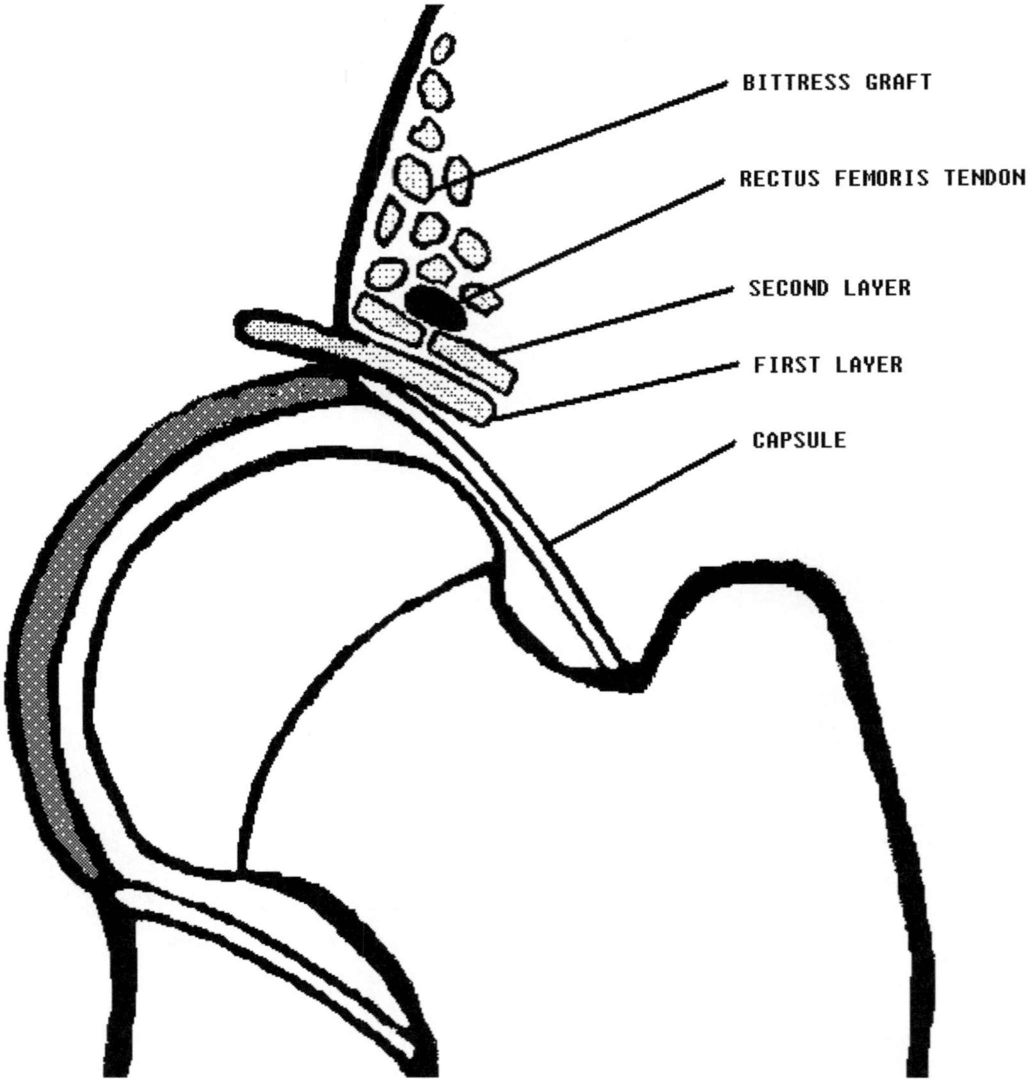

Fig. 6. The slotted acetabular augmentation operative technique.

2.3 Postoperative treatment

A single hip spica cast was applied with the hip in 15 degrees of abduction, 20 degrees of flexion and in neutral rotation position. The median hospital stay was ten days (6-17). After six weeks the cast was removed and the patients started passive and active range of motion exercises. No weight bearing was permitted for six weeks postoperatively. After removal of the cast, the patients were allowed to bear 1/5 of body weight on the affected extremity for next three months.

Radiographs were taken prior to surgery (Fig. 7) and at the latest follow-up (Fig. 8); a 10 % magnification rate was taken into account.

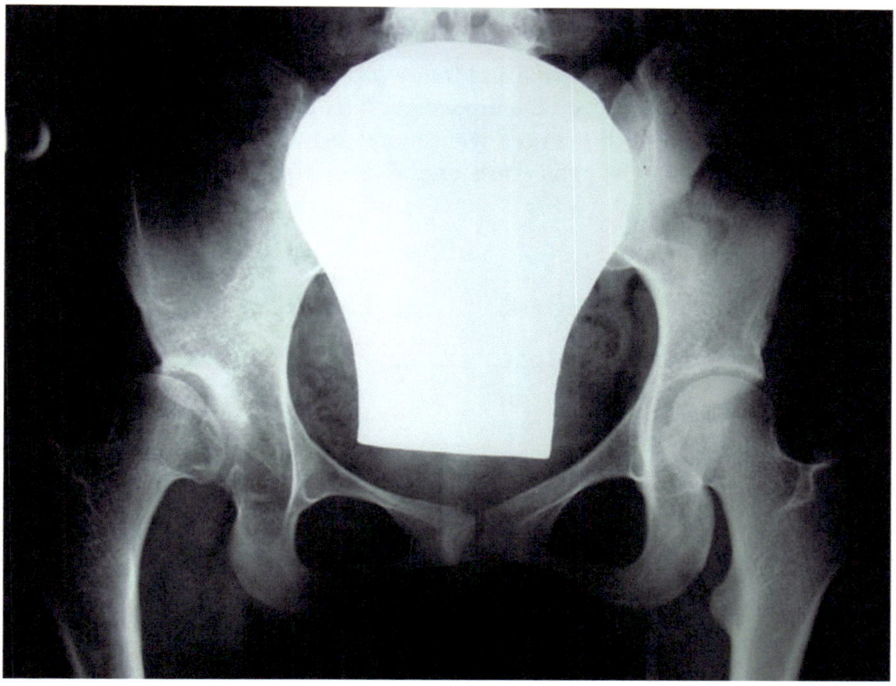

Fig. 7. Radiographs of a 19-year-old woman with the Wiberg angle of 1° on the right, taken before the operation.

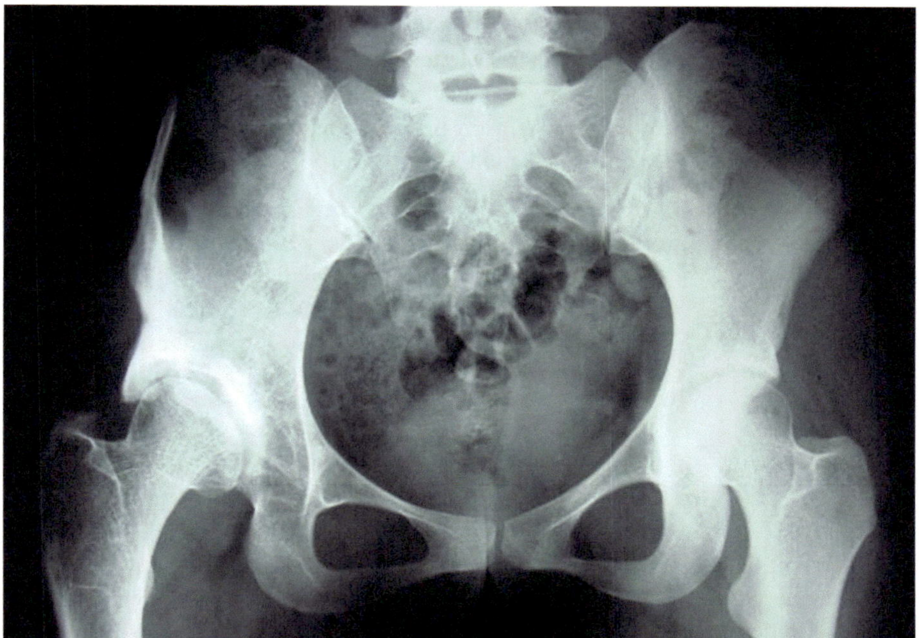

Fig. 8. Radiographs of the same woman 4 years after the slotted acetabular augmentation. The Wiberg angle increased to 42°.

3. Results

Table 1 shows the median preoperative and follow-up values and the ranges for the centre-edge angle of Wiberg, peak stress on the hip weight-bearing area and the clinical Harris Hip Score. Statistically significant differences were found between preoperative and follow-up values of the centre-edge angle, peak stress on the hip weight-bearing area and Harris Hip Score ($p < 0.001$).

	ϑ_{CE} **(degress)**	P_{max} **(MPa)**	**HHS (points)**
PREOPERATIVE	9	14,9	60
	min. 1; max. 26	min. 6,3; max. 28,1	min. 45; max. 98
AT FOLLOW-UP	43	4,1	93
	min. 31; max. 55	min. 3; max. 6,1	min. 49; max. 100

Table 1. Median values and ranges before the operation and at the latest follow-up. ϑ_{CE}; centre-edge angle of Wiberg, P_{max} ; peak stress on the weight bearing area of the hip, *HHS;* Harris Hip Score. The differences between preoperative and at follow-up values are highly significant ($P < 0.001$).

The median joint-space width was 5 (3-9) mm prior to surgery, and 4 (2-6) mm at the latest follow-up. The difference was not statistically significant ($p = 0.2$).

Postoperatively, all patients experienced less pain in performing activities of daily living. Complete pain relief was reported by three patients (four SAAs), and less pain in performing activities of daily living by eight patients (nine SAAs). Pain experienced postoperatively by one patient (one SAA) was due to retrotrochanteric bursitis and was relived after an injection. Six patients (eight SAAs) were very satisfied, and six patients (six SAAs) were satisfied with the outcome. None of the patients reported dissatisfaction with the procedure.

4. Discussion

From 1987 to 1995, the Bernese periacetabular osteotomy was the preferred method for the treatment of residual congruent dysplastic hips at this Department (Kralj et al., 2005). Since 1997, SAA has been used in the treatment of adult females with residual dysplasia of the hip demonstrating spherical congruency, although the technique was originally indicated for the treatment hips with aspherical congruence in children and adolescents (Staheli 1981; Staheli & Chew, 1992). There were no male patients with residual hip dysplasia in our series.

In this study the classification system of the Commission for the study of hip dysplasia of the German Society for Orthopaedics and Thraumatology was used (Tönnis et al., 1985). Their evaluation scheme is based on the grades of deviation from normal. All hips evaluated in our study had a ϑ_{CE} of less than 30°, thereby meeting the criteria for hip dysplasia. Preoperatively, two hips were grade 2, eight hips grade 3 and four hips grade 4. After the operation, all hips were grade 1. In two patients (three hips) a decreased range of motion in flexion and in abduction was found after the operation, which may be due to overcorrection of the acetabular roof with the consequential femoroacetabular impingement. This poor outcome can be attributed to an avoidable mistake. The aim of the operation is to increase the angle of Wiberg and we should avoid acetabular overcoverrage exceeding 40°.

The tendon suturing over the grafts, and spica cast immobilisation seem to afford adequate immobilisation as indicated by the absence of radiographic graft displacement, and good graft incorporation and remodelling. The cast was well tolerated by the patients. Lengthy immobilisation in a spica cast appears to be a major drawback of the SAA technique compared with redirectional and periarticular acetabular osteotomies, which in the majority of cases require no spica cast immobilisation. No complications related to internal osteosynthesis are to be expected in the SAA patients. Moreover, SAA requires no osteotomy, which tends to be the main source of complications in redirectional and periarticular acetabular osteotomies, such as nerve palsy, pseudarthosis, pain, intraarticular fracture and iatrogenic worsening of arthrosis, necessitating total hip replacement (Staheli, 1991).

In SAA, the capsule under the bony shelf is supposed to undergo metaplasia into the fibrocartilage (Moll, 1982). No significant changes of the joint-space width medial to the shelf, i.e. the original acetabular roof, were noted in our study, which suggests that no significant joint cartilage degeneration occurred during the follow-up period. Reduction in the median peak stress on the hip weight-bearing area was obtained in SAA and Bernese osteotomy with the use of the above described mathematical model (Daniel et al., 2001; Iglič & Kralj-Iglič, 1999; Iglič et al.,2002). The greatest influence on the peak stress is exerted by the radius of the femoral head, followed by the interhip distance, the position of the attachment point of the muscles on the greater trochanter and the pelvic height and width. Furthermore, the method has proved to be clinically relevant for evaluating the long-term clinical status of hips after osteotomies for aseptic necrosis of the femoral head (Dolinar et al., 2003) and after Bernese osteotomy (Kralj et al., 2005). This method has also been used to analyse the effect of the Salter innominate osteotomy (Vengust et al., 2001), and the Imhauser and Dunn-Fish operations for severe slipped capital femoral epiphysis (Zupanc et al., 2001).

In SAA and in Bernese osteotomy it was assumed that additional femoral head coverage was round (Iglič et al., 1993a). The postoperative values decreased to the level observed in healthy adult hips (Mavčič et al., 2002). SAA is therefore considered to be an adequate alternative to the redirectional and periarticular osteotomies of the acetabulum. No reports on the SAA treatment of hip dysplasia in adults have yet been published, but good outcomes have been reported with other augmentation techniques in adults (Courtois et al., 1987; Love et al., 1980; Migaud et al., 2004). The severity of preoperative arthrosis and the congruency have been identified as the main factors impairing survivorship in these patients (Fawzy et al., 2005).

We believe that with small number of patients with residual dysplasia the simplicity and safety of the SAA technique outweigh the advantages of the relatively highrisk Bernese periacetabular osteotomy.

5. Conclusion

In our series, the procedure has proved reliable and safe. Its advantages include symptomatic pain relief, adequate acetabular roof coverage and reduced peak stress on the weight bearing area of the hip. It can be used to postpone the development of hip arthrosis in adults with acetabular dysplasia.

6. Acknowledgements

The authors thank Veronika Kralj-Iglič, Aleš Iglič, Blaž Mavčič and other creators of the computer program HIPSTRES. The computer programs HIPSTRESS can be obtained from the web page http://physics.fe.uni-lj.si free of charge in order to use them for scientific purposes.

7. References

Armand M, Lepistö J, Tallroth K. Outcome of periacetabular osteotomy: joint contact pressure calculation using standing AP radiographs, 12 patients followed for average 2 years. Acta Orthop, 2005; 76: 303–13

Brinckmann P, Frobin W, Hierholzer E. Stress on the articular surface of the hip joint in healthy adults and persons with idiopathic osteoarthrosis of the hip joint. J Biomech 1981;14:149–56

Chiari K (1953) Beckenosteotomie zur Pfannendachplastik. Wien Med Wochenschr 103(38):707–714

Courtois B, Le Saout J, Lefevre C, Kerboul B, Robin L, Miroux D, Lagdani R (1987) The shelf operation for painful acetabular dysplasia in adults. A continous series of 230 cases. Int Orthop 11(1):5–11

Daniel M, Antolič V, Iglič A, Kralj-Iglič V (2001) Determination of contact hip stress from nomograms based on mathematical model. Med Eng Phys 23(5):347–357

Dolinar D, Antolič V, Herman S, Iglič A, Kralj-Iglič V, Pavlovčič V (2003) Influence of contact hip stress on the outcome of surgical treatment of hips affected by avascular necrosis. Arch Orthop Trauma Surg 123:509–513

Durnin CW, Ganz R, Klaue K. The acetabular rim syndrome—a clinical presentation of dysplasia of the hip. J Bone Joint Surg 1991;73B:423–9

Fawzy E, Mandellos G, De Steger R, McLardy-Smith P, Benson MKD, Murray D (2005) Is there a place for shelf acetabuloplasty in the management of adult acetabular dysplasia? A survivorship study. J Bone Joint Surg (Br) 87(9):1197–1202

Genda E, Iwasaki N, Li G. Normal hip joint contact pressure distribution in single-leg standing - effect of gender and anatomic parameters. J Biomech, 2001; 34: 895–905

Ganz R, Klaue K, Vinh TS, Mast JW (1988) A new periacetabular osteotomy for the treatment of hip dysplasia. Technique and preliminary results. Clin Orthop 232:26–36

Hadley NA, Brown TD, Weinstein SL (1990) The effect of contact pressure elevations and aseptic necrosis on the long-term clinical outcome of congenital hip dislocation. J Orthop Res 8(4):504–513

Hipp JA, Sugano N, Millis MB, Murphy SB (1999) Planning acetabular redirection osteotomies based on joint contact pressures. Clin Orthop Rel Res 364:134–143

Hsin J, Saluja R, Eilert RE. Evaluation of the biomechanics of the hip following a triple osteotomy of the innominate bone. J Bone Joint Surg Am, 1996; 78: 855–62

Iglič A, Srakar F, Antolič V. Influence of the pelvic shape on the biomechanical status of the hip. Clin. Biomech. 1993b;8:233–4.

Iglič A, Daniel M, Kralj-Iglič V, Antolič V, Jaklič A. Peak hip joint contact stress in male and female population. J. Musculoskeletal Res. 2001;5:17–21

Iglič A, Kralj Iglič V, Antolič V, Srakar F, Stanič U (1993a) Effect of the periacetabular osteotomy on the stress on the human hip joint articular surface. IEEE Trans Rehabil Eng 1:207–212

Iglič A, Kralj-Iglič V (1999) Computer system for determination of hip joint contact stress distribution from antero-posterior pelvic radiograph. Radiol Oncol 33:263–266

Iglič A, Kralj-Iglič V, Daniel M, Maček-Lebar A (2002) Computer determination of contact stress distribution and size of weight bearing area in the human hip joint. Comput Methods Biomech Biomed Eng 5(2):185–192

Ipavec M, Brand RA, Pederson DR, Mavčič B, Kralj-Iglič V, Iglič A (1999) Mathematical modelling of stress in the hip during gait. J Biomech 32:1229–1235

Kersnič B, Iglič A, Kralj-Iglič V, Srakar F, Antolič V. Increased incidence of arthrosis in women could be related to femoral and pelvic shape. Arch. Orthop. Trauma Surg. 1997;116:345–7

Kralj M, Mavčič B, Antolič V, Iglič A, Kralj-Iglič V (2005) The Bernese periacetabular osteotomy: clinical, radiographic and mechanical 7–15-year follow-up of 26 hips. Acta Orthop 76(6):833–840

Kummer B. Biomechanischer Aspekt der Luxationshu¨fte. Orthopadie 1988;17:452–62

Kummer B. Die klinische Relevanz biomechanischer Analysen der Huftregion. Z. Orthop. 1991;129:285–94.

Legal H. Introduction to the biomechanics of the hip. In: Tonnis D, editor. Congenital dysplasia and dislocation of the hip. Berlin: Springer-Verlag; 1987. p. 26–57

Li G, Sakamoto M, Chao EYC: A comparison of different methods in predicting static pressure distribution in articulating joints. J Biomech, 1997; 30: 635–38

Love BR, Stevens PM, Williams PF (1980) A long-term review of shelf arthroplasty. J Bone Joint Surg (Br) 62(3):321–325

Malvitz TA, Weinstein SL. Closed reduction of congenital dysplasia of the hip. J. Bone Joint Surg. 1994;76A:1777–91

Mavčič B, Pompe B, Antolič V, Daniel M, Iglič A, Kralj-Iglič V (2002) Mathematical estimation of stress distribution in normal and dysplastic human hips. J Orthop Res 20(5):1025–1030

Maxian TA, Brown TD, Weinstein SL (1995) Chronic stress tolerance levels for human articular cartilage: two nonuniform contact models applied to long term follow up of CDH. J Biomech 28(2):159–166

Michaeli DA, Murphy SB, Hipp JA: Comparison of predicted and measured contact pressures in normal and dysplastic hips. Med Eng Phys, 1997; 19: 180–86

Migaud H, Chantelot C, Giraud F, Fontaine C, Dequennoy A (2004) Long-term survivorship of hip shelf arthroplasty and Chiari osteotomy in adults. Clin Orthop 418:81–86

Moll FK Jr (1982) Capsular change following Chiari inominate osteotomy. J Pediatr Orthop 2(5):573–576

Pauwels F. Biomechanics of the normal and diseased hip. Berlin: Springer-Verlag, 1976

Pemberton PA (1965) Pericapsular osteotomy of the ilium for treatment of congenital subluxation and dislocation of the hip. J Bone Joint Surg (Am) 47:65–86

Pompe B, Daniel M, Sochor M, Vengust R, Kralj-Iglič V, Iglič A. Gradient of contact stress in normal and dysplastic human hips. Med Eng Phys, 2003; 25: 379–85

Salter RB, Hansson G, Thompson GH (1984) Innominate osteotomy in the management of residual congenital subluxation of the hip in young adults. Clin Orthop 182:53–68

Staheli LT (1981) Tehnique: slotted acetabular augmentation. J Pediatr Orthop 1(3):321–327

Staheli LT (1991) Surgical management of acetabular dysplasia. Clin Orthop Rel Research 264:111–121

Staheli LT, Chew DE (1992) Slotted acetabular augmentation in children and adolescence. J Pediatr Orthop 12(5):569–580

Steel HH (1973) Triple osteotomy of the innominate bone. J Bone Joint Surg (Am) 55(2):343–350

Sutherland DH, Greenfield R (1977) Double innominate osteotomy. J Bone Joint Surg (Am) 59(8):1082–1091

Tönnis D, et al (1985) Die operative Behandlung der Hüftdysplasie. Technik und Ergebnisse. Bücherei des Orthopäden, Enke, Stuttgart, Bd 44

Vengust R, Daniel M, Antolič V, Zupanc O, Iglič A, Kralj-Iglič V (2001) Biomechanical evaluation of hip joint after Salter innominate osteotomy: a long-term follow-up study. Arch Orthop Trauma Surg 40:511–516

Zupanc O, Antolič V, Iglič A, Jaklič A, Kralj-Iglič V, Stare J, Vengust R (2001) The assessment of contact stress in the hip joint after operative treatment for severe slipped capital femoral epiphysis. Inter Orthop 25:9–12

Part 4

Knee

6

Opening Wedge High Tibial Osteotomy

Cristiano Hossri Ribeiro, Nilson Roberto Severino
and Ricardo de Paula Leite Cury
*Knee Surgery Division, Department of Orthopedics and Traumatology,
Faculdade de Ciências Médicas da Santa Casa de São Paulo,
Brazil*

1. Introduction

Tibial osteotomy is a procedure that is used to correct misalignment of the lower limb. It aims to improve the pain and/or knee functions, through the correction of varus deformity. The technique has been used for many years, and is now consecrated in medical circles.

In the literature, we find descriptions of the technique dating back to the 50s, with Jackson (Jackson, 1958). However, it was not until the 70s, with the publications of Conventry (Coventry, 1969 and 1973) and Insall (Insall, 1975), that proximal tibial osteotomy became common practice. At that time, closing wedge osteotomies were performed, despite the greater technical difficulty and risks involved, as there were no fixation materials available that could enable opening wedge osteotomy. Only after the development of medial wedge plate fixation that opening wedge osteotomy became applicable (Puddu, 2004).

Proximal tibial osteotomy has been increasingly used, because it is no longer indicated exclusively for the treatment of medial arthrosis resulting from primary varus. This technique is currently indicated for patients with other varus deformities, independent of the presence of arthrosis, such as lesions of the cartilage, meniscus, and ligaments (double and triple varus).

Patients with varus deformity generally have asymmetrical wear of the knee joint. This is due to the concentration of axial force in the medial compartment, which causes greater impact on the subchondral bone of this compartment, intravenous hypertension, and microfractures of the subchondral bone. Over time, this overload results in the deformity and pain that characterize arthrosis (Lobenhoffer et al., 2003).

2. Indications

2.1 Primary varus

The classical indication of valgizing osteotomy of the tibia is osteoarthritis of the medial compartment of the knee, associated with varus deformity (Murphy, 1994) (primary varus). In this situation, patients complain of pain in the medial compartment, and varus deformity is observed in the clinical examination. In recent years, osteotomy has no longer been an indication that is restricted to cases of primary varus. Patients with joint injuries affecting the medial compartment, with lesions of the medial meniscus and osteochondral injury associated with genu varum (bow-leggedness) require correction of the leg misalignment, in order to treat the injuries. Another common indication is cases of ligament instability associated with genu varus.

2.2 Double varus

Double varus consists of the presence of varus bone deformity accompanied by injury of the central ligament and/or lateral collateral injury, which presents lateral pivot shift of the lateral condyle. Clinically, an opening of the lateral compartment when stress is placed on it is observed in joint varus (Noyes et al., 2000).

2.3 Triple varus

Triple varus is characterized by the association of varus deformity with central ligament insufficiency (anterior and posterior cruciate ligaments, ACL and PCL), and failure of the posterolateral corner (Noyes et al., 2000). In this situation, there is an increase in external rotation of the limb during walking, with the presence of recurvatum.

In cases of double and triple varus, opening wedge tibial osteotomy should be carried out simultaneously to the ligament treatment, or in an initial operation (Franco et al., 2002). Correction in a single operation is long and tiring, involving greater risks for the patient. It is preferable to correct the bone in the first operation, as in some cases, an adaptive retensioning of the lateral structures is observed. It should be emphasized that it is common for patients submitted to ligament reconstruction to develop instability due to the failure to correct the mechanical axis (Noyes et al., 2000).

3. Contraindications

Osteotomy is contraindicated in patients with signs of tricompartmental arthrosis, injury in the lateral compartment (meniscus and/or osteochondral injury), deformities greater than 20 degrees, extension deficit, or a range of movement of less than 90 degrees. The following are considered relative contraindications: obesity, smoking and patellofemoral pain. Generally, upper tibial osteotomy provides beneficial results, when carried out at the start of evolution of the process of arthrosis in younger individuals. Thus, the procedure is contraindicated in individuals aged over 60 years with a low level of physical activity. These patients would benefit more from arthroplasty (Hernigou et al., 1987).

4. Surgical technique

The most common techniques used in tibial osteotomy are: opening wedge, closing wedge, cupuliform and biplanar. This chapter addresses opening wedge osteotomy, as it is the most commonly used and the most widely-cited technique in the recent literature, according to the results of a search on the Pubmed database using the terms "osteotomy", and "genu varus".

Closing wedge tibial valgization osteotomy was frequently used in the 1970s and 1980s, but lost space with the popularization of open wedge osteotomy(Esenkaya and Elmali, 2006,

Benzakour et al, 2010). The procedure consists of making a subtractive wedge in the lateral and proximal region of the tibia (metaphysiary region), which provides correction of major deformities, without requiring a bone graft. However, besides the higher risk of neurovascular lesion due to the lateral access route, it also has the disadvantage that it requires osteotomy of the fibula (Magyar et al., 1999, Gaasbeek et al, 2010).

Opening wedge high tibial osteotomy (HTO) has become popular in recent years because it enables a medial approach, which minimizes the risks of neurovascular lesion and the need for dissection of the soft tissues. It enables the wedge to be opened and closed during the procedure, giving a better end result. Another advantage of this technique is that it enables earlier mobility and immediate weight-bearing, depending on the implant used (Esenkaya and Elmali, 2006).

The main disadvantages of opening wedge are: increased height of the patella, the need to introduce a bone graft, which adds risks of pseudoarthrosis, and delayed consolidation (Puddu, 2000).

4.1 Preoperative planning

The preoperative planning consists of radiographic evaluation of the knee in the anterior-posterior profile and axial views of the patella, lateral view of the knee and panoramic view with full weight-bearing.

In the radiographs, we observe the degree of arthrosis (Ahlbäck, 1968) of the medial compartment, the height and signs of arthrosis of the patella, and the integrity of the lateral compartment, in cases of primary varus (Fig. 1). In patients who present double and triple varus, panoramic radiography can show a larger opening in the lateral compartment, compared with the normal side, due to ligament insufficiency of the lateral structures of the knee.

4.2 Determination of the mechanical axis

Panoramic radiography with full weight-bearing is essential, as it determines the **mechanical axis** of the limb and enables the opening wedge to be calculated. The mechanical axis is measured by drawing a line from the center of the femoral head to the center of the knee, and from this point to the center of the ankle. The intersection of the lines on the knee gives the degree of varism (Dugdale et al., 1992).

Nuclear magnetic resonance imaging is an important complementary exam that should be requested, as it provides important and detailed information on the degree of impairment of the patellofemoral joint cartilage of the medial and lateral compartment. As stated above, the presence of lesion of the cartilage in the lateral compartment or lateral meniscal lesion contraindicates osteotomy for correction of primary varus. Furthermore, in cases of double and triple varus, magnetic resonance imaging helps in the diagnosis of peripheral and central ligament lesions, contributing to the surgical planning (Murphy, 1994).

4.3 Calculation of the opening wedge

The opening wedge is calculated using the method of Dugdale, with the objective of transferring the axis of weight-bearing to 62% of the surface of the tibia laterally, in cases of primary varus. This correction enables a final angle of 3 to 6 degrees of valgus from the mechanical axis to be obtained (Dugdale et al., 1992). This calculation is done using panoramic radiography with full weight-bearing.

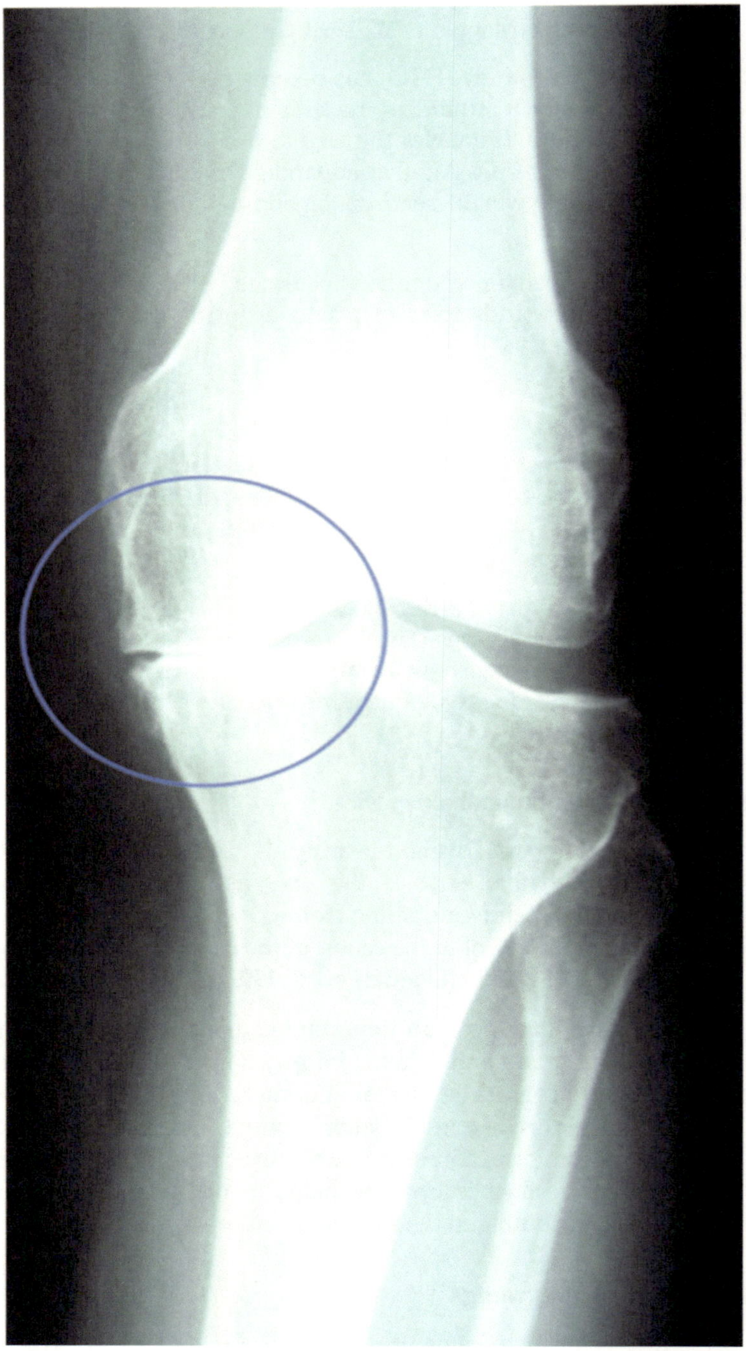

Fig. 1. Radiography of the knee with medial osteoarthrosis and varus deformity

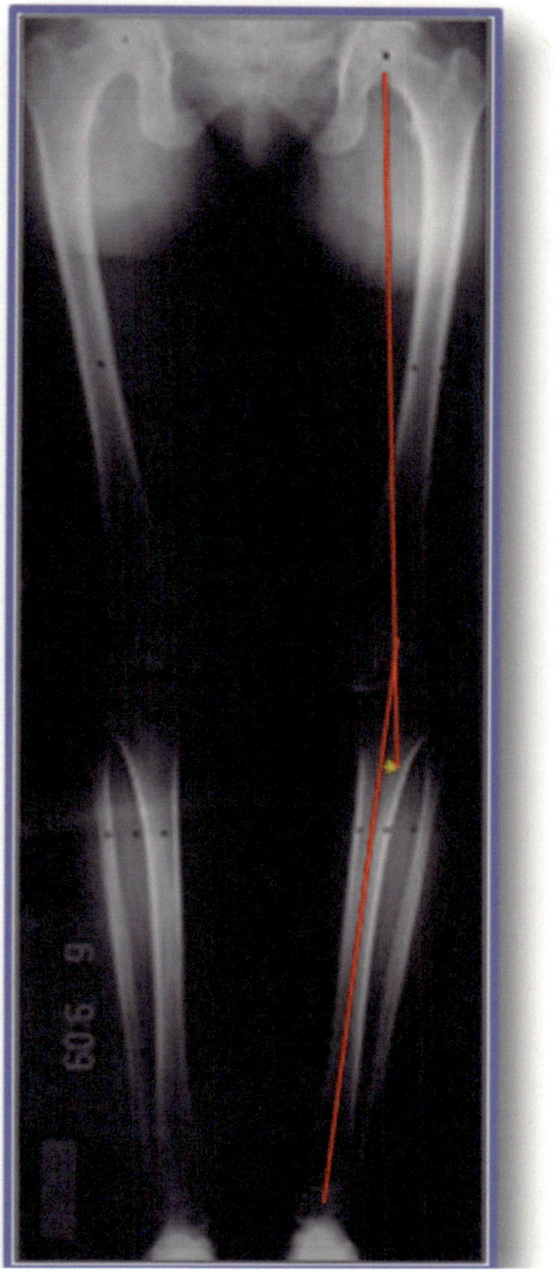

Fig. 2. Panoramic radiography with full weight-bearing on the lower limbs with measuring of the mechanical axis

The **angle of correction** is obtained from the intersection between a line drawn from the center of the femoral head to the point previously found on the surface of the knee for transfer of the axis of weight-bearing (62%) and another line from this point to the center of the ankle (Fig.3) (Dugdale et al., 1992).

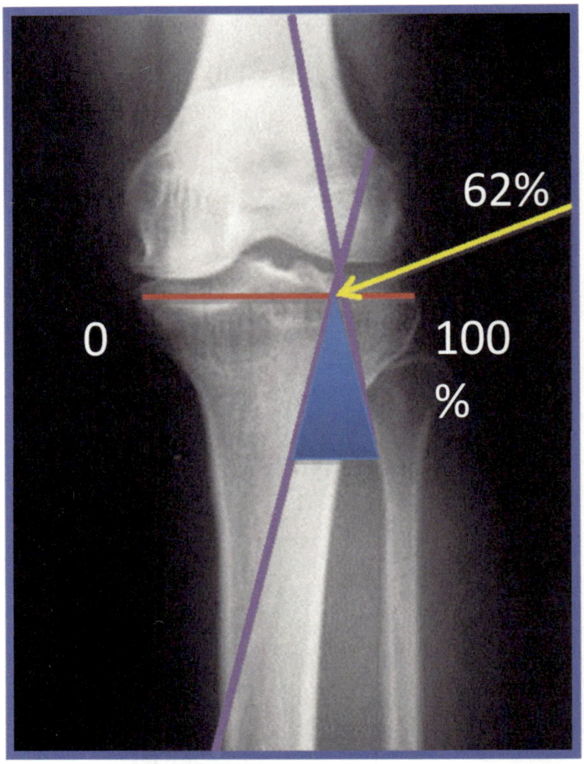

Fig. 3. Measuring the opening wedge

It is important to clarify that the degree of correction influences the final result of the surgery (Hernigou et al., 1987). Hypocorrection gives unsatisfactory clinical results (Insall et al., 1984; Amendola, 2003), as does hypercorrection, which can compromise the lateral compartment more than desired.

In patients with double and triple varus, the aim of calculating the opening wedge is to transfer the axis of weight-bearing to the center of the knee, i.e. to achieve a final mechanical angle of 0 degrees (Noyes et al., 2000). This is done in the same way as in cases of primary varus, but the line from the center of the ankle and from the head of the femur cross in the center of the knee, forming the angle of correction.

4.4 Description of the surgical technique

The surgical procedure is done with the patient in dorsal decubitus, under rachianesthesia. Before osteotomy, arthroscopy of the knee should be performed to treat the joint lesions: meniscus, cartilage and removal of loose bodies.

Opening wedge osteotomy is done with the aid of radioscopy. First, a longitudinal incision is made in the proximal and medial third of the tibia. This is followed by dissection of the pes anserinus (goose's foot) and superficial medial collateral ligament. Two parallel Kirshner wires are passed from medial to lateral in the direction of the head of the fibula, taking care to pass over the anterior tuberosity of the tibia. After confirming that the wires are in the correct position, the bone is cut, leaving the lateral cortical intact. The wedge opening calculated in the preoperative planning is then performed. The alignment obtained can be checked during the surgery, with the navigation system (Song et al., 2007) or by means of a metallic guide that enables the axis of weight bearing of the knee to be verified, through radioscopy.

For fixation of the osteotomy, there is great variety of plates available that provide stabilization. These differ in terms of design, use of wedge and angular blocking system.

Bone graft is indicated in opening wedges larger than 7.5 degrees (Puddu, 2000), to give added stability and consolidation potential. The graft may be homologous or artificial. The advantages of artificial graft are the shorter surgery time and lower risk for the patient. But we observe, in the radiographic evolution, a longer integration time of this graft compared with homologous graft, which does not influence the time to liberation of weight-bearing for the patient (data not published, submitted to publication).

After the procedure, the patients are not immobilized, and are encourage to become mobile earlier. Partial weight-bearing is allowed at six weeks with full weight-bearing at 10 weeks, on average, accompanied by radiographic consolidation.

5. Complications

Various complications of osteotomy have been cited in the literature (Esenkaya & Elmali, 2006; Paccola & Fogagnolo, 2005), such as: fracture of the lateral cortical, intra-articular fracture, hypo or hypercorrection, alteration in tibial slope, infection, pseudoarthrosis, deep vein thrombosis and infection.

5.1 Lateral cortical fracture

Lateral cortical fracture is a severe complication that can occur during the surgical act, decreasing axial resistance (47%) and rotational resistance (54%) of the osteotomy (Puddu, 2000). It occurs when the lateral tibial cortex is perforated or cut by the chisel. We also observed this complication when we opened the osteotomy wedge with the anterior and posterior cortexes intact. It is diagnosed during surgery through the observation of subluxation of the osteotomy. When this complication occurs, it is necessary to add a lateral fixation (screw or hook) at the apex of the opening wedge, to increase the stability of the osteotomy (Paccola & Fogagnolo, 2005) (Fig. 4).

5.2 Intra-articular fracture

Intra-articular fracture is a rare complication arising from an incorrectly positioned osteotomy cut. Excessive slope in the articular direction, or a cut in which a very thin proximal fragment is left increase the risk of this type of complication (Fig. 5).

To avoid this, it is necessary to pass the guide wires distally on the medial surface of the tibia, 4 cm from the joint surface, positioned towards the head of the fibula, with observation by fluoroscopy. In the case of fracture with deviation, it must be reduced and fixed with screws.

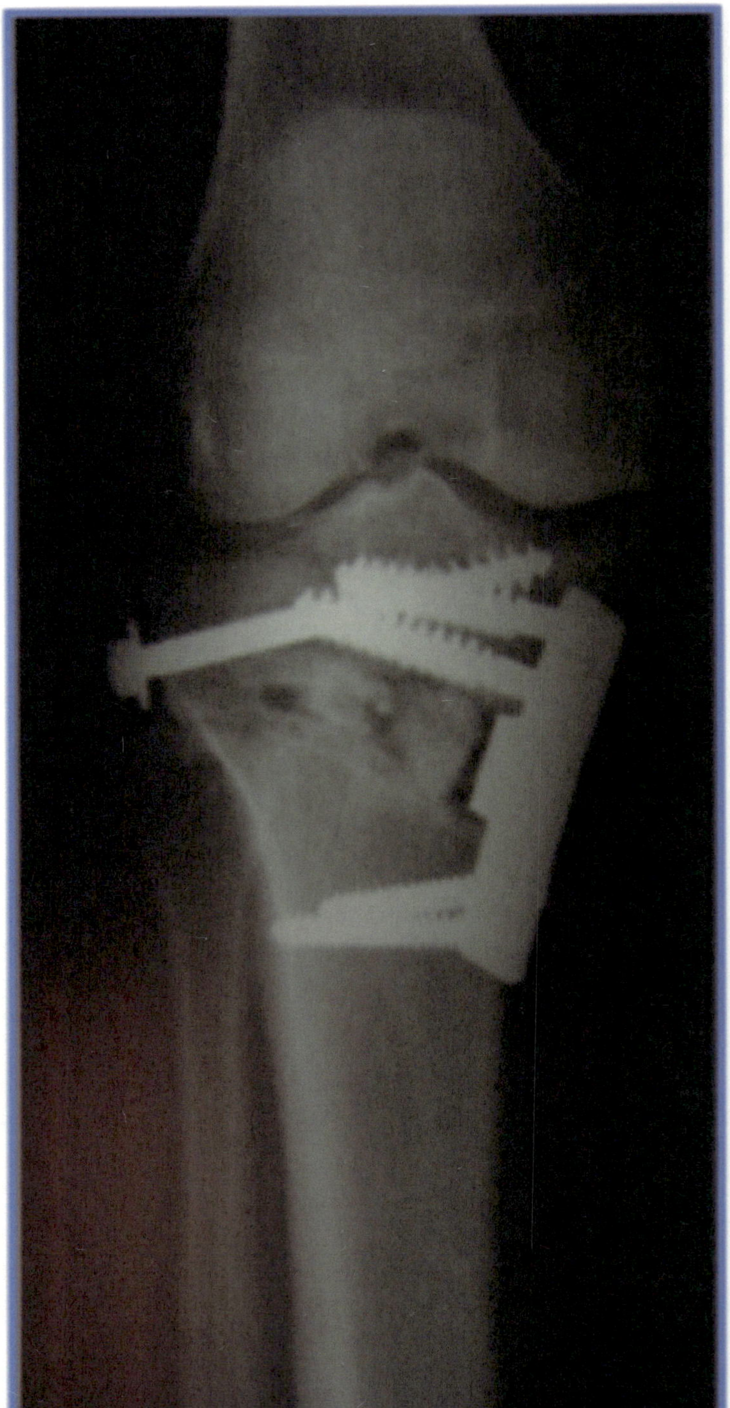

Fig. 4. Screw fixation in fracture of the lateral cortex

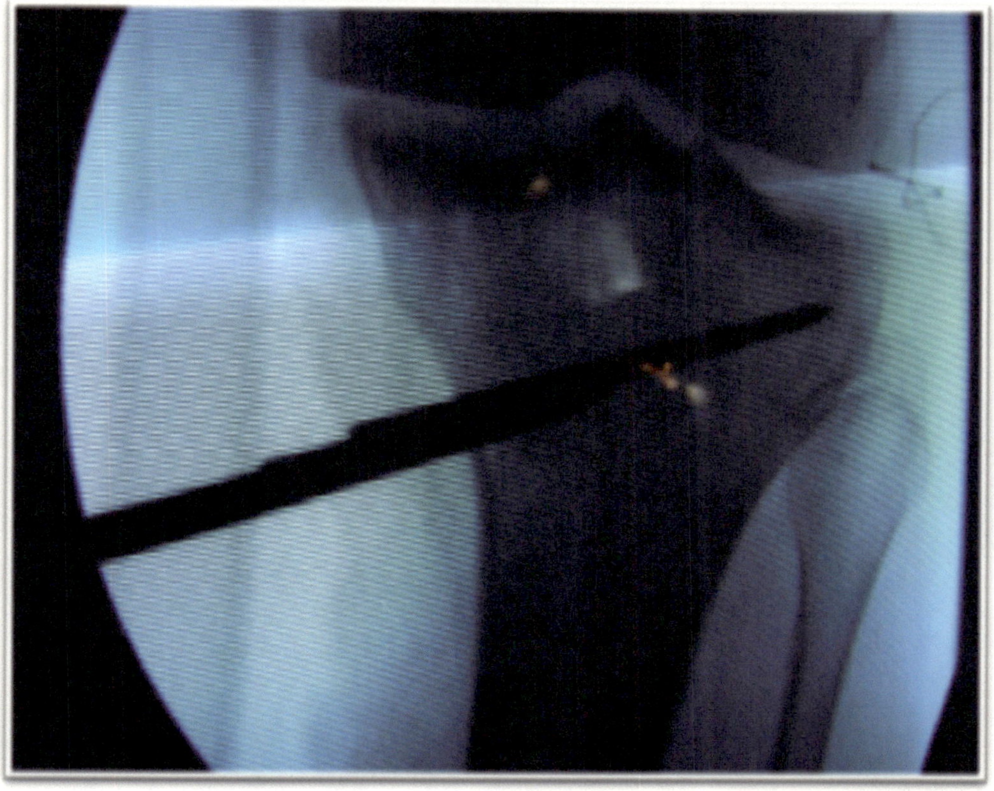

Fig. 5. Correct position of the tibial osteotomy

5.3 Hypo- and hypercorrection

Hypo- and hypercorrection in opening wedge valgizing tibial osteotomy are undesirable complications observed in most cases, following surgery (Rinonapoli et al., 1998). This gives an unsatisfactory result, as the level of final correction is directly linked to the end result of the osteotomy (Rinonapoli et al., 1998, Benzakour et al, 2010). Various techniques are used before and during surgery to increase the likelihood of achieving precisely the desired correction. Preoperative planning with radiographies, as described earlier in this chapter, is of great value, and should always be used. During surgery, clinical observation of alignment is used, as well as the technique of guide wire which, positioned by the surgeon on the anatomical points of the lower limb, indicates the site of the weight-bearing axis in the knee, under observation of radioscopy. Recently, we used the navigation system as the main instrument for controlling the degree of correction of the osteotomy (Song et al., 2007). Navigation in the osteotomy adds greater accuracy and precision, despite the longer surgery time (Gebhard et al., 2011).

5.4 Slope

The tibial slope is, on average 10 degrees of posterior inclination Clarke et al., (2001). Opening wedge tibial osteotomy enables this slope to be altered. In the vast majority of cases, we see an undesirable increase in tibial slope, which causes a loss of knee extension, and also an overload in the anterior cruciate ligament (Song et al., 2007). Patients who present insufficiency of this ligament evolve with worsening instability (Song et al., 2007). The best way to control the tibial slope is through observation of the osteotomy wedge opening. This should present an anterior opening of two thirds of the size of the posterior (Song et al., 2007), forming a trapezoidal opening wedge at the medial border of the tibia (Fig. 6). The navigation system is of great help in controlling the mechanical axis and also the tibial slope (Hart et al., 2007).

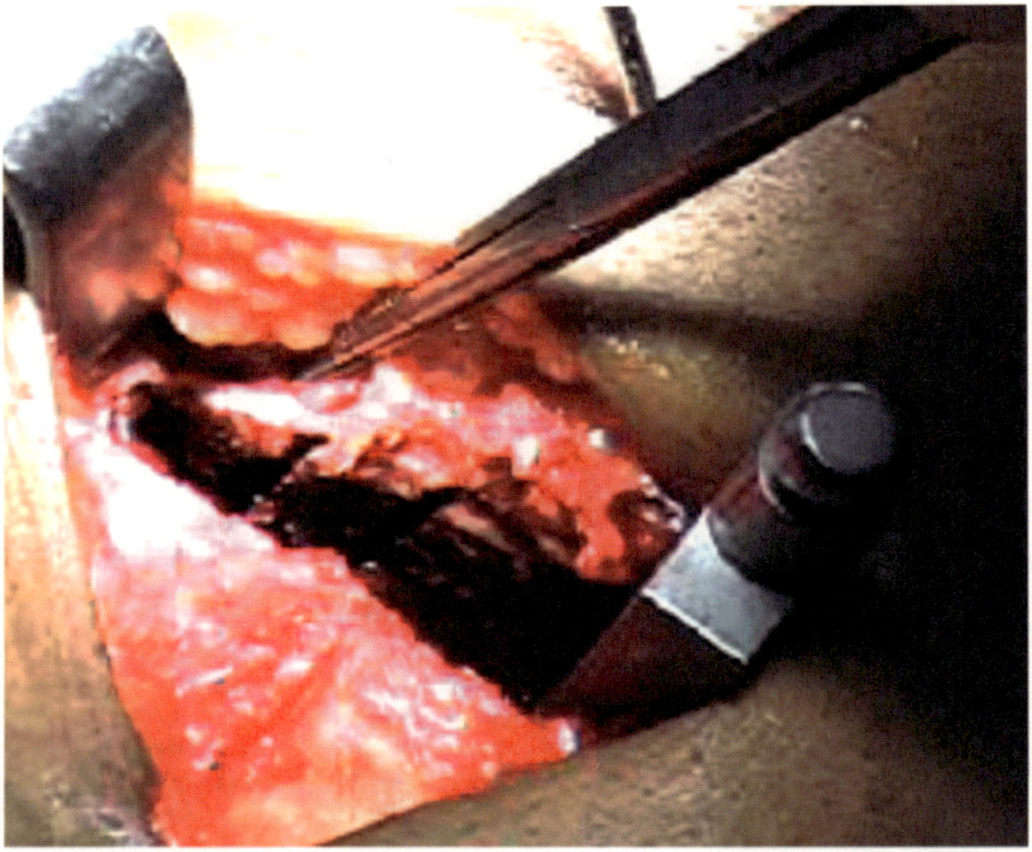

Fig. 6. Opening wedge in trapezoidal form

5.5 Pseudoarthrosis

Pseudoarthrosis is a rare complication that occurs in up to 5% of cases (Miller et al, 2009, Meidinger et al,2011, Valkering et al, 2009). It mainly occurs when no stability is added at the osteotomy site, or in the absence of bone graft in the opening wedge (Noyes et al., 2000). It recognizes the introduction of bone graft in openings greater than 7.5 mm (Puddu, 2004).

Deep vein thrombosis and infection are inherent complications to any surgical procedure. Prophylactic care should be followed, according to the clinical criteria of each patient.

Few complications of HTO are described in the literature (Jackson and Waugh, 1974, Rinonapoli et al., 1998; Song et al., 2007; Gebhard et al., 2011, Hart et al., 2007, Ribeiro et al., 2009, Miller et al., 2009, Meidinger et al, 2011, Gaasbeek et al, 2010). However, due to the continuous development of the technique and of new synthesis materials, new studies should be undertaken in order to evaluate the complication rates according to each modality of HTO.

6. Recent advances

In recent years, we have seen an increase in the number of publications on the use of the computerized navigation system in osteotomy (Gebhard et al., 2011; Hart et al., 2007). Its purpose is to help obtain the ideal final mechanical axis. Navigation works through the implantation of positioning sensors in the thigh, knee and leg. It provides a very accurate measurement of the mechanical axis of the tibial slope during the surgical procedure. As mentioned earlier, the final mechanical axis obtained directly influences the result of the osteotomy. Simple clinical observation and/or the use of the scalpel handle in the radioscopy do not show great precision (Noyes et al., 2000). But the navigation system gives accuracy and precision to the osteotomy, despite the increased surgery times and the risk of fracture of the femur and tibia (Song et al., 2007; Gebhard et al., 2011; Hart et al., 2007).

7. Final considerations

The precise indication for HTO is essential to obtain good results. Clearly, the satisfactory result of the HTO is directly related to the final correction obtained, therefore it is important to carry out preoperative planning and intraoperative follow-up with the navigation or radioscopy. The technical precautions should be carefully observed, to avoid the surgical complications described here.

8. References

Ahlbäck, S. (1968). Osteoarthrosis of the knee. A radiographic investigation. *Acta Radiologica: Diagnosis (Stockh)*, Vol.Suppl 277, (January 1968), pp. 7–72, ISSN 0567-8056.

Amendola, A. (2003) Unicompartimental osteoarthritis in the active patient: the role of high tibial osteotomy. *Arthroscopy*, Vol.19, No.Suppl 1, (December 2003), pp. 109–16, ISSN 0749-8063.

Benzakour, T, Hefti, A, Lemseffer, M, El Ahmadi, JD, Bouyarmane, H & Benzakour A. (2010). High tibial osteotomy for medial osteoarthritis of the knee: 15 years follow-up. *International orthopaedics,* Vol.34, No.2, (January 2010), pp. 209-15, ISSN 0341-2695.

Clarke, HD, Scott, WN, Insall, JN, Pedersen, HB, Math, KR, Vigorita, VJ & Cushner, FD. (2001). Anatomy. In: *Surgery of the Knee*. Insall, JN & Scott, N, Eds, pp. 13-76, ISBN 978-14-377-1503-3.

Coventry, MB (1969). Stepped staple for upper tibial osteotomy. *The Journal of Bone and Joint Surgery. American volume*, Vol.51, No.5, (July 1969), pp. 1011, ISSN 0021-9355.

Coventry, MB. (1973). Osteotomy about the knee for degenerative and rheumatoid arthritis. *The Journal of Bone and Joint Surgery. American volume*, Vol.55, No.1, (January 1973), pp. 23–48, ISSN 0021-9355.

Dugdale, TW, Noyes, FR & Styer, D. (1992). Preoperative planning for high tibial osteotomy. The effect of lateral tibiofemoral separation and tibiofemoral length. *Clinical Orthopaedics and Related Research*, No.274, (January 1992), pp. 248–64, ISSN 0009-921X.

Esenkaya, I & Elmali, N. (2006). Proximal tibia medial open-wedge osteotomy using plates with wedges: early results in 58 cases. *Knee Surgery, Sports Traumatology, Arthroscopy: Official Journal of the ESSKA*, Vol.14, No.10, (October 2006), pp. 955–61, ISSN 0942-2056.

Franco, V, Cerullo, G, Cipolla, M, Gianni, E & Puddu, G. (2002). Open wedge high tibial osteotomy. *Techniques in Knee Surgery*, Vol.1, No.1, (September 2002), pp. 43–53, ISSN 1536-0636.

Gaasbeek, RD, Nicolaas, L, Rijnberg, WJ, van Loon, CJ & van Kampen, A. (2010). Correction accuracy and collateral laxity in open versus closed wedge high tibial osteotomy. A one-year randomised controlled study. *International orthopaedics*, Vol.34, No.2, (August 2009), pp. 201-7, ISSN 0341-2695.

Gebhard, F, Krettek, C, Hüfner, T, Grützner, PA, Stöckle, U, Imhoff, AB, Lorenz, S, Ljungqvist, J, Keppler, P & AO CSEG. (2011). Reliability of computer-assisted surgery as an intraoperative ruler in navigated high tibial osteotomy. *Archives of Orthopaedic and Trauma Surgery*, Vol.131, No.3, (March 2011), pp. 297–302, ISSN 0936-8051.

Hart, R, Stipcák, V, Kucera, B, Filan, P & deCordeiro, J. (2007). Präzise computergestützte Beinachsenkorrektur mit öffnender valgisierender Tibiakopfosteotomie. [Precise, computed-assisted leg angle correction with open-wedge high tibial osteotomy]. Der *Orthopäde*, Vol.;36, No.6, (June 2007), pp. 577-81, ISSN 0085-4530.

Hernigou, P, Medevielle, D, Debeyre, J & Goutallier, D. (1987). Proximal tibial osteotomy for osteoarthritis with varus deformity. A ten to thirteen-year follow-up study. *The Journal of Bone and Joint Surgery. American volume*, Vol.69, No.3, (March 1987), pp. 332–54, ISSN 0021-9355.

Insall, JN, Joseph, DM & Msika, C. (1984). High tibial osteotomy for varus gonarthrosis. A long- term follow-up study. *The Journal of Bone and Joint Surgery. American volume*, Vol.66, No.7, (September 1984), pp. 1040–8, ISSN 0363-5465.

Insall, JN. (1975). High tibial osteotomy in the treatment of osteoarthritis of the knee. *Surgery Annual*, Vol.7, pp. 347-59, ISSN 0081-9638.

Jackson, JP & Waugh, W. (1974). The technique and complications of upper tibial osteotomy A review of 226 operations. *The Journal of Bone and Joint Surgery. British volume*, Vol.56, No.2, (May 1974), pp. 226-45, ISSN 0301-620X.

Jackson, JP. (1958). Osteotomy for osteoarthritis of the knee. Proceedings and Reports of Universities Colleges, Councils And Associations, United States of America,

March 1958. *The Journal of Bone and Joint Surgery. British volume*, Vol.40, No.4, November 1958), pp. 826, ISSN 0301-620X. Retrieved from: <URL: http://web.jbjs.org.uk/cgi/reprint/40-B/4/817>

Lobenhoffer, P & Agneskirchner, JD. (2003). Improvements in surgical technique of valgus high tibial osteotomy. *Knee Surgery, Sports Traumatololy, Arthroscopy: Official Journal of the ESSKA*, Vol.11, No.3, (May 2003), pp. 132–8, ISSN 1433-7347.

Magyar, G, Ahl, TL, Vibe, P, Toksvig-Larsen, S & Lindstrand, A. (1999). Open-wedge osteotomy by hemicallotasis or the closed-wedge technique for osteoarthritis of the knee. A randomised study of 50 operations. *The Journal of Bone and Joint Surgery. British volume*, Vol.81, No.3, (May 1999), pp. 444–8, ISSN 0301-620X.

Meidinger, G, Imhoff, AB, Paul, J, Kirchhoff, C, Sauerschnig, M & Hinterwimmer, S. (2011). May smokers and overweight patients be treated with a medial open-wedge HTO? Risk factors for non-union. *Knee surgery, sports traumatology, arthroscopy: official journal of the ESSKA*, Vol.19, No.3, (December 2010), pp. 333-9, ISSN 0942-2056.

Miller, BS, Downie, B, McDonough, EB & Wojtys, EM (2009). Complications after medial opening wedge high tibial osteotomy.*Arthroscopy*, Vol.25, No.6, (June 2009), pp. 639-46, ISSN 0749-8063.

Murphy, SB (1994). Tibial osteotomy for genu varum. Indications, preoperative planning, and technique. *The Orthopedic Clinics of North America*, Vol.25, No.3, (July 1994), pp. 477–82, ISSN 0030-5898.

Noyes, FR, Barber-Westin, SD & Hewett, TE. (2000). High tibial osteotomy and ligament reconstruction for varus angulated anterior cruciate ligament-deficient knees. *The American Journal of Sports Medicine*, Vol.28, No.3, (May-June 2000), pp. 282-96, ISSN 0363-5465.

Paccola, CA & Fogagnolo, F. (2005). Open-wedge high tibial osteotomy: a technical trick to avoid loss of reduction of the opposite cortex. *Knee Surgery, Sports Traumatololy, Arthroscopy: Official Journal of the ESSKA*, Vol.13, No.1, (January 2005), pp. 19-22, ISSN 1433-7347.

Puddu, G & Franco, V. (2000). Femoral antivalgus opening wedge osteotomy. *Operative Techniques in Sports Medicine*, Vol. 8, No.1, (January 2000). Retrieved from: <URL: http://www.deepdyve.com/lp/elsevier/femoral-antivalgus-opening-wedge-osteotomy-G5nZoP3YAX>

Puddu, G. (2004). High tibial osteotomy. The arthritic knee in the young athlete, SYM 15. *Proceedings of 11th ESSKA 2000 Congress and 4th World Congress on Sports Trauma*, Athens, Greece, May 2004. pp. 446–7.

Ribeiro, CH, Severino, NR, Cury, Rde P, de Oliveira, VM, Avakian, R, Ayhara, T & de Camargo OP. (2009). A new fixation material for open-wedge tibial osteotomy for genu varum. *The Knee*, Vol.16, No.5, (February 2009), pp. 366-70, ISSN 0968-0160.

Rinonapoli, E, Mancini, GB, Corvaglia, A & Musiello S. (1998). Tibial osteotomy for varus gonarthrosis. A 10- to 21-year followup study. *Clinical Orthopaedics and Related Research*, No.353, (August 1998), pp. 185–93, ISSN 0009-921X.

Song, EK, Seon, JK & Park, SJ. (2007). How to avoid unintended increase of posterior slope in navigation-assisted open-wedge high tibial osteotomy. *Orthopedics*, Vol.30, No.10 Suppl, (October 2007), pp. S127–31, ISSN 0147-7447.

Valkering, KP, van den, Bekerom MP, Kappelhoff, FM & Albers GH. (2009) Complications after tomofix medial opening wedge high tibial osteotomy. *The journal of knee surgery*, Vol.22, No.3 (July 2009), pp. 218-25, ISSN 1538-8506.

7

High Tibial Osteotomy

Michael Donnelly, Daniel Whelan and James Waddell
St. Michael's Hospital, Toronto, Ontario, University of Toronto, Canada

1. Introduction

High tibial osteotomy (HTO) has been used for many years to correct angular deformity about the knee, however, it's use in the treatment of knee arthritis was not described in the English language literature until 1958 (Jackson 1958). This report presented at the Sheffield Regional Orthopaedic Club detailed Jackson's experience of fourteen osteotomies 'to correct a lateral deformity of the knee accompanied by osteoarthritis'. Six were supracondylar femoral osteotomies and eight were high tibial osteotomies, he concluded that range of motion was better after HTO and overall there was a 'reasonable chance of relieving pain'. HTOs had however, been in use in France for many years before this (Hernigou 1987).

This idea of using a HTO to offload a diseased knee compartment has since been embraced and widely used with multiple techniques employed with varying degrees of success achieved and reported. Typically, high tibial lateral closing wedge osteotomy (HTLCWO) or high tibial medial opening wedge osteotomies (HTMOWO) are used in the management of isolated medial compartment disease with high tibial medial closing wedge osteotomies and distal femoral osteotomies, either lateral opening or medial closing wedge, employed in the setting of lateral compartment disease. Dome osteotomies of the proximal tibia are also occasionally used. As our understanding of knee pathology and biomechanics has changed so to have our indications for HTO usage. Current indications include but are not limited to varus or valgus malalignment with associated symptomatic isolated medial or lateral compartment early degenerative disease respectively, to offload compartments with isolated meniscal or articular cartilage loss, to offload compartments before meniscal or articular cartilage replacement or regeneration surgeries, to attempt to change the natural history and symptomatology of conditions such as spontaneous osteonecrosis of the knee and osteochonditis dessicans, and in the management of knee ligament deficiency.

1.1 Lower limb alignment and axes

Prior to embarking on any surgical intervention to realign or offload a compartment a thorough understanding of the normal mechanical and anatomic axes about the knee is required. The following is a brief description of some of the important axes and angles about the knee. The mechanical axis of a bone is represented by a straight line passing through the centre of the joints above and below that bone, the centre of the hip joint equates to the centre of the femoral head, the centre of the knee to the centre of the tibial spines and the centre of the ankle to the centre of the tibial plafond. The anatomic axis corresponds to the mid-diaphyseal line, which therefore maybe curved as in the case of the femur in the saggital plane. Usefully, the tibial anatomic and mechanical axes are parallel in the frontal plane, whereas the femoral axes subtend an angle of 7+/- 2 degrees, in the normal population. In order to quantify pre-operative discrepancies and plan correction, the knee joint lines of the femur and tibia must be identified – in the frontal plane these correspond to a straight line drawn between the apices of the convexities of the distal femoral condyles and a straight line between the apices of the concavities of the tibial plateaus respectively. This allows estimation of the lateral distal femoral angle relative to the mechanical and anatomic axes of the femur, 88^0 ($85\text{-}90^0$) and 81^0 ($79\text{-}83^0$) respectively. The medial proximal tibial angle is 87^0 ($85\text{-}90^0$) relative to the tibial anatomic and mechanical axes by virtue of the fact that both are parallel in the frontal plane of the tibia. Overall, this results in lower limb tibio-femoral mechanical alignment in 1.3^0 of varus and tibio-femoral anatomic alignment in 6.8^0 of valgus. In the saggital plane the joint line angle of the femur is the straight line that connects the two points of the anterior and posterior meta-diaphyseal junctions, creating a posterior distal femoral angle of 83^0 ($79\text{-}87^0$), with the distal femoral anatomic axis in the saggital plane. In the saggital plane the joint line angle of the tibia is drawn along the subchondral bone of the tibial plateau, creating a posterior proximal tibial angle of 81^0 ($77\text{-}84^0$), with the tibial anatomic axis (Palley 2002). Using these angles and axes the site of the deformity and the site and degree of correction can be planned pre-operatively.

2. Specific indications for high tibial osteotomy

2.1 Medial compartment arthritis with varus limb malalignment

Isolated medial compartment arthritis with associated varus lower limb malalignment is the most common indication for HTO. The success of this procedure is premised on the fact that seventy per cent of the load generated by the joint reaction force is borne by the medial compartment if the mechanical axis passes through the centre of the knee, whereas this reduces to fifty per cent if the knee is in four degrees of valgus and to forty per cent if the knee is in six degrees of valgus (Kettelkamp et al., 1976). Adequate valgus correction is required to ensure survival of the HTO (Pfahler et al, 2003) this has led most to recommend correction to between two and eight degrees of valgus (Coventry 1993, Hernigou 1987, Jakob 1992), with some advocating correction to between eight and fifteen degrees of anatomic valgus (Aglietti 2003, Koshino 1979, 2004).

Surgical indications include active physiologically young patients with a varus arthritic knee, progressive symptoms unresponsive to six months of conservative treatment, greater than ninety degrees of flexion, less than ten degrees of fixed flexion contracture, intact collateral and cruciate ligaments, no tibio-femoral subluxation and degenerative changes which do not exceed Kellgren-Lawrence grade three. Ideally, the patient should have a body mass index below thirty kg/m^2, should not smoke, and caution should be employed in the setting of diabetes mellitus or medication usage which may delay healing of the osteotomy. Contraindications include lateral compartment degenerative disease, previous subtotal or total lateral meniscectomy, greater than 3mm of medial tibial bone loss, symptomatic patellofemoral disease, inflammatory arthropathy, patient unwillingness to accept the anticipated post operative appearance of the limb (in valgus) (Wright 2005). Mild to moderate asymptomatic patellofemoral degenerate disease is typically not a contraindication to HTO.

The ideal patient should have a normal lateral compartment before transferring load to it in performing the osteotomy, however, while consensus exists regarding the need to assess the lateral compartment, consensus does not exist regarding the means by which the compartment is assessed pre or intra-operatively. A thorough history and physical examination should focus on excluding pain generators within the lateral compartment. Radiological evaluation should include weight bearing plain radiographs. A schuss view taken PA with the patient weight-bearing with the knees at thirty degrees of flexion should be considered pre-operatively as it has been shown to be more sensitive than standard AP weight bearing radiographs in identifying patients with loss of joint space in the lateral compartment in particular (Ritchie 2004). MRI scanning is also utilized to assess the integrity of the lateral compartment, specifically the lateral meniscus and as technologies improve, the quality of the articular cartilage. Some routinely perform arthroscopy as part of the surgery to assess the lateral compartment (Song 2010). Intra-operative arthroscopy facilitates assessment and management of medial meniscal tears, which are common in this patient population, aswell as aiding in accurate assessment of a tibial plateau fracture, should one occur.

When a patient is deemed suitable for a HTO the next question is what type of osteotomy to use. As outlined above, a dome osteotomy, although very effective in correcting deformity and shifting the mechanical axis, is less commonly used now, hence this chapter will concentrate on the pros and cons of medial opening and lateral closing wedge osteotomies. Often the decision is based on surgeon preference for one type of osteotomy over the other; however, individual patient factors should also be considered during the pre-operative plan. A patient with a limb length discrepancy resulting in the affected lower limb being longer pre-operatively may be more appropriately considered for a HTLCWO rather than a HTMOWO which will further lengthen the leg, with the former shown to shorten the leg by 2.7 +/- 4mm and the latter shown to lengthen the leg by 5.5 +/- 4.4mm (Magnusson 2011). Similarly, the patella height on the pre-operative radiograph should also be assessed and the patient with patella baja considered for a lateral closing wedge and early post operative mobilization as opposed to a medial opening wedge osteotomy which has been shown to reduce patellar height (Wright 2001). Careful analysis of the pre-operative radiographs is a critical in determining the degree of planned correction. Using full length standing radiographs, the mechanical axis is outlined by drawing a line from the centre of the femoral head to the centre of the ankle joint. Once it has been determined that the varus deformity is on the tibial side, the planned angular correction is determined by drawing a line from the centre of the femoral head to a point at sixty two per cent of the total width of the tibial plateau measured from medial to lateral, known as the Fujisawa point (Fujisawa 1979). A second line is then drawn from the centre of the ankle joint to this point - the angle subtended by these two lines is the angular correction required to bring the mechanical axis to this Fujisawa point in the lateral compartment thereby offloading the medial compartment. Using medial opening wedge techniques the degree of correction can be adjusted intra-operatively as outlined below however, using closing wedge techniques the angular correction must be planned and converted to millimeters at the site of the closing wedge osteotomy on pre-operative imaging measured at a set distance from the joint line so as to ensure the correct size wedge is osteotomised for the desired correction. If using this technique when performing closing wedge surgery the soft tissue component of the deformity must be taken into account by subtracting one degree for every millimeter of additional lateral compartment opening in the standing view of the varus knee, from the planned wedge, so as not to over-correct resulting in excessive valgus once the patient weight bears (Noyes 2000). Opinions differ as to the exact amount of correction required or likely to be cosmetically acceptable to the individual patient, hence the actual point chosen is typically somewhere between the Fujisawa point and the lateral border of the lateral tibial spine.

2.1.1 Surgical technique – High tibial medial opening wedge osteotomy

The patient is positioned supine on a radiolucent operating table allowing intra-operative fluoroscopic visualization from the centre of the femoral head to the centre of the ankle joint. The chosen anesthetic and antibiotics are administered. A thigh tourniquet is applied to the operative limb and standard prep and drape is performed. A vertical incision, eight centimeters in length, is made over the centre of the medial tibial plateau. The sartorial fascia is incised just proximal to and inline with the gracilis tendon. The superficial medial collateral ligament is identified. A 1.8mm threaded k-wire is passed obliquely under image guidance from the metaphyseal flare of the proximal medial tibia towards the head of the fibula - ensuring it exits fifteen to twenty millimeters below the lateral tibial plateau. A second threaded K-wire is then passed obliquely, from a point one to two centimeters postero-inferior to the first k-wire, ensuring it is parallel to the first k-wire in the coronal plane, and that a line drawn between these k-wires is parallel to the slope of the proximal tibia in the saggital plane. Using intra-operative AP imaging this can be verified by measuring the angle of the posterior slope of the tibia on the pre-op radiograph, then flexing the knee to this amount should cause superimposition of one wire over the other on AP imaging if the planned posterior slope has been replicated. The medial collateral ligament is then sharply divided along the planned osteotomy site, just distal to and paralleling these two wires. Care must be taken to ensure the MCL is completely divided especially posteriorly to ensure it does not act as a tether preventing opening of the osteotomy posteriorly thereby potentially increasing the posterior tibial slope.

Then knee is then flexed and a Cobb or broad tissue elevator is then passed subperiosteally along the posterior tibia in the direction of the planned osteotomy. A saggital saw is then passed under image guidance from medial to within five to ten millimeters of the lateral cortex staying in direct contact with the two k-wires so as not to deviate from the planned osteotomy path. The posterior cortex is osteotomised in the same plane, guided by the k-wires and the broad tissue elevator being key to protecting the posterior neurovascular structures throughout the procedure. A fifteen degree oblique osteotomy posterior to the tibial tuberosity in an anterior proximal to posterior distal direction is then performed using the saggital saw taking care to protect the patellar tendon throughout. If however, the medial tibial opening wedge osteotomy is utilized in a patient with patella baja or in whom a significant correction is anticipated, the tibial tuberosity is osteotomised obliquely from the level of the osteotomy to distal, maintaining the tuberosity in continuity with the proximal fragment thereby not altering the spatial relationship between the patella and the proximal tibia (Gaasbeek 2004).

At all times when using the saggital saw, saline lavage is employed to prevent local soft tissue or bone necrosis. The osteotomy of the anteromedial and anterolateral cortices of the proximal tibia are then completed using an osteotome. A 3.2mm drill is then passed from medial to lateral to the intact lateral cortex which is then drilled in three different sites from anterior to posterior again in line with the k-wires. This serves to weaken the lateral hinge and allow it open by plastic deformation rather than fracture during the remainder of the procedure. The osteotomy is then slowly opened using stacked osteotomes slowly inserted under image guidance from medial to lateral to within five to ten millimeters of the lateral cortex until the desired degree of opening, as per pre-operative planning, is obtained. The first two broad osteotomes are inserted with additional osteotomes thereafter inserted between these two. A laminar spreader is then inserted as posterior as possible to hold the osteotomy in this position as the osteotomes are removed. The osteotomy should be opened twice as much posteriorly as it anteriorly to ensure alteration of the posterior slope does not occur. The adequacy of the correction is then assessed using fluoroscopy, by positioning the proximal end of the diathermy cable over the centre of the femoral head and the distal end of the cable under tension over the centre of the ankle, where this passes through the extended knee under image intensification corresponds to the new mechanical axis, which can easily be adjusted using the laminar spreaders so that it crosses the desired point between the lateral border of the lateral tibial spine and the Fuijisawa point.

At this point the osteotomy can be fixed by a variety of means, the one described here uses a proximal tibial locking compression plate, TomoFix® (Synthes GmbH; Solothurn, Switzerland) which is applied to the proximal tibia, with a two millimeter spacer in the most distal of the four proximal locking screw holes and another in the most distal of the four distal screw holes. These spacers prevent soft tissue necrosis under the plate, particularly of the pes anserinus tendons and periosteum adjacent to the osteotomy. A 2.0mm k-wire is passed through the middle of the proximal three locking drill guide sleeves, parallel to the joint to hold the plate in position while the remaining anterior and posterior proximal locking screws are inserted. This k-wire is then removed and replaced by a screw. The most proximal of the four screw holes distal to the osteotomy site is then drilled to accommodate a cortical screw to reduce the tibial shaft to the plate. The middle two distal screw holes are then filled with unicortical locking screws. The two spacers and then the cortical screw are removed at this point and replaced by locking screws.

A variety of graft options exist to fill the osteotomy site including autograft, allograft, synthetic bone graft substitutes and synthetic bone scaffolds, studies exist to support each. Using the above technique increasingly no bone graft is used to fill the osteotomy with satisfactory results reported to date (Staubli 2010). This avoids the morbidity associated with autograft harvesting sites, allograft infection risks and the difficulties in achieving boney union associated with the use of synthetic graft materials, but does require that the plate remain in situ for eighteen months post-operatively.

The skin and subcutaneous tissue are closed over a non-suction drain using interrupted sutures. A standard dressing applied. Range of motion is commenced on day one following removal of the drain. Partial weight bearing of fifteen kilograms is allowed until the wound is fully healed, generally between ten and fourteen days, at which point weight bearing as tolerated is permitted, with the patient mobilizing without crutches from six weeks post-op. Although opinions vary, this protocol may be applicable to medial tibial opening wedge osteotomies using the above described fixation technique, however, the post-op protocol should be tailored to the stability of the fixation technique used so as to prevent loss of fixation.

2.1.2 Surgical technique – High tibial lateral closing wedge osteotomy

The lateral tibial closing wedge osteotomy was originally described and popularized by Coventry (Coventry 1965), since then the operation has undergone a number of technical variations especially in relation to dealing with the proximal tibio-fibular joint and fibular osteotomy, in an effort to avoid complications relating to the peroneal nerve in particular.

The patient is position supine on the radiolucent operating table allowing intra-operative fluoroscopic visualization from the centre of the femoral head to the centre of the ankle joint. The chosen anesthetic and antibiotics are administered. A thigh tourniquet is applied to the operative limb and standard prep and drape is performed. An arthroscopic evaluation of the joint may be performed at this point.

A curved oblique incision is utilized extending from the tip of the fibula to the tibial tuberosity anteriorly before descending approximately three centimeters long the lateral border of the tibial tuberosity. The tibialis anterior insertion is released as a z-plasty to facilitate later repair, the tibialis anterior and long toe extensor musculature is taken down using a large periosteal elevator to expose the lateral proximal tibial metaphysis. The proximal tibio-fibular joint is then opened to allow mobilization of the proximal fibula. A 1.8mm threaded k-wire is passed under image guidance from lateral to medial twenty millimeters below and parallel to the joint line, with its starting point as far posterior as possible. A second k-wire is then passed two centimeters anterior and parallel to the first. This k-wire should be superimposed on the first on imaging with the knee in extension. To mark the distal osteotomy a k-wire is passed obliquely from medial to lateral at the desired distance from the proximal osteotomy site as per pre-operative planning again with its starting point as posterior as possible, to converge with the proximal osteotomy wires at the medial cortex. A second k-wire is then passed from a starting point one to two centimeters anterior to and parallel to the first, again superimposition is checked on fluoroscopy with the knee in extension. A Cobb or large periosteal elevator is passed posterior to the proximal tibia to protect the posterior structures as the osteotomy is performed. Similarly, a right angle retractor is placed posterior to the patellar tendon to protect it while the osteotomy is performed. The proximal osteotomy is performed first using a saggital saw passed distal to but in direct contact with the k-wires at all times from lateral to medial leaving the posterior tibial cortex intact. Image guidance is used to ensure the saggital saw is taken to within five to ten millimeters only of the medial cortex. The distal osteotomy is then performed with the saggital blade resting on the proximal surface of the distal osteotomy marker k-wires, again converging on the proximal k-wires but staying five to ten millimeters from the medial cortex. The distal osteotomy includes the posterior cortex along its length. The wedge is then removed with osteotomes; a curette is used to ensure cancellous bone is removed from the posterior cortex which has been left intact on the proximal fragment to add stability to the construct at completion (Coventry 1965). A 3.2mm drill is then passed from lateral to medial three times through different points on the medial cortex from posterior to anterior to weaken this medial hinge and allow it deform without fracturing. A valgus load is then slowly applied using a large reduction clamp on the lateral side to close the osteotomy. Using the diathermy cable as outlined in the medial opening wedge technique discussion above the new mechanical axis is assessed, if it is deemed satisfactory the osteotomy is held reduced with two staples on the lateral side. The capsule of the proximal tibio-fibular joint and anterior compartment musculature are then repaired using interrupted sutures. The skin is closed. Standard dressings are applied. Epidural anesthesia should be avoided post-operatively as it may mask the development of a compartment syndrome which should be carefully watched for. Range of motion rehab and partial weight bearing are commenced day one post operatively due to the inherent stability of the construct. Early range of motion rehab is crucial to prevent patella baja (Billings 2000). Earlier papers have recommended the use of long leg casting for six weeks and partial weight bearing to maintain alignment when staples are employed for fixation if the boney contact within the osteotomy site is less than 50% (Harrison 1987).

2.2 Lateral compartment arthritis with valgus malalignment

A much less common indication for osteotomy relates to the valgus knee with lateral compartment arthritis. Similar indications and contra-indications as in the setting of the varus knee as outlined above are utilized. Clinical exam should include careful assessment of other joints to outrule an as yet undiagnosed rheumatologic condition which may be driving the valgus deformity and indicative of tri-compartmental disease within the joint. Similarly, it is important to outrule any hip adduction contracture as this will create a valgus moment about the knee and likely lead to recurrence of the deformity over time.

The use of a HTO to correct valgus malalignment or to offload the lateral compartment requires careful consideration particularly with regard to the anatomy of the involved knee. Where a valgus knee is boney in origin the problem typically lies on the femoral side, most often due to dysplasia of the lateral femoral condyle. The resultant knee valgus is apparent clinically in both flexion and extension. This presents the surgeon with the difficult decision as to which side of the knee joint to perform the osteotomy on. A HTO in this setting, particularly if the proximal tibia is not contributing to the deformity will correct the deformity in both flexion and extension but will, by necessity, create joint line obliquity. A distal femoral osteotomy, on the other hand, while not changing the obliquity of the joint line will usually only correct the deformity in the coronal plane, resulting in persistent valgus in flexion.

2.2.1 Surgical technique – High tibial medial closing wedge osteotomy

Pre-operative planning as described is utilized to determine the size of the wedge required at the level of the osteotomy to achieve the desired correction, of 0-2 degrees of mechanical tibio-femoral varus. The osteotomy is performed just proximal to the tibial tubercle. As in section 2.1.1 above, the same technique is utilized to expose the medial proximal tibia. The hamstring tendons are identified and retracted, the superficial MCL is identified and its fibres, which are often lax in this setting, are elevated off bone and retracted posteriorly at the level of the planned osteotomy. Two 1.8 mm threaded k-wires are passed, as guidewires, from medial to lateral parallel to the joint line and each other, in both the coronal and saggital planes, to exit the lateral tibia just proximal to the proximal tibio-fibular joint. The proximal tibial fragment should measure at least 2 cms at its thinnest point. Fluoroscopy is used to ensure correct guidewire positioning as per pre-operative planning. The knee is then flexed and a wide periosteal elevator is passed along the posterior cortex of the proximal tibia along the line of the planned osteotomy and its position again checked under fluoroscopy. The patellar tendon is retracted. A saggital saw is used to osteotomise the proximal tibia just distal to, but staying in contact with the already positioned guidewires. The osteotomy should include the anterior and posterior cortices and should extend to but not through the lateral cortex. The thickness of the planned resection wedge is measured on the medial cortex and two further 1.8 mm threaded guidewires are then passed from medial to lateral to converge with the two proximal guidewires just medial to the lateral cortex. When measuring the medial wedge thickness allowance must be made for the thickness of the saw blade, being utilized, to reduce the risk of over-correction. These two guidewires should be parallel to the proximal two guidewires in the saggital plane so as not to change the posterior tibial slope. The wide elevator again is used to protect the posterior structures before the osteotomy is performed using the saggital saw just distal to but in contact with these two distal guidewires, again the osteotomy extends to but not through the lateral cortex. The resection wedge is removed and a 3.2 mm drill is used to perforate and weaken the lateral cortex as required to allow gentle varus directed force close the osteotomy site. The diathermy cable under tension is passed from the centre of the femoral head to the centre of the ankle joint and fluoroscopy used to ensure the new mechanical axis passes through the centre of the knee. The osteotomy is then held reduced with two bones staples. The superficial MCL is assessed and a decision made as to whether to double breast suture it over itself or whether to excise a redundant portion of its fibres and re-oppose its edges at an appropriate tension. The tissues are closed over one deep drain. Early partial weight bearing is allowed in this setting due the stable nature of this construct and broad metaphyseal surfaces for boney healing.

2.2.2 Surgical technique – Distal femoral medial closing wedge osteotomy

When the required valgus deformity correction exceeds 12 degrees, that correction is best performed through a distal femoral medial closing wedge osteotomy(Figure 1); in order to avoid excessive joint line obliquity as would likely occur with a correction of this magnitude on the tibial side (Coventry 1987). As outlined above pre-operative planning is again of paramount importance. First the angular magnitude of the required correction is determined to bring the mechanical axis of the limb through the centre of the knee. The osteotomy site is then identified radiologically such that it will be as distal as possible without compromising the patellofemoral joint. The width of the osteotomy at this site in millimeters is then determined.

The patient is positioned supine on a radiolucent operating table allowing intra-operative fluoroscopic visualization from the centre of the femoral head to the centre of the ankle joint. The chosen anesthetic and antibiotics are administered. A thigh tourniquet is applied to the operative limb and standard prep and drape is performed. An arthroscopy is performed in particular to assess the medial compartment for any degenerate changes and to treat meniscal or chondral pathology in the lateral compartment. A vertical paramedian incision, approximately 2 cms medial to a midline incision is utilized extending proximally for 15 cms from the level of the joint line. A subvastus approach thereafter is used to elevate the vastus medialis obliquus (VMO) off the medial intermuscular septum to facilitate exposure of the medial distal femur. The medial superior geniculate vessels are identified and ligated as required. A guidewire is passed from anteromedial to posterolateral, parallel to and 2 cms proximal to the joint line under image guidance. This serves as a marker for the blade plate insertion site, which should be approximately 2 cms distal to the proposed osteotomy site, a second guidewire is then passed 1.5 cms anterior to the first such that the wires are parallel to the joint line in the coronal plane and perpendicular to the long axis of the femur in the saggital plane, so that when the blade plate is inserted it will lie on the femoral shaft.

A 4.5 mm drill is used to perforate the medial femoral cortex between these 2 guidewires, the blade plate chisel with the plate holder attached is inserted parallel to the guidewires under image guidance again ensuring that the plate holder remains parallel with the long axis of the femur. The chisel is removed, to mark the proposed distal limb of the osteotomy site, as defined on the preoperative plan, two threaded 1.8mm guidewires are passed from medial to lateral, approximately 2 cms proximal to and parallel to the first two guidewires, which can then be removed. Two guidewires are used at all times to maintain visuospatial awareness of the correction in the saggital plane so as to avoid building flexion or extension into the correction. The patellofemoral joint should be assessed to ensure it will not be breached by the distal osteotomy. A broad periosteal elevator is passed along the posterior cortex of the femur with the knee in flexion to protect the neurovascular structures and a homann retractor is placed anteriorly to protect the quadriceps tendon. A broad saggital saw is used to perform the distal limb of the osteotomy just proximal to but in direct contact with the guidewires. The osteotomy extends to but not through the lateral cortex.

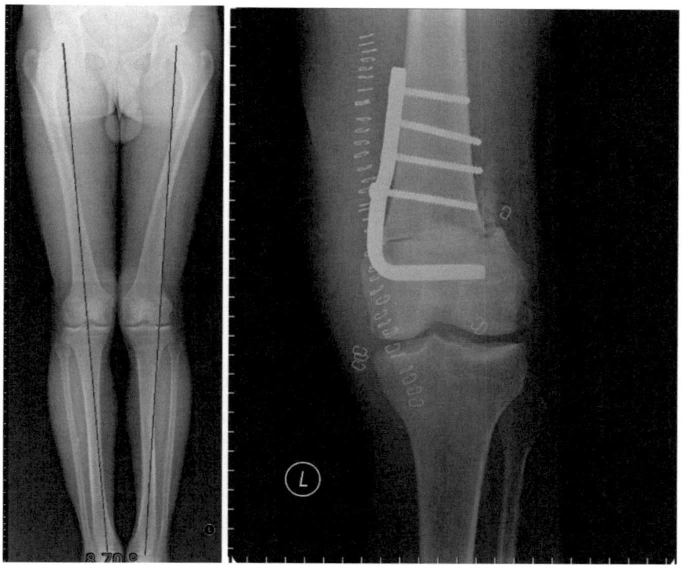

Fig. 1. Pre-operative 3 foot standing film showing significant left knee valgus with the mechanical axis passing through the centre of the lateral compartment, with adjacent post-operative film following medial distal femoral closing wedge osteotomy with correction of the deformity.

The planned width of the resection wedge is measured on the medial cortex and two 1.8 mm threaded guidewires passed from medial to lateral such that they converge just medial to the distal osteotomy guidewires in the coronal plane but are parallel to them in the saggital plane. The broad periosteal elevator and homann retractor are replaced and the proximal limb of the osteotomy is completed in similar fashion staying just distal to but in direct contact with the proximal osteotomy limb guidewires. The wedge of bone is removed and the intact lateral cortex weakened using a 3.2 mm drill bit to facilitate closure of the osteotomy without fracture of the lateral hinge. Fluoroscopy is used to check that the new mechanical axis passes through the centre of the knee. A five hole 95 degree plate with a 50-60mm blade is then bent to 90 degrees so as to allow complete osteotomy reduction and compression along a line perpendicular to the femoral shaft (Wang 2005). The blade is impacted into the distal femur along the pre-chiseled path. The bone of the medial distal femur just proximal to the blade is compressed by the plate if soft or impacted using a punch to allow seating of the plate within the cortex of the distal femur until the plate lies on the femoral shaft, without requiring medialisation of the shaft which would compromise the correction and disrupt the continuity of the lateral cortex. This is also the reason for choosing a shorter blade and negates the need for the use of offset blade plates which are bulky, can compromise postoperative range of motion and often require removal due to pain. Consideration at this stage, based on bone and osteotomy fixation quality, can be given to using a derotation screw either through the plate or outside the plate to cross the osteotomy and aid in controlling rotation of the distal fragment and facilitate earlier range of motion rehabilitation (Wang 2005). The wound is closed in layers using interrupted sutures. Toe touch weight bearing only is permitted for the first six weeks, thereafter weight bearing is gradually re-introduced.

3. High tibial osteotomy for ligamentous insufficiency

Prior to embarking on ligamentous or joint preserving surgeries about the knee careful attention must be paid to the alignment of the limb as well as the actual joint involved – namely the knee in this chapter. If malalignment has contributed to meniscal, cartilage or ligamentous injury and that malalignment is not corrected prior to or at the time of a planned reconstructive surgery – that reconstruction will be subject to the same stresses which resulted in the failure of the native tissues in the first place resulting in higher failure rates in the reconstructed tissues also. The importance of the history and physical examination in this setting cannot be overplayed. A precise history of pre-injury function, pain, range of motion, previous injuries or surgeries are crucial to elucidate, prior to enquiring as to the exact injury mechanism leading to the current consultation. Relatively innocuous injury, previous failed surgery for the same condition or bilaterality should alert the physician to the possibility of fundamental structural malalignment which may contribute to early failure of a repair or reconstruction.

The clinical exam is critical and must start with assessing limb alignment during gait to look for dynamic instability in the knee joint under load, before looking at alignment in standing and the status of individual ligaments. While walking, a varus thrust or knee hyperextension gait must be carefully sought out, as isolated ligamentous reconstructions of the anterior or posterior cruciate ligaments respectively in these settings will likely result in poor surgical outcomes. Standing alignment and old surgical scars should be noted prior to a thorough examination of the individual ligaments of the knee looking for increased lateral opening at 30° of knee flexion when a varus directed force is applied, increased external or posterolateral rotation at 30° and 90° of flexion, increased subluxation on the reverse pivot-shift test, increased anterior translation on the lachman and anterior drawer tests, and increased posterior translation on the posterior drawer test for a posterior cruciate ligament (PCL)-deficient knee all compared with the normal contralateral knee.

Radiological assessment involves careful analysis of the current mechanical axes on the three foot standing films, as well as joint space narrowing on the medial side and opening on the lateral side. The lateral x-ray is used to assess the patellar height and the posterior tibial slope, the angle subtended by two lines, one drawn parallel to the long axis of the tibial diaphysis and the other from the anterior proximal tibia to the posterior proximal tibia, to give a normal value of between 7 and 10 degrees. The importance of the posterior tibial slope has been highlighted by numerous investigators who have shown that with increasing posterior tibial slope comes increased anterior translation of the tibia on the femur (Giffin 2004), with some advocating reduction of the slope if it is greater than 10 degrees in the ACL deficient knee (Dejour 1994). The common finding of posteromedial wear in the ACL deficient knee and cadaveric studies showing increased pressure transmitted to the osteotomised knee with increased posterior slope further highlight the importance of this point (Rodner 2006). The opposite applies to the PCL deficient knee in which increasing the posterior tibial slope may indeed be beneficial by reducing the posterior sag in flexion.

3.1 Anterior cruciate ligament deficiency and the varus knee

One of the commonest elective orthopaedic operations performed is reconstruction of the torn anterior cruciate ligament (ACL) in the knee. Much modern debate and literature centers on graft selection, tunnel placement and graft fixation methods. However, perhaps more important than any of these debates is patient selection and pre-operative assessment, so as to identify that patient who is predisposed to failure of an isolated reconstruction of the ACL. A patient who gives a history of previous ACL reconstruction on the other or same side, who has had a previous medial meniscectomy or longstanding instability warrants careful assessment for varus malalignment. Noyes has written extensively on the subject, breaking down the varus ACL deficient knee into three categories, namely, primary, double and triple varus. Primary varus is used to define the patient with osseous tibio-femoral varus alignment, which may or may not be worsened by medial meniscal or medial compartment articular cartilage loss. Where varus in this setting has resulting in attenuation of the lateral soft tissue restraints with lateral compartment widening the term double varus is used and finally triple varus is encountered in the knee that due to chronic or acute injury adopts a varus recurvatum posture (Noyes 2000).

When double or triple varus is encountered it is recommended that ACL reconstruction be performed in conjunction with or after high tibial osteotomy, with posterolateral soft tissue reconstruction added in the setting of triple varus. The type of HTO utilized is usually either a HTMOWO or a HTLCWO, with every effort made to avoid increasing the posterior tibial slope, in order to avoid increasing stresses transmitted to the ACL graft. Important subtleties in lateral closing wedge surgery in this setting relate to ensuring the new mechanical axis passes through the Fujisawa point and avoidance of disruption of the proximal tibio-fibular joint so as not to further defunction the lateral ligamentous restraints. Osteotomy of the fibula should be performed at the level of the neck with removal of a wedge of bone to allow compression as the tibial osteotomy is closed (Noyes 2000). A HTMOWO should be considered where patella alta pre-exists, where concomitant MCL surgery is required, and where limb length discrepancy with the operative limb being shorter is encountered. Similarly, if the HTO and ACL reconstruction are being performed simultaneously - both can be performed with relative ease through the one anteromedial incision (Amendola 2004) (Figure 2). This single stage combined technique has demonstrated excellent medium term survival and return to function. In a French retrospective study of 30 ACL deficient knees with early medial compartment arthritic changes, in 29 patients of mean age 30 years who underwent single stage ACL reconstruction and HTO (25 closing wedge and 5 opening wedge), at mean follow up of 12 years, 47% were still involved in intense sporting activity namely skiing, tennis and soccer, while a further 36% described their involvement in sporting activity as moderate. Radiologically only 17% of this cohort had progressed one grade at final follow-up (Bonin 2004).

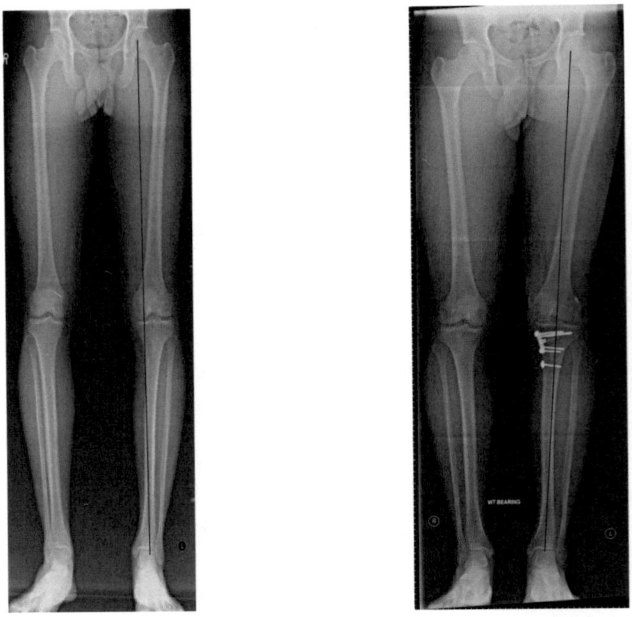

Fig. 2. Mechanical axis pre and post combined HTMOWO and ACL reconstruction.

3.1.1 Surgical technique – Single stage HTO and ACL reconstruction

A careful stepwise approach however, is required to avoid complications. The steps involved include, arthroscopy to assess the articular surfaces, debridement or repair of meniscal injuries, notch preparation, anteromedial incision over the proximal tibia, hamstring harvest and preparation, passage of two 1.8 mm threaded guide wires along the path of the medial opening wedge tibial osteotomy, paying careful attention to the saggital alignment of these wires so as not to increase the posterior tibial slope through the osteotomy, if anything the slope of the line joining these wires in the saggital plane should be less than the current posterior tibial slope of the patient. Next the femoral tunnel is drilled through an anteromedial tunnel followed by tibial tunnel drilling proximal to the osteotomy site guide wires with consideration given to ultimate proximal tibial locking plate and screw placement, as well as the position of the tibial tubercle osteotomy step cut. The medial opening wedge osteotomy is then performed using standard techniques as outlined above ensuring that the osteotomy is opened using laminar spreaders, twice as much posteriorly as it is anteriorly, so as not to increase the tibial slope (Noyes 2005). The final drill used for the tibial tunnel is re-introduced by hand into the tibial tunnel and left in situ while the proximal tibial locking plate is applied across the osteotomy and provisionally held with k-wires through the proximal locking holes to ensure the ACL tibial tunnel will not be compromised by the proximal locking screws from the plate. The k-wires in the locking plate are replaced by screws to fully stabilize the osteotomy. The ACL graft is then passed and fixed on the femoral side, cycled and fixed on the tibial side using dual fixation, however, the proximal tibial locking plate should not be used as a means of secondary fixation for the tibial graft as it occasionally requires removal at a later date. The arthroscope is re-inserted into the knee - the lateral tibial plateau is examined for evidence of iatrogenic fracture and the tension within the ACL graft is checked, the knee is thoroughly washed out and the wounds closed using interrupted sutures. Rehabilitation should commence the following day with patellar mobilization, early knee range of motion; isometric quadriceps strengthening and toe touch weight bearing for six weeks.

3.2 Chronic posterolateral instability and the varus knee

With improved understanding of the anatomy and biomechanics of the structures of the posterolateral corner of the knee has come a trend towards early repair or reconstruction of these structures with a view to returning the patient to pre-injury function as soon as possible. Nonetheless, many of these patients are not seen 'early', within 2-3 weeks of injury, by a surgeon with a specialist interest in treating these injuries, and therefore are seen or present on a delayed basis.

When a patient with chronic posterolateral instability of the knee is seen a careful assessment of the alignment of that knee is once again warranted. The fact that two convex surfaces, the lateral femoral condyle and lateral tibial plateau, articulate within a compartment bounded by a mobile lateral meniscus adds to the instability of the compartment placing increased stresses on the posterolateral structures for stability. Varus malalignment will place continued stress across any planned reconstruction and likely ultimately lead to failure of that reconstruction. Biomechanical studies have shown reductions in lateral compartment opening when a varus moment is applied and tibial external rotation when an external rotation torque force is applied to a posterolateral corner deficient cadaveric knee following HTMOWO. It should be noted that, unlike in the technique described previously in this chapter, the superficial MCL was left intact at the level of the osteotomy in this study and was thought to add to the stability of the knee through tightening of the posteromedial structures through its attachments to the deep MCL and posterior oblique ligaments. However, the effect of this statistically significant increase in tension in the superficial MCL, when both varus moments and external rotation torques were applied, on the articular cartilage of the medial compartment is, as yet, unknown (LaPrade 2008). These findings of increased stability in the posterolateral corner deficient cadaveric knee following HTMOWO have been backed up by clinical studies showing that 38% of patients with combined varus malalignment and posterolateral corner insufficiency treated initially with HTMOWO did not require subsequent reconstruction of their concomitant posterolateral corner insufficiency. This study of 21 patients with a mean follow up of 37 months concluded that those patients with isolated chronic posterolateral corner insufficiency, low energy injury mechanisms and higher pre-operative knee function scores were least likely to require secondary posterolateral corner reconstruction following HTMOWO to correct varus malalignment (Arthur 2007).

4. Complications of high tibial osteotomy

General complications of any surgical intervention can be broken down into acute intra-operative, acute post-operative (within hours), early post-operative (within days to weeks) and delayed post-operative (within months to years). Broadly speaking, in this setting, acute intra-operative complications include direct neurovascular injury when performing the tibial or fibular osteotomies, intra-articular proximal tibial fracture, fracture of the medial or lateral tibial cortical hinge, tibial tubercle fracture with disruption of the patellar tendon and extensor mechanism, failure to adequately correct the deformity, intra-articular placement of fixation screws or staples.

Acutely post-operatively neurovascular complications predominate with compartment syndrome, bleeding from the osteotomy site or from direct vascular injury occasionally encountered, similarly neural palsies typically declare themselves during this time frame. Infection, thrombo-embolic events, stiffness and pain predominate during the early post-operative phase, while delayed union, non-union, recurrence of deformity, osteonecrosis of the proximal tibia, varus instability, patella baja and less commonly patella alta, hardware breakage, loosening or hardware related pain are encountered during the delayed post-operative period.

Rates of the more common complications include infection of 0.8 – 10.4%, symptomatic deep venous thrombosis of 2-5% in most series (Tunggal 2010), deep venous thrombosis by venography of 41%(Turner 1993), intra-articular fractures during HTLCWO of 0-20%(Tunggal 2010) and during HTMOWO of up to 11%(Hernigou 1987), lateral cortical hinge fracture of 35%, medial cortical hinge fracture of 55-82%, delayed union and non-union of closing wedge osteotomies of 4-8.5%and <1-5% respectively, peroneal nerve palsy post closing wedge osteotomy of 0-20% with up to 50% resulting in permanent deficit of varying severity (Tunggal 2010), less common complications include popliteal and anterior tibial artery injuries and compartment syndrome. Compartment pressures especially in the anterior compartment have been shown to increase following HTO, these pressures can be reduced by the use of a drain, thereby reducing the risk of compartment syndrome, which is therefore recommended (Gibson 1986).

The specific complications related to HTO typically compare the two most commonly used techniques, namely HTMOWO and HTLCWO, and the various means of fixation utilized. Broadly speaking, medial opening wedge is favored by some due to the reduced risk of neurovascular complications associated with the fibular osteotomy required during lateral closing wedge surgery, the reduced prevalence of compartment syndrome as the anterior compartment is not violated, and the fact that it is easier to perform through one incision allowing careful alteration of the extent of the correction intra-operatively prior to definitive fixation. Of 186 knees which underwent HTMOWO surgery and stabilization with a Tomofix® plate 10 (5.4%) went on to non-union. The identified risk factors for non-union were smoking, elevated body mass index and fracture of the lateral cortical hinge (Meidinger 2011). The lateral closing wedge is favored by others on the basis that the direct bone on bone contact provides earlier stability, faster osteotomy healing and permits earlier weight-bearing.

Individual studies report varying but nonetheless significant complication rates in association with these surgeries, for instance, in a prospective cohort study of 40 patients comparing HTMOWOs stabilized with a modified Puddu plate and grafted using tricalcium phosphate to HTLCWOs stabilized with an AO/ASIF L-plate, the overall complication rate was 55% in the Puddu plate group and 20% in the AO/ASIF L-plate group. This statistically significant difference in complications between the groups included 7 tibial non-unions and 6 hardware failures in the Puddu plate group and is accounted for by the rehabilitation protocol which permitted full weight-bearing in both groups at 6 weeks. The authors suggest that a fixed angle device such as a TomoFix® plate might be a more suitable device for osteotomy fixation when an opening wedge technique is utilized (van den Bekerom 2008).

A single surgeon series of 194 osteotomies comparing HTLCWOs stabilized with two stepped staples and HTMOWOs stabilized with Aescula opening wedge plates, demonstrated overall and major complication rates of 27.9% and 16.4% in the closing wedge patients respectively, compared to 20.0% and 11.1% in the opening wedge patients. The actual major complications in the closing wedge group were 7 peroneal nerve injuries, 2 cases of compartment syndrome, one deep infection, 2 non-unions, one failure of fixation, 2 cases of loss of correction and 2 cases of varus instability. While the major complications in the opening wedge group consisted of two failures of fixation, 2 cases of loss of correction and 6 lateral tibial plateau fractures. These differences, however, did not reach statistical significance; nonetheless the authors recommend using the opening wedge technique. Obesity (BMI>27.5kg/m^2) was found to be the only independent predictor of a major complication in this study, which excluded smokers (Song 2010).

Similarly, in an, in press, meta-analysis of 12 papers from 9 clinical trials comparing outcomes in opening (n=324) versus closing (n=318) wedge high tibial osteotomy surgeries, no difference in the incidence of infection, deep vein thrombosis, peroneal nerve palsy, non-union or rates of revision to knee arthroplasty could be demonstrated. No significant difference was found for any clinical outcome including pain, functional score or complications, medial opening wedge osteotomies, however, resulted in superior anatomical correction whilst simultaneously resulting in greater reductions in patellar height and greater increases in posterior tibial slope compared to closing wedge surgeries. The authors point out, that the reason no clinical difference in outcomes may have been identified may be due to type 2 error, failure to blind assessors and inadequate follow-up (Smith 2010).

5. Results of high tibial osteotomy

Apart from analysis of complications associated with the surgery itself probably the best, although crude, means available currently to assess the results of HTO surgery are through analysis of reported survival rates and patient satisfaction scores. Once again the largest series pertain to the patient with medial compartment overload treated with a HTMOWO or HTLCWO.

Lateral closing wedge surgery in 413 patients using a Krakow staple for stabilization yielded survival rates of 95%, 79% and 56% at 5, 10 and 15 years respectively, with 85% of patients being enthusiastic or satisfied with the surgery and 84% willing to undergo the surgery again at mean of 12 year follow up. Multivariate regression analysis also showed that patients aged less than 50 years, BMI < 25kg/m^2 and ACL deficiency were all associated with increased odds of survival (Hui 2011).

In a study of 54 patients who underwent 55 HTOs, being either lateral closing wedge using a modified Weber technique and stabilized with a bent half tubular plate and 2 screws or medial opening wedge facilitated by release of the MCL and stabilized using a plate over a tricortical iliac crest bone graft, the 5, 10 and 15 year survival rates were 98%, 92% and 71%

respectively. The median follow up was 16.5 years (interquartile range (IQR) 14.5-17.9 years) satisfaction index was 80% (IQR 63-89), median knee injury and osteoarthritis outcome score was 71 (IQR 49-82) and median Western Ontario and McMaster university osteoarthritis index was 82 (IQR 66-96). There was no difference in survival rates or outcome scores when HTMOWO was compared to HTLCWO in this study but once again the study was likely underpowered to show any potential difference with fewer patients in the former group compared to the latter (Schallberger 2011).

One hundred patients retrospectively analyzed following HTLCWO surgery with stabilization using 2 staples exhibited a survival rate of 75% at 10 years with regression analysis showing higher likelihood of conversion to total knee arthroplasty (TKA) in females and patients whose Ahlback grade was ≥ 2 pre-operatively (van Raaij 2008).

Using Kaplan-Meier survivorship analysis, 73% of patients at 5 years, 51% of patients at 10 years, 39% at 15 years, and 30% at 20 years after high tibial osteotomy had not required conversion of a HTLCWO to a TKA; in 106 osteotomies in 85 patients with a minimum follow up of 10 years. Highlighting the importance of careful patient selection, on subset analysis of these patients, those under 50 years of age with a pre-operative flexion arc of greater than 120 degrees demonstrated much improved survival rates of 95% at 5 years, 80% at 10 years, and 60% at 15 years (Naudie 1999).

A HTLCWO stabilized using a Blount staple and AO semi-tubular plate and screws was used in 301 osteotomies available for follow-up at a mean of 18 years. The 20 year survival was 85% with revision as the end-point most likely in those patients aged greater than 50 years and with Ahlback arthritis grade ≥ 3 pre-operatively. Knee function was considered satisfactory in 77% of patients at final follow-up (Flecher X 2006).

HTLCWO has long been the gold standard and therefore the volume of literature currently available is weighted in its favour, however, this technique requires a fibular osteotomy and or disruption of the proximal tibio-fibular joint with their inherent risks to the peroneal nerve, lateral compartment muscle origin disruption, bone stock loss from the proximal tibia and a potentially more difficult conversion to TKA, for these reasons medial opening wedge techniques have gained popularity over recent years, especially since the development of fixed angled locking plates.

Using a medial opening wedge technique stabilized with a plate and screws and the gap filled posteriorly with a wedge of acrylic bone cement, Hernigou et al, demonstrated survival rates of 94% at 5 years, 85% at 10 years and 68% at 15 years, in 245 osteotomies in 197 patients with a mean age of 60 years (Hernigou 2001).

One hundred and twenty four HTMOWO osteotomies, performed in 110 patients with mean age of 53 years and mean follow-up of 10.4 years, grafted using a tricalcium phosphate wedge and stabilized using an AO T-plate, demonstrated survival rates of 89% at 5 years and 74% at 10 years. At final follow-up 88% classified themselves as satisfied or very satisfied with their outcome (Saragaglia 2011).

Two Japanese studies have shown superior survival rates at long term follow up; the exact role of cultural and ethnic factors in these studies is unclear, the results in this population nonetheless, speak for themselves. The first study used HTLCWOs stabilized using a Giebel plate, aiming for 10 degrees of anatomic valgus or placement of the mechanical axis within the centre of the lateral compartment, in 118 knees in patients of mean age 62.9 years, whose mean flexion contracture was 7.7 degrees, with mean follow-up of 14.4 years. Using Kaplan-Meier survival analysis, the probability of survival was 99.3% at 5years, 97.6% at 10 years and 90.4% at 15 years. The mean Hospital for special surgery score at final follow up was also deemed good or excellent in 73.7% of patients. Range of motion < 100 degrees and BMI > 27.5 kg/m^2 were associated with early failure, but interestingly, a pre-operative flexion contracture > 15 degrees and maximum flexion < 120 degrees showed a significant association with long term survival of the osteotomy (Akizuki 2008). The second study of 75 knees (60 female and 15 male) in 53 patients, in patients with a mean age of 59.6 years and mean fixed flexion contracture of 6 degrees, using HTLCWOs stabilized with either Charnley's external fixation clamps or a dual plating technique using a blade plate on the lateral side, demonstrated Kaplan -Meier survival rates of 97.8% at 5 years, 96.2% at 10 years and 93.2% at 15 years. In all patients walking distance was limited to less than 500m due to pain pre-operatively but had improved to greater than 1km without pain in 94.3% at 15-28 year follow up, at which time 98%were satisfied with their outcome (Koshino 2004).

6. High tibial osteotomy and conversion to total knee arthroplasty

One of the difficulties related to the decision as to whether to proceed with an osteotomy as against a primary arthroplasty procedure relates to concerns about conversion of that post-osteotomy patient to an arthroplasty should the patient require same in the future. This is based on the knowledge that osteotomy outcomes gradually deteriorate with time and therefore if a patient lives long enough they will likely require conversion to a TKA, which will be a more technically demanding operation than the standard primary TKA.

The difficulties encountered in converting a post-osteotomy patient to a TKA include initially ensuring there was no history of infection related to the metalwork required for fixation of the osteotomy. If there was a history of infection be it superficial or otherwise at the time of the osteotomy surgery it would be prudent to stage the conversion to TKA with removal of all retained metal work, appropriate culture of local soft tissue samples and normalization of blood work prior to proceeding with the definitive arthroplasty.

If there was no history of infection pre-operative planning should include templating to assess the need for removal of retained hardware. If removal of hardware is deemed unnecessary for tibial component placement, all tools for removal of retained hardware should be available at the time of surgery should the need arise. Whether hardware removal should be staged or not is often dictated by surgeon preference as opposed to hard data.

Pre-operatively, the knee range of motion should be assessed so that the surgeon will have an idea as to whether or not the patient might require an extensile procedure such as a quadriceps snip or tibial tubercle osteotomy to facilitate exposure of the joint. Similarly, patellar tracking and patellar mobility should aid in deciding on the need for lateral retinacular release or not. The previous incision should be taken into account when planning the approach to the knee, if a HTMOWO had been performed, this incision should not compromise the approach, however, when a lateral incision has been used for a previous HTLCWO care must be taken to ensure that either an adequate skin bridge is planned for or the two incisions converge at an angle no less than 60 degrees.

Radiographic analysis should examine the current alignment, with lateral or medial compartment opening on weight bearing perhaps indicative of ligamentous incompetence and raising the requirement for the availability of more constrained components at the time of surgery. The bone stock within the proximal tibia particularly on the lateral side, when a patient has had a HTLCWO should be carefully assessed; this should alert the surgeon to the possibility of the need for lateral augments and therefore stemmed tibial components. The geometry of the planned primary tibial component must be taken into account when analyzing the pre-operative radiograph to ensure the keel or pegs will not abut or breach the lateral cortex due to the relative medialisation of the medullary canal following HTLCWO, if this is likely to be a problem consideration should be given to, downsizing and medialising the tibial component, use of a system with shorter tibial pegs or studs or the use of stemmed revision components to offset the tibial tray from the stem. The lateral radiograph is important in assessing the posterior tibial slope and the height of the patella, with patella baja alerting the surgeon to possible difficulties in everting the patella; this is especially relevant when the patient has had a HTLCWO and immobilization post-operatively. Restoration of the posterior tibial slope is important in ensuring flexion and extension gap symmetry as well as in preventing impingement of the tibial component keel on the anterior cortex of the tibia in the case of excessive posterior slope.

Most of these problems are less of an issue following HTMOWO, due to the fact that bone stock is preserved, the fibula has not been disrupted or osteotomised and therefore gives a definite guide to joint line restoration and tibial component rotation, the medullary canal has not been medialised and as long as care has been taken to ensure the primary correction at the time of the osteotomy occurred through opening of the wedge posteriorly, patella baja should also be minimized.

Even though these technical difficulties are present during the conversion of a post-osteotomy knee to a TKA, studies to date have failed to show that this has a deleterious effect on outcomes. In a systematic review of the published literature up to September 2007, 17 studies met the inclusion criteria but pooling of the data was not possible due to the heterogeneity of the studies. Malalignment and instability are major causes of early failure following TKA with most revisions performed within 5 years, with a median follow-up of 5 years in eight included studies reporting on revision surgery no significant differences in TKA failure for the patients receiving TKA after previous osteotomy compared to primary TKA was identified in this review. This review concluded that the use of HTO postpones primary TKA for a median of 7 years in younger patients. Six studies that reported knee range of motion reported median reductions of 10 degrees for patients receiving TKA after HTO compared to primary TKA patients. At mid-term follow-up in eight out of nine studies reviewed significant differences in overall function evaluated by standard knee clinical scores could not be shown between the groups (van Raaij 2009). Since this review a number of studies as outlined below, detailing similar findings, have been published.

A study of 29 knees in 24 patients, who underwent 19 HTLCWOs and 10 HTMOWOs, matched to a control group of 28 patients with 29 knee arthroplasties for age, pre-operative American knee society score and radiographic AP alignment aswell as length of follow-up (97 months), failed to show any difference in patient satisfaction between the groups with

96.5% of patients in both groups having a good or excellent result at this time point. The authors report that prior HTO did not adversely affect component fixation, but at final follow-up there were significantly more radiolucent lines under the tibial components on lateral radiographs in the study group and one patient had gone on to revision at 37 months for aseptic loosening. Additional techniques to facilitate exposure were required in 7 patients being 3 quadriceps snips, 3 lateral releases and 1 tibial tubercle osteotomy. The Caton index was also significantly reduced in the study group post-operatively, in which 3 patients required subsequent patella resurfacing at 18, 19 and 27 months with the authors suggesting that primary patella resurfacing be considered in these patients to reduce rates of anterior knee pain (Amendola 2010).

In a study of 48 patients who underwent TKA after HTLCWO with a mean follow-up of 13.3 years, the mean knee society score increased from 90 pre-operatively to 160 post-operatively, with the authors concluding that prior HTLCWO did not affect the clinical and radiological results of TKA in the longer term (Treuter 2011).

From an original study group of 39 patients who underwent bilateral TKA using cruciate retaining components, at a mean of 8.7 years post unilateral HTLCWO, 20 patients had died leaving 19 patients available for follow up at a mean of 14 years post total knee replacement. There was no significant difference in Knee society or pain scores between the knees, no femoro-tibial revisions had been performed in any knee at final follow-up (Meding 2011).

Matched-pair analysis was used to minimize the effect of variables such as age, gender, follow-up, etiology and prosthetic design in comparing the results of 41 primary TKA patients with 41 patients who underwent TKA using a cemented posterior stabilized design without patella resurfacing, following HTLCWO. Although 3 patients required lateral releases and 1 a medial tightening there was no difference in mean operative time between the groups. Complication rates of 19.5% in the study group (including 4 patients with wound necrosis at the level of the previous lateral incision) and 4.8% in the control group were not statistically different. At final follow-up, at a mean of 82 months in the study group and 85 months in the control group, range of motion was reduced in the study group compared to controls (pre arthroplasty range of motion was not available for either group) and other than a reduced knee score of the knee society score there was no difference in VAS, WOMAC, Lequesne, UCLA, Feller's Patellar Score and SF-36 scores. There was no difference in component alignment or rate of radiolucencies detected at final follow up between the groups and no patient had undergone femoral or tibial component revision (Efe 2010).

7. Conclusions

High tibial osteotomy is an effective and successful procedure; it demands meticulous surgical technique to limit complications and achieve correct post-operative alignment. Where these techniques and goals are adhered to enduring long term results and high satisfaction rates in carefully selected patients are to be expected. It's use should not be avoided by the surgeon for fear of difficulties relating to conversion to total knee arthroplasty especially if medial opening wedge techniques are used, since to date outcomes are comparable in primary arthroplasty patients when compared to those undergoing arthroplasty following high tibial osteotomy.

8. References

Akizuki S, Shibakawa A, takizawa T, Yamazaki I, Horiuchi H (2008). The long-term outcome of high tibial osteotomy, A ten to 20 year follow-up. J Bone Joint Surg (Br) 2008; 90: 592-596.

Aglietti P, Buzzi R, vena LM, Baldini A, Mondaini A (2003). High tibial valgus osteotomy for medial gonarthrosis; a 10 to 21 year study. *Journal of Knee Surgery* 2003; 16: 21-26.

Amendola A, Fowler PJ, Litchfield R, Kirkley S, Clatworthy M (2004). Opening wedge high tibial osteotomy using a novel technique: early results and complications. *J Knee Surg*. 2004; 17: 164-169.

Amendola L, Fosco M, Cenni E, Tigani D (2010). Knee joint arthroplasty after tibial osteotomy. Int Orthop 2010; 34: 289-295.

Arthur A, LaPrade R, Agel J (2007). Proximal Tibial Opening Wedge Osteotomy as the Initial Treatment for Chronic Posterolateral Corner Deficiency in the Varus Knee: A Prospective Clinical Study Am J Sports Med 2007; 35: 1844-1850.

Billings A, Scott D, Camargo M, Hofmann A (2000). High Tibial Osteotomy with a Calibrated Osteotomy Guide, Rigid Internal Fixation, and Early Motion. Long-Term Follow-up**J Bone Joint Surg (Am)* 2000; 82(1): 70-79.

Bonin N, Ait Si Selmi T, Donell S, Dejour H, Neyret P (2004). Anterior cruciate reconstruction combined with valgus upper tibial osteotomy: 12 years follow-up. *The Knee* 2004; 11: 431– 437.

Coventry MB (1965). Osteotomy of the upper portion of the tibia for degenerative arthritis of the knee. A preliminary report. J Bone Joint Surg(Am) 1965; 47(5): 984–990.

Coventry MB (1987). Proximal tibial varus osteotomy for osteoarthritis of the lateral compartment of the knee. *J Bone Joint Surg (Am)* 1987; 69: 32-38.

Coventry MB, Ilstrup DM, Wallrichs SL (1993). Proximal tibial osteotomy. A critical long-term study of eighty seven cases. *Journal of Bone and Joint Surgery (Am)* 1993; 75: 196-201.

Dejour H, Neyret P, Boileau P, Donell ST (1994). Anterior cruciate ligament reconstruction combined with valgus tibial osteotomy. *Clin Orthop Relat Res.* 1994; 299: 220-228.

Efe T, Heyse TJ, Boese C, Timmesfeld N, Fuchs-Winkelmann S, Schmitt J, Theisen C, Schofer MD (2010). TKA following high tibial osteotomy versus primary TKA--a matched pair analysis. *BMC Musculoskelet Disord.* 2010 Sep 14; 11: 207.

Flecher X, Parratte S, Aubaniac JM, Argenson JN (2006). A 12-28 year follow-up study of closing wedge high tibial osteotomy. *Clin Orthop Relat Res.* 2006; 452: 91-6.

Fujisawa Y, Masuhara K, Shiomio S (1979). The effect of high tibial osteotomy on osteoarthritis of the knee. An arthroscopic stuy of 54 knee joints. Orthop Clin North Am. 1979;10: 585–608.

Gaasbeek RD, Sonneveld H, van Heerwaarden RJ, Jacobs WC, Wymenga AB (2004). Distal tuberosity osteotomy in open wedge high tibial osteotomy can prevent patella infera: a new technique. *Knee* 2004;11:457-61.

Gibson M, Barnes M, Allen M, Chan R (1986). Weakness of foot dorsiflexion and changes in compartment pressures after tibial osteotomy. *J Bone Joint Surg* 1986; 68: 471-475.

Giffin JR, Vogrin TM, Zantop T, Woo S, Harner CD (2004). Effects of increasing tibial slope on the biomechanics of the knee. *Am J Sports Med.* 2004; 32: 376-382.

Harrison MM, Waddell JP (1987). A comparison of plate versus staple-and-cast fixation in maintaining femoral tibial alignment after valgus tibial osteotomy. *Canadian Journal of Surgery* 2005; 48(1): 33-38.

Hernigou p, Medeville D, Debeyre J, Goutallier D (1987). Proximal tibial osteotomy for osteoarthritis with varus deformity. *Journal of Bone and Joint Surgery (Am)* 1987; 69: 332-354.

Hernigou P, Ma W. Open wedge tibial osteotomy with acrylic bone cement as bone substitute. *The Knee* 2001; 8: 103-110.

Hui C, Salmon LJ, Kok A, Williams HA, Hockers N, van der Tempel WM, Chana R, Pinczewski LA (2011). Long-term survival of high tibial osteotomy for medial compartment osteoarthritis of the knee.

Am J Sports Med. 2011 ; 39(1): 64-70.

Jackson JP (1958). Osteotomy for osteoarthritis of the knee. *Journal of Bone and Joint Surgery (Br)* 1958; 40: 826.

Jakob RP, Murphy SB (1992). Tibial osteotomy for varus gonarthrosis: indication, planning and operative technique. Instr Course Lect 1992; 41: 87-93.

Kettelkamp DB, Wenger DR, Chao EY, Thompson C (1976). Results of proximal tibial osteotomy. The effects of tibiofemoral angle, stance-phase flexion-extension, and medial plateau force. *Journal of Bone and Joint Surgery (Am)* 1976; 58: 952-960.

Koshino T, Tsuchiya K (1979). The effect of high tibial osteotomy on osteoarthritis of the knee. Clinical and histological observations. *International Orthopaedics* 1979; 3: 37-45.

Koshino T, Yoshida T, Ara Y, Saito I, Saito T (2004). Fifteen to twenty-eight years' follow-up results of high tibial valgus osteotomy for osteoarthritic knee. *The Knee* 2004; 11: 439- 444.

LaPrade R, Engebretsen L, Johansen S, Wentorf F, Kurtenbach C (2008). The Effect of a Proximal Tibial Medial Opening Wedge Osteotomy on Posterolateral Knee Instability: A Biomechanical Study Am J Sports Med 2008; 36: 956-960.

Magnussen RA, Lustiq S, Demey G, Neyret P, Servien E (2011). The effect of medial opening and lateral closing high tibial osteotomy on leg length. *Am J Sports Med* 2011; 39(9): 1900-1905.

Meding JB, Wing JT, Ritter MA (2011). Does high tibial osteotomy affect the success or survival of a total knee replacement? *Clin Orthop Relat Res.* 2011; 469(7): 1991-1994.

Meidinger G, Imhoff AB, Paul J, Kirchhoff C, Sauerschnig M, Hinterwimmer S (2011). May smokers and overweight patients be treated with a medial open-wedge HTO? Risk factors for non-union. *Knee Surg Sports Traumatol Arthrosc.* 2011; 19(3): 333-9.

Naudie D, Bourne RB, Rorabeck CH, Bourne TJ (1999). Survivorship of the high tibial valgus osteotomy: a 10 to 22 year follow-up study. *Clin Orthop* 1999; 367: 18-27.

Noyes F, Barber-Westin S, Hewett T (2000). High Tibial Osteotomy and Ligament Reconstruction for Varus Angulated Anterior Cruciate Ligament-Deficient Knees. The American Journal of Sports Medicine 2000; 28(3): 282-296.

Noyes FR, Goebel SX, West J. Opening wedge tibial osteotomy: the 3-triangle method to correct axial alignment and tibial slope (2005). Am J Sports Med. 2005; 33: 378-387.

Paley D (2002). Principles of deformity correction (First edition). Springer, ISBN 3-540-41665-x, New York.

Pfahler M, lutz C, Anetzberger H, Maier M, Hausdorf J, Pellengahr C, Refior HJ (2003). Long term results of high tibial osteotomy for medial osteoarthritis of the knee. Acta Chir Belg 2003; 103: 603-606.

Ritchie JF, Al-Sarawan M, Worth R, Conry B, Gibb P (2004). A parallel approach: the impact of schuss radiography of the degenerate knee on clinical management. *The Knee* 2004; 11(4): 283-287.

Rodner C, Adams D, Diaz-Doran V, Tate J, Santangelo S, Mazzocca A, Arciero R (2006). Medial Opening Wedge Tibial Osteotomy and the Sagittal Plane: The Effect of Increasing Tibial Slope on Tibiofemoral Contact Pressure Am J Sports Med 2006; 34: 1431-1441

Saragaglia D, Blaysat M, Inman D, Mercier N. Outcome of opening wedge high tibial osteotomy augmented with a Biosorb® wedge and fixed with a plate and screws in 124 patients with a mean of ten years follow-up. *Int Orthop.* 2011; 35(8): 1151-1156.

Schallberger A, Jacobi M, Wahl P, Maestretti G, Jakob R (2011). High tibial valgus osteotomy in unicompartmental medial osteoarthritis of the knee: a retrospective follow-up study over 13–21 years. *Knee Surg Sports Traumatol Arthrosc* 2011; 19: 122–127.

Smith TO, Sexton D, Mitchell P, Hing C (2010). Opening- or closing-wedged high tibial osteotomy: A meta-analysis of clinical and radiological outcomes, *Knee* (2010), doi:10.1016/j.knee.2010.10.001.

Song EK, Seon J, Park S, Jeong M (2010). The complications of high tibial osteotomy; closing – verus opening – wedge methods. *Journal of Bone and Joint Surgery (Br)* 2010; 92-B: 1245-1252.

Staubli AE, Jacob H (2010). Evolution of open-wedge high-tibial osteotomy: experience with a special angular stable device for internal fixation without interposition material. *Int Orthop.* 2010; 34(2): 167–172.

Treuter S, Schuh A, Hönle W, Ismail MS, Chirag TN, Fujak A (2011). Long-term results of total knee arthroplasty following high tibial osteotomy according to Wagner. *Int Orthop.* 2011 Oct 9. [Epub ahead of print].

Tunggal J, Higgins G, Waddell J (2010). Complications of closing wedge high tibial osteotomy. *International Orthopaedics* 2010; 34: 255-261.

Turner RS, Griffiths H, Heatley FW(1993). The incidence of deep-vein thrombosis after upper tibial osteotomy. A venographic study. *J Bone Joint Surg (Br)* 1993; 75: 942-944.

Van den Bekerom M, Patt T, Kleinhout M, Van der Vis H, Rob Albers G (2008). Early complications after high tibial osteotomy. A comparison of two techniques. *J Knee Surg* 2008; 21(1): 68-74.

Van Raaij T; Reijman M; Brouwer RW; Jakma TS; Verhaar JN (2008) Survival of closing-wedge high tibial osteotomy: good outcome in men with low-grade osteoarthritis after 10-16 years. *Acta Orthopaedica,* 2008; 79 (2): 230-4.

Van Raaij TM, Reijman M, Furlan AD, Verhaar JA (2009). Total knee arthroplasty after high tibial osteotomy. A systematic review. *BMC Musculoskelet Disord.* 2009 Jul 20; 10: 88.

Wang J, Hsu C (2005). Distal Femoral Varus Osteotomy for Osteoarthritis of the Knee Surgical Technique *Journal of Bone and Joint Surg (AM)* 2005; 87: 127-133.

Wright JM, Heavrin B, Begg M, Sakyrd G, Sterett W (2001). Observations on patellar height following opening wedge proximal tibial osteotomy. *Am Journal of Knee Surgery* 2001; 14: 163-173.

Wright JM, Heber C, Slawski D, Madsen M, Windsor R (2005). High Tibial Osteotomy. *Journal Am Acad Orthop Surg* 2005; 13: 279-289.

8

Computer-Assisted High Tibial and Double Level Osteotomies for Genu Varum Deformity

Dominique Saragaglia[1] and Sam Hakki[2]
[1]*Department of Orthopaedic Surgery and Sport Traumatology, Grenoble South Teaching Hospital, Échirolles,*
[2]*Bay Pines Health Care System Hospital, St Petersburg, Florida*
[1]*France*
[2]*USA*

1. Introduction

Medial compartment knee osteoarthritis is not uncommon and high tibial osteotomy (HTO) was described for the first time more than 50 years ago (Jackson, JP & Waugh, W 1961; Judet, R &Dupuis, JF & Honnard, F 1964; Merle d'Aubigné, R & Ramadier, JO 1961). Nowadays, it remains a good option (Coventry, MB & Ilstrup, DM & Wallrichs, SL 1993; Hernigou, Ph & Medevielle, D & Debeyre, J 1987; Jenny JY & Tavan, A & Jenny, G, et al 1998; Lerat, JL 2000; Lootvoet, L & Massinon, A & Rossillon, R, et al 1993; Papachristou, G & Pleassa, S & Sourlas, J & Levidiotis, C & Chronopoulos, E & Papachristou, C 2006; Rinonapoli, E & Mancini, GB & Corvaglia, A, et al 1998; Saragaglia, D & Blaysat, M & Inman, D & Mercier, N 2010; Yasuda, K & Majima, T & Tsuchida, T, et al 1992) despite the large expansion of total knee replacement (TKR) or the revival of unicompartmental knee prosthesis boosted by the less-invasive surgery concept. Ideally, HTO is indicated for active patients who are less than 65 years of age with moderate arthritis (narrowing joint line up to 100% without any bone wear or joint instability). Nevertheless, special attention should be paid to joint line orientation which can be distorted by excessive over or under correction which will eventually lead to earlier failure (Saragaglia, D & Blaysat, M & Inman, D & Mercier, N 2010) due to obliquity of joint line (Fig.1). This oblique joint line corresponds to an excessive valgus of the tibial mechanical axis (Babis, GC & An, KN & Chao, E. YS, et al 2002). Moreover, varus knee deformity may be a result of both tibial and femoral deformities. Correction of combined (femoral and tibial) varus deformity at the tibia level by (3° to 6°) to achieve a good clinical result may worsen the obliquity of knee joint line.

We have considered combined femoral and tibial osteotomy as a solution to avoid excessive joint line obliquity. However, prior to the advent of computer navigation this was only performed on a limited basis because of the difficulty in obtaining an accurate mechanical axis in relation to joint line plane.

Drawing on our experience with TKR and HTO navigation (Picard, F & Leitner, F & Raoult, A, et al 1999; Saragaglia, D & Pradel, Ph & Picard, F 2004; Saragaglia, D & Picard, F &

Chaussard, et al 2001; Saragaglia, D & Roberts, J 2005; Saragaglia, D & Rubens-Duval, B & Chaussard, C 2007; Hakki, S & Saleh, K & Bilotta, V et al) we used the principles of computer-assisted surgery for double level osteotomy (DLO) hoping to increase the accuracy of this difficult procedure. Our experience is based on 42 DLO performed between August 2001 and June 2010, out of 370 computer-assisted knee osteotomies for genu varum deformities (11.3%).We will present first, the preoperative radiological assessment, the computer-assisted operative procedure and the indications of HTO, DLO and distal femoral osteotomy (DFO). Then we will present the rationale behind this way of thinking and our results.

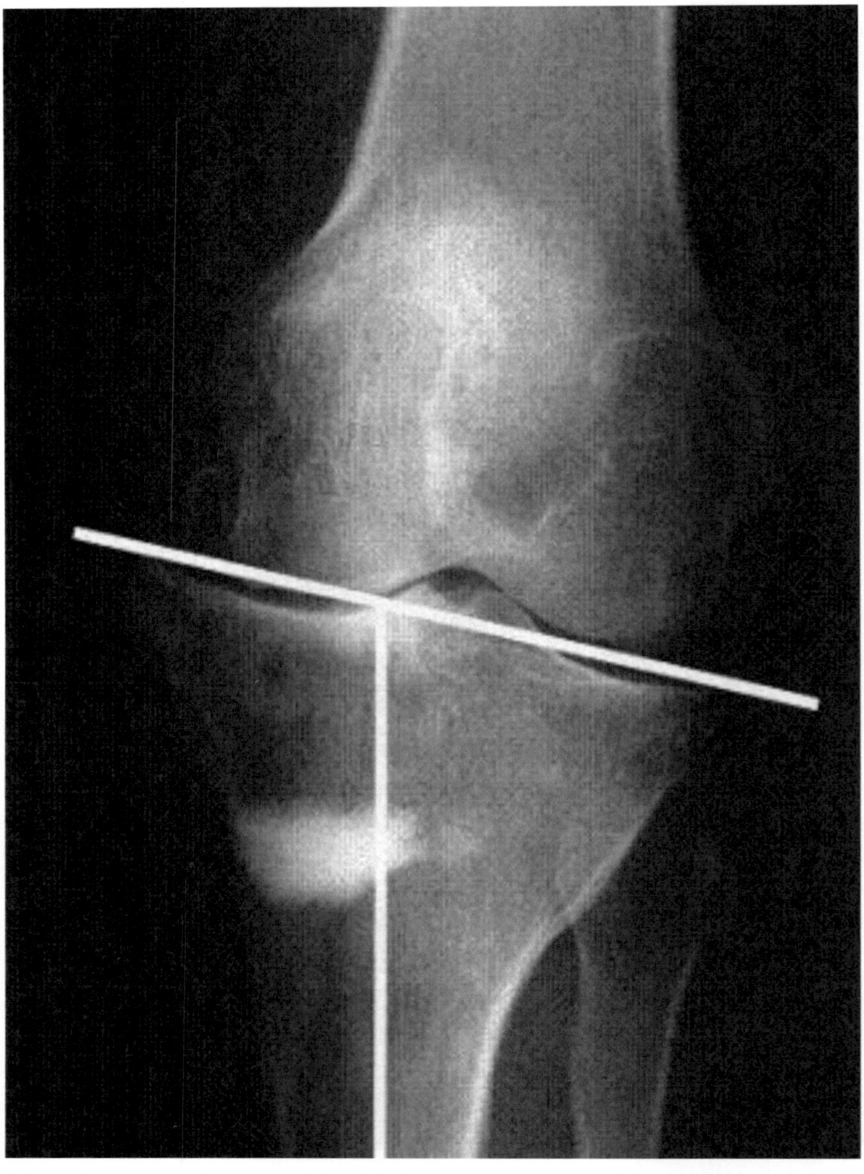

Fig. 1. Although varus deformity of the left knee was corrected the joint line remained in excessive valgus. This will lead to early failure HTO in this case.

2. Radiological assessment

Preoperatively Standing AP, lateral, and 45 degree PA weight bearing (Rosenberg) views are obtained. In addition, it is essential to obtain AP long leg standing x-rays to assess the hip knee ankle (HKA) angle for preoperative planning. Ramadier's protocol (Ramadier, JO & Buard, JE & Lortat-Jacob, A, et al 1982) allows these measurements to be reproducible pre and postoperatively. This protocol can be described as follows: first, to determine accurately the frontal plane by looking for a true lateral view of the knee which is obtained when the posterior margins of the condyles are superimposed; secondly, to turn 90° around the knee the image intensifier to obtain an accurate long leg AP standing view, the x-ray being perpendicular to the frontal plane; finally, to draw the foot print on a cardboard in order to reproduce the same rotation of the lower leg pre and postoperatively. Using this cardboard by placing the foot in the print, it is easy to do the same view as much as one wants. The long leg film is critical since the deformity may not be visible on standard knee films (Fig. 2a and 2b). One must measure the HKA angle, the medial distal femoral mechanical angle (MDFMA) and the medial proximal tibial mechanical angle (MPTMA)(Fig. 3a and 3b) in order to plan the level of the osteotomy femoral, tibial, or both. (Fig 3c)

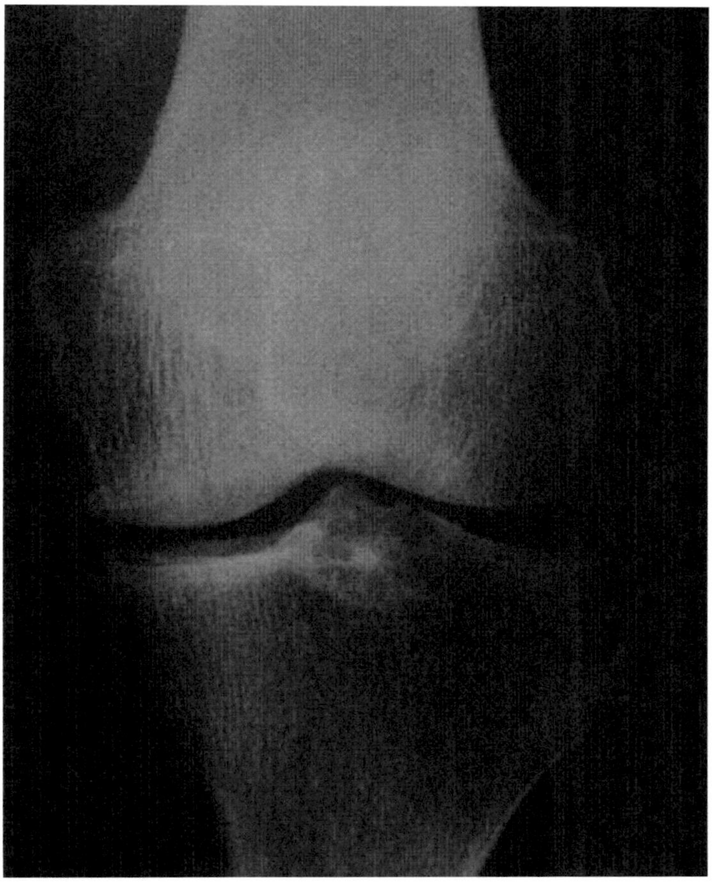

Fig. 2. a: Standard non weight bearing knee films does not show the significant varus deformity this patient has.

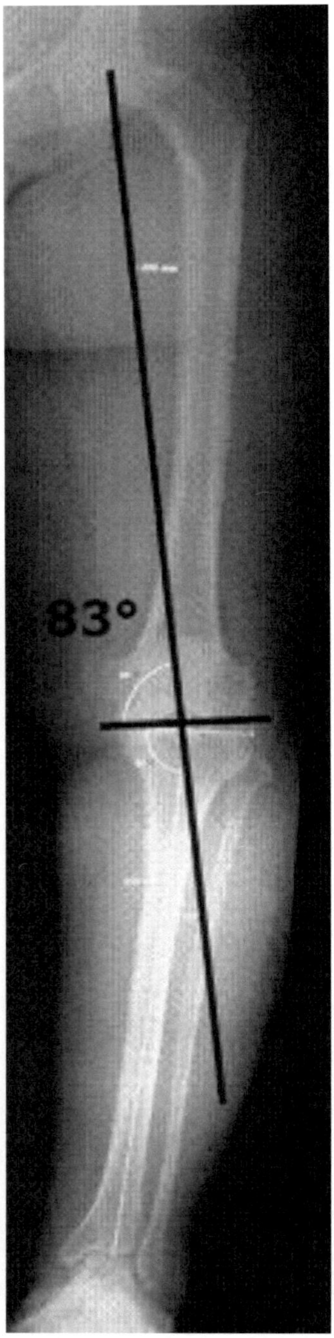

Fig. 2. b: The weight bearing long films serve many purposes: 1 - It shows significant varus deformity in comparison to figure 2a of the same patient. 2 - Quantitative measurements can be made of the severity of varus deformities in relation to the mechanical axis.
3 - Determines where the joint line is. 4 - Quantifies the deformity whether its femoral, tibial, or both.

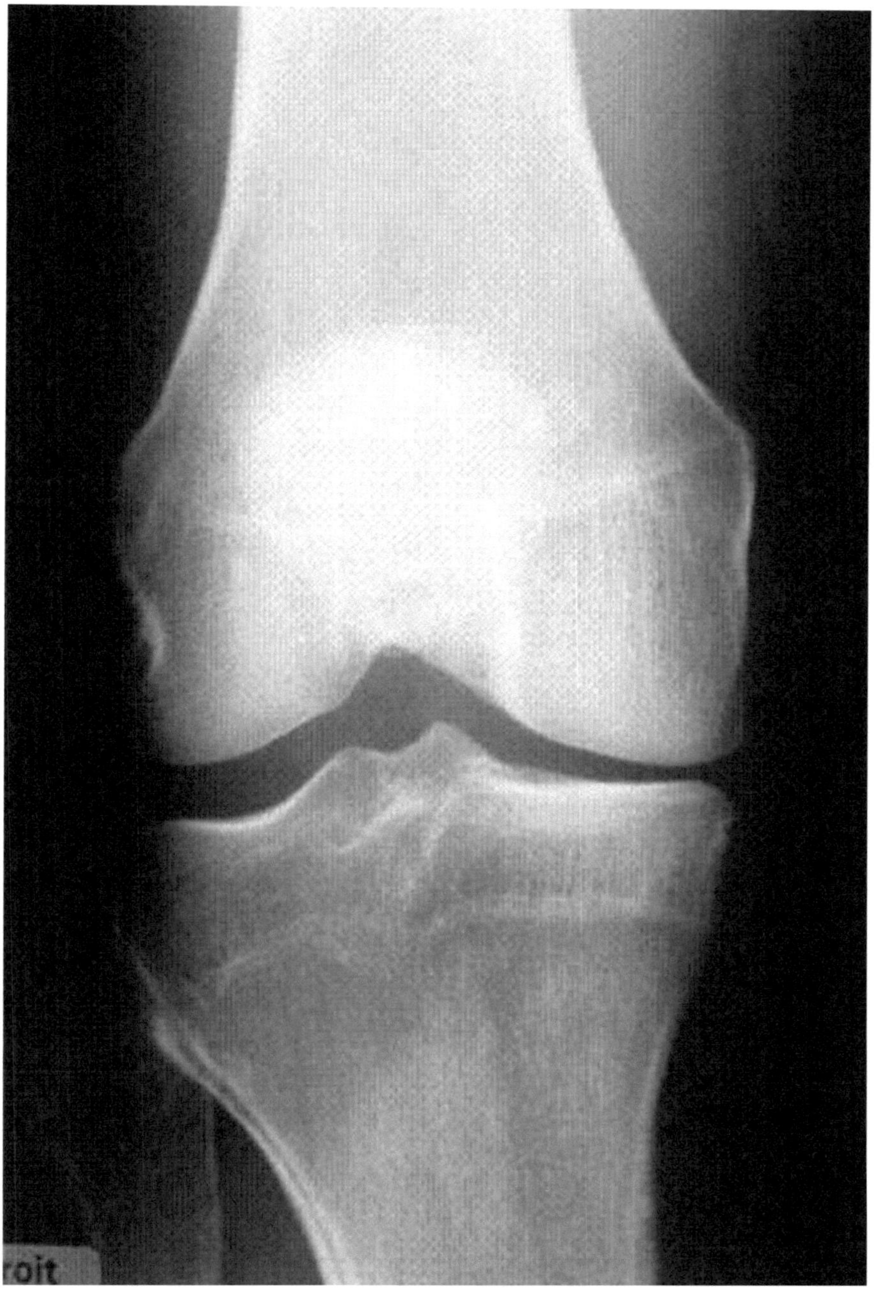

Fig. 3. a: 42 year old female with what seems to be mild tibia varus deformity

Grading of osteoarthritis is performed typically using the modified Ahlbäck classification (Saragaglia, D, Roberts, J 2005) (grade I, < 50% joint space narrowing; grade II, 50-100%; grade III, 100% narrowing without any bone wear; grade IV, bone wear but no lateral instability; grade V, bone wear with lateral compartment degeneration with or without posterolateral subluxation).

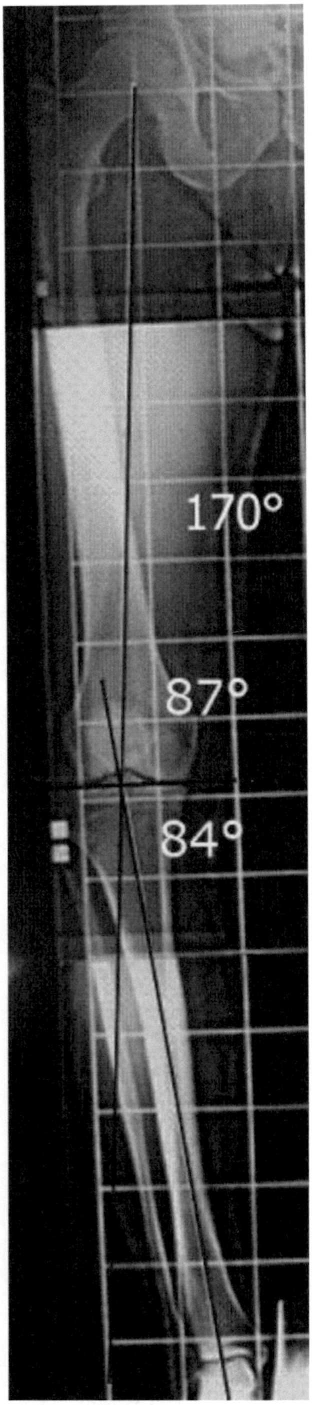

Fig. 3. b: Pre-operative long weight bearing x-ray in the same patient as 3a showing 6^0 of femoral and 6^0 of tibial varus deformity. Correction of one bone will not restore the joint line.

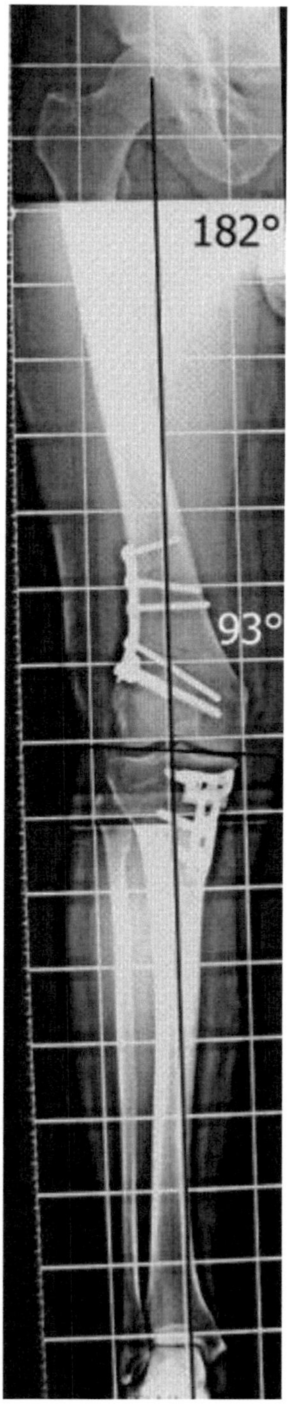

Fig. 3. c: Post operative x-ray film showing correction of both femoral and tibial varus deformity with restoration of the joint line and correction of varus deformity to a 2^0-3^0 valgus angle.

3. Surgical technique

3.1 Opening wedge HTO computer-navigated

The software is a derivative of the one used for TKA which has been fully described elsewhere (Picard, F & Leitner, F & Raoult, A etal 1999; Hakki, S & Saleh, K & Bilotta, V, et al.) (Orthopilot® Navigation System, B-Braun-Aesculap, Tuttlingen, Germany). The same principal of real time acquisition of the rotation centre of the hip, knee and ankle centres and of the anatomical landmarks at the level of the knee joint line and ankle is applied. They allow the mechanical axis of the lower limb to be shown dynamically on the computer screen, i.e. the axis of the lower limb to be seen both pre and post osteotomy and to check if the pre-planned correction has been established.

The rigid body markers are fixed percutaneously at the level of the distal femur and proximal tibia allowing acquisition of the centres of the hip, knee and ankle (Fig.4). The lower limb mechanical axis then appears on the screen and can be compared with the pre-operative radiological goniometry.

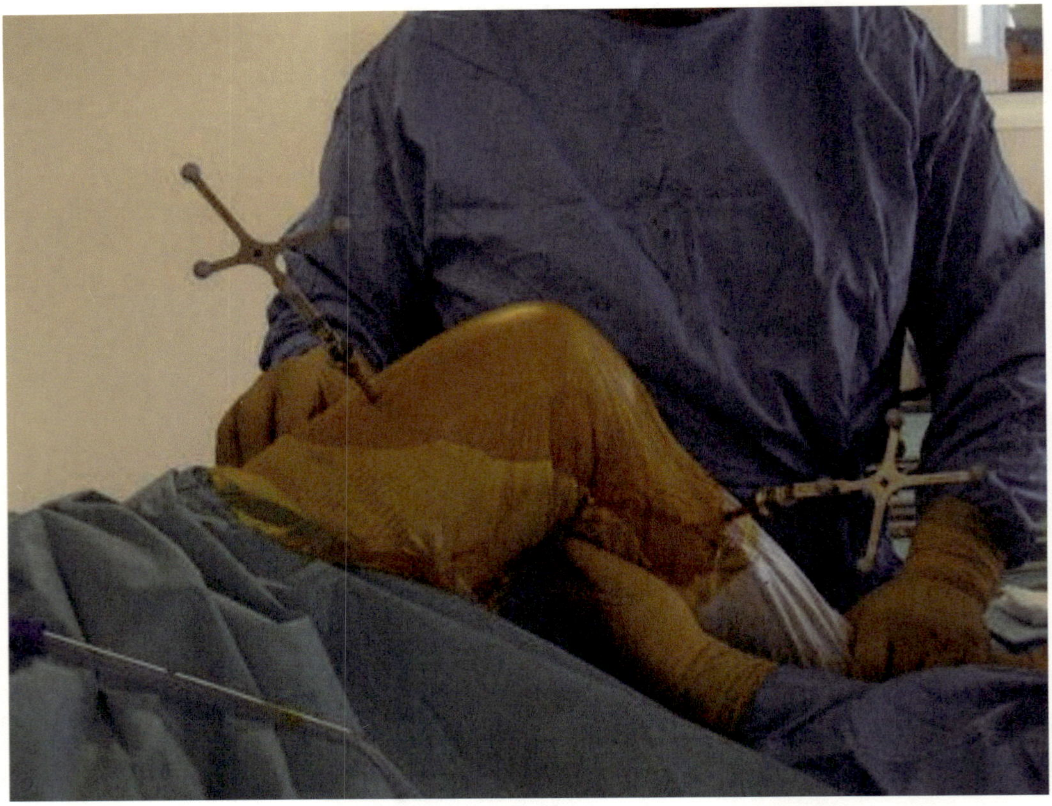

Fig. 4. Computer navigation is used to accurately quantify the deformity in all range of motion of the left knee.

A 5 to 6 centimeter long incision is made on the medial upper end of the tibia just at the level of the anterior tuberosity of the tibia. The pes anserinus is incised just above the gracilis tendon and a retractor is placed against the postero medial corner of the tibia (Fig.5).

Then, the superficial medial collateral ligament is released from its tibial insertion to allow an adequate opening of the osteotomy.

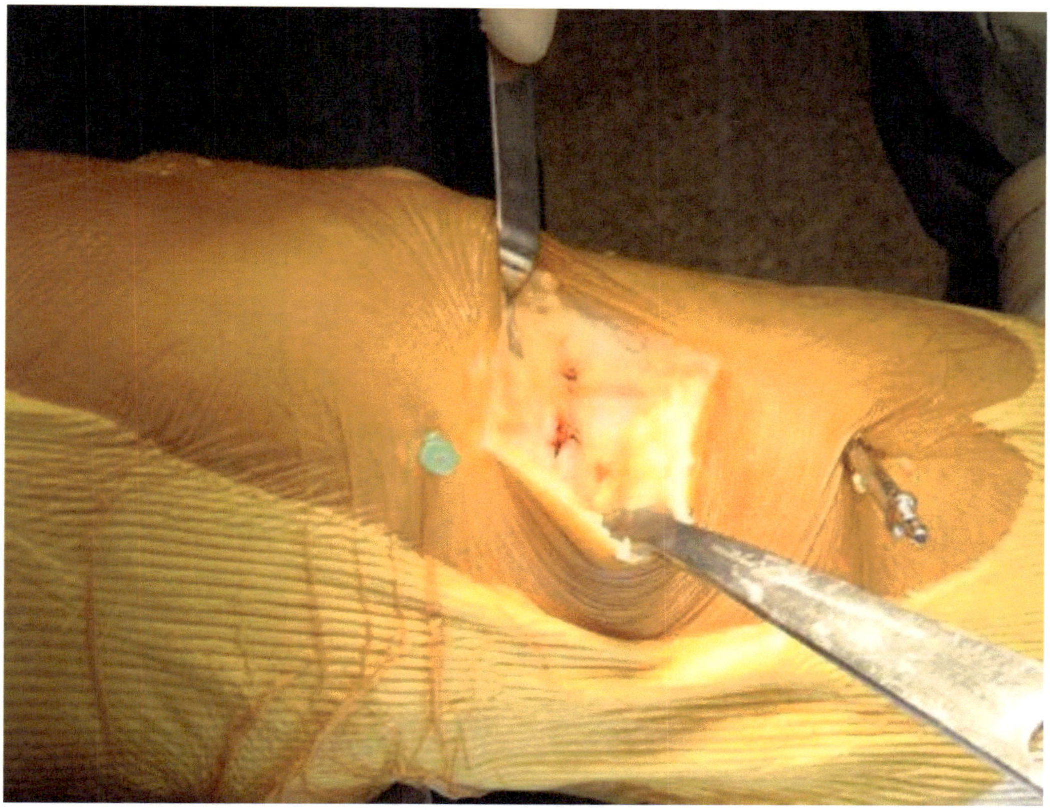

Fig. 5. Incision is made proximal to the tracker of the tibia at the level of tibia tuberosity. Note: pes anserinus is incised just above the gracilis tendon.

The HTO is then performed 3cm below the level of the medial joint line, the level of which is confirmed by placing an intra-articular needle. The osteotomy is directed at the fibula head, keeping the saw as horizontal as possible to avoid fracturing the lateral tibial plateau. With the aid of 2 Pauwels osteotomes inserted along the tract of the saw cut, the tibia is placed into valgus (Fig.6).

These are then replaced by a metal spacer, which is inherently stable and allows the amount of correction to be accurately checked. If there was 8° of varus one would try a 10-11 mm spacer and check to make sure an appropriate hypercorrection is produced real time on the computer screen (Fig. 7). If this is insufficient we try a thicker spacer and the reverse if the correction is too great.

The metallic spacer is then replaced with a bio-absorbable β Tricalcium phosphate wedge (Biosorb®R, SBM, Lourdes, France) of the desired thickness (Fig.8), and the intervention completed by plating the proximal tibia (Fig.9 and 10 a,b,c). Then the accuracy of the osteosynthesis is checked with the image intensifier and the wound is closed.

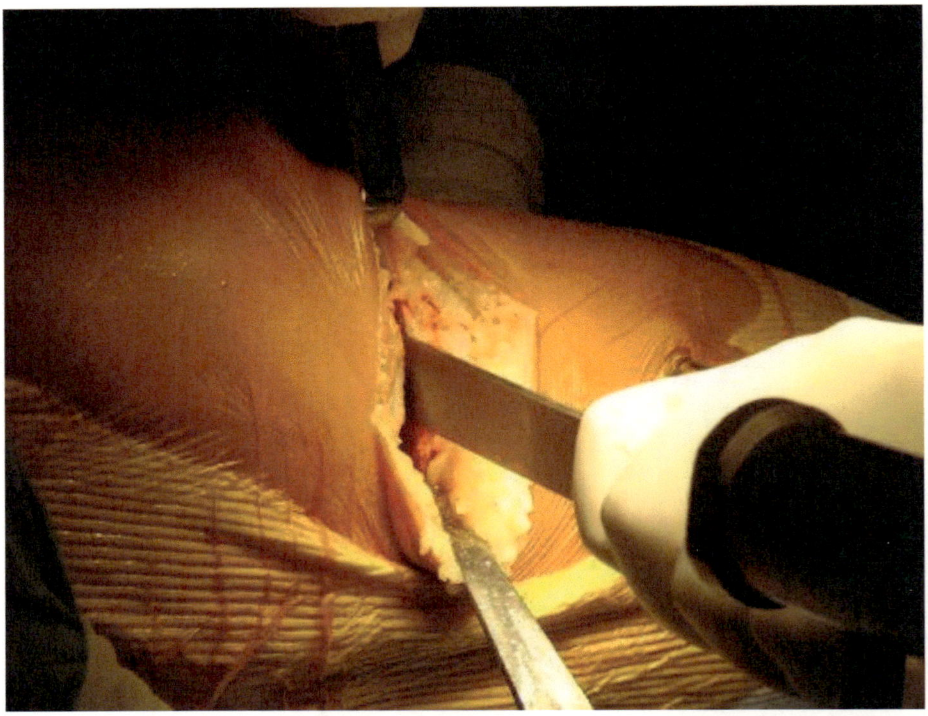

Fig. 6. The superficial part of medial collateral ligament is released to allow opening of the wedge osteotomy.

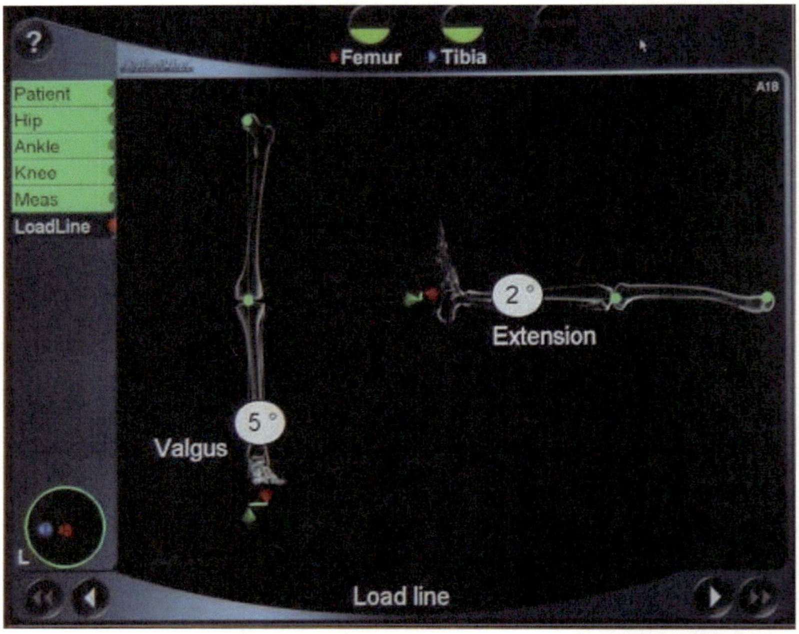

Fig. 7. The real time, exact degree of varus correction is shown on the screen. This will help surgeons to avoid over or under correction of varus deformities.

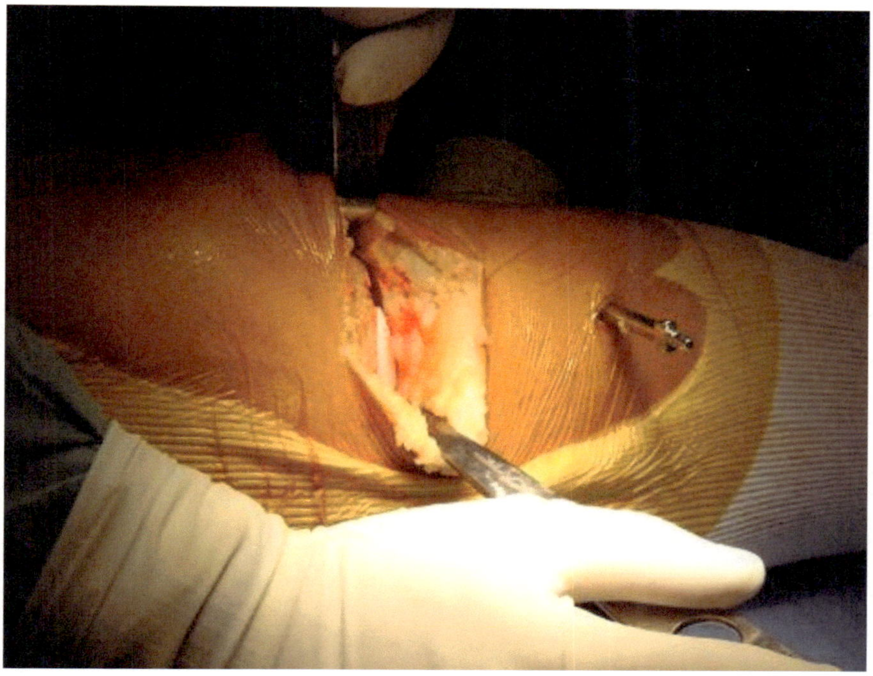

Fig. 8. The exact size of bio-absorbable spacer is determined by computer navigation reading.

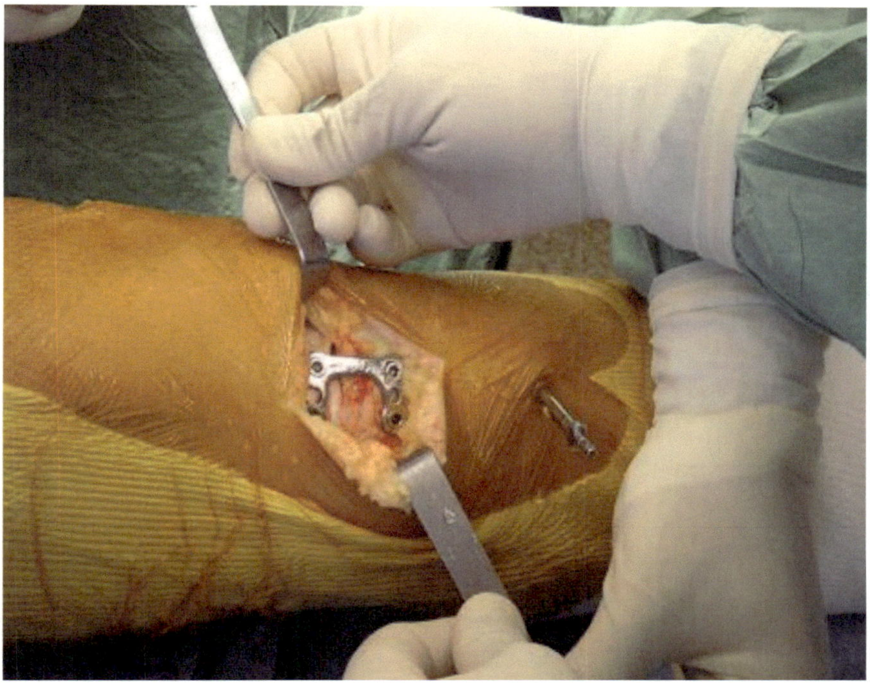

Fig. 9. Plate and screws are used to maintain the correction at the desired angle as determined by the computer. Long film Röntgenogram may also be used to confirm alignment.

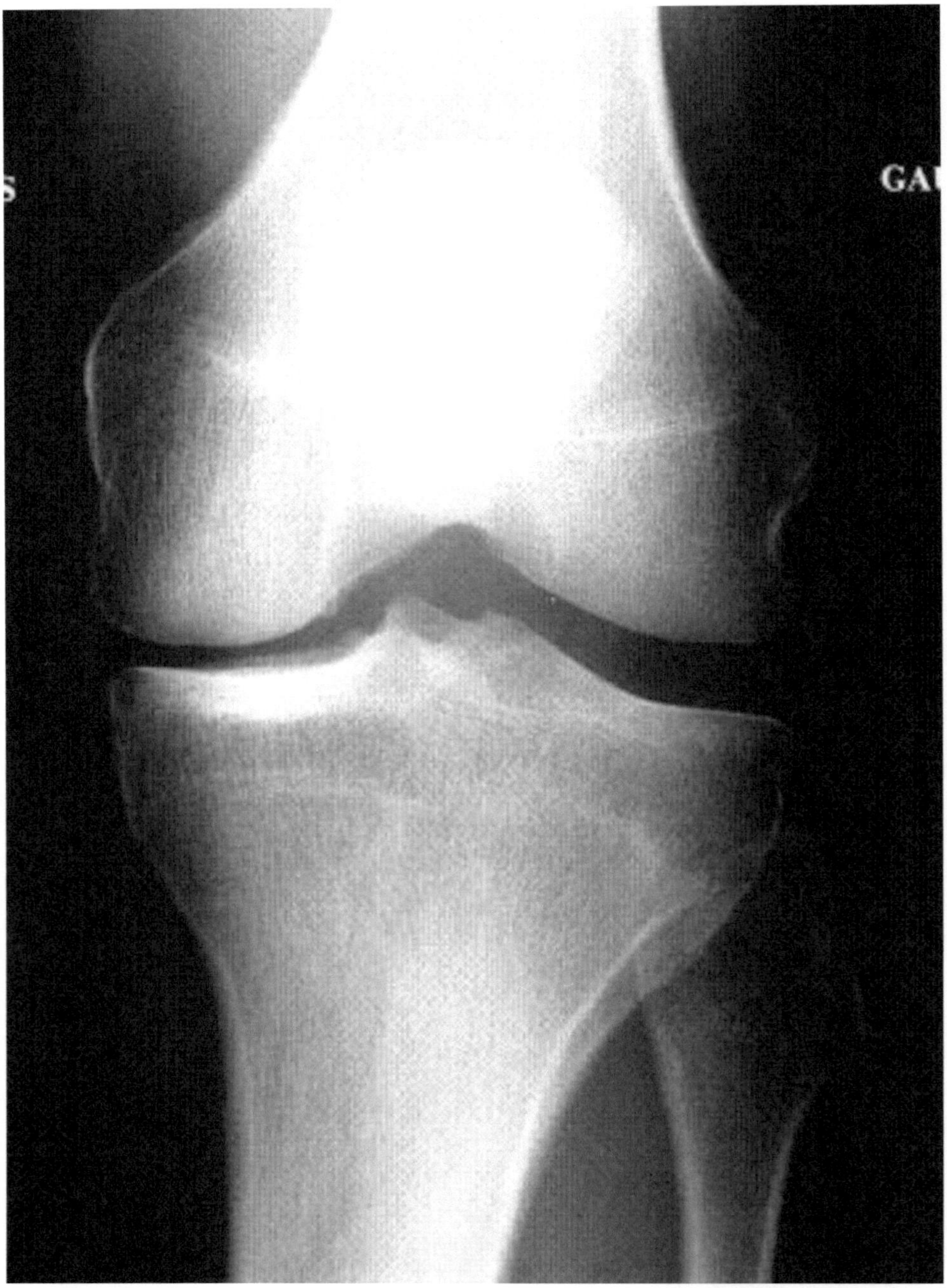

Fig. 10. a: Preoperative standard left knee film showing varus deformity of left knee

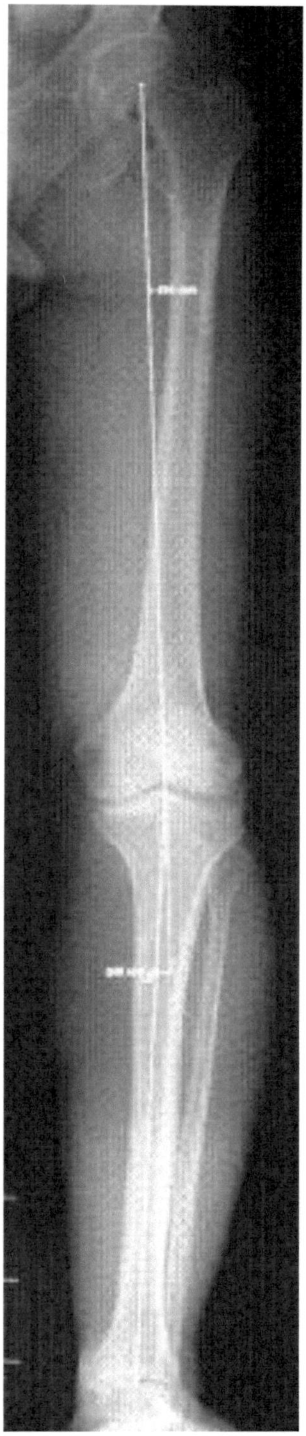

Fig. 10. b: Weight bearing long film determined that the varus deformity is only in the tibia. Joint line and femur were anatomical.

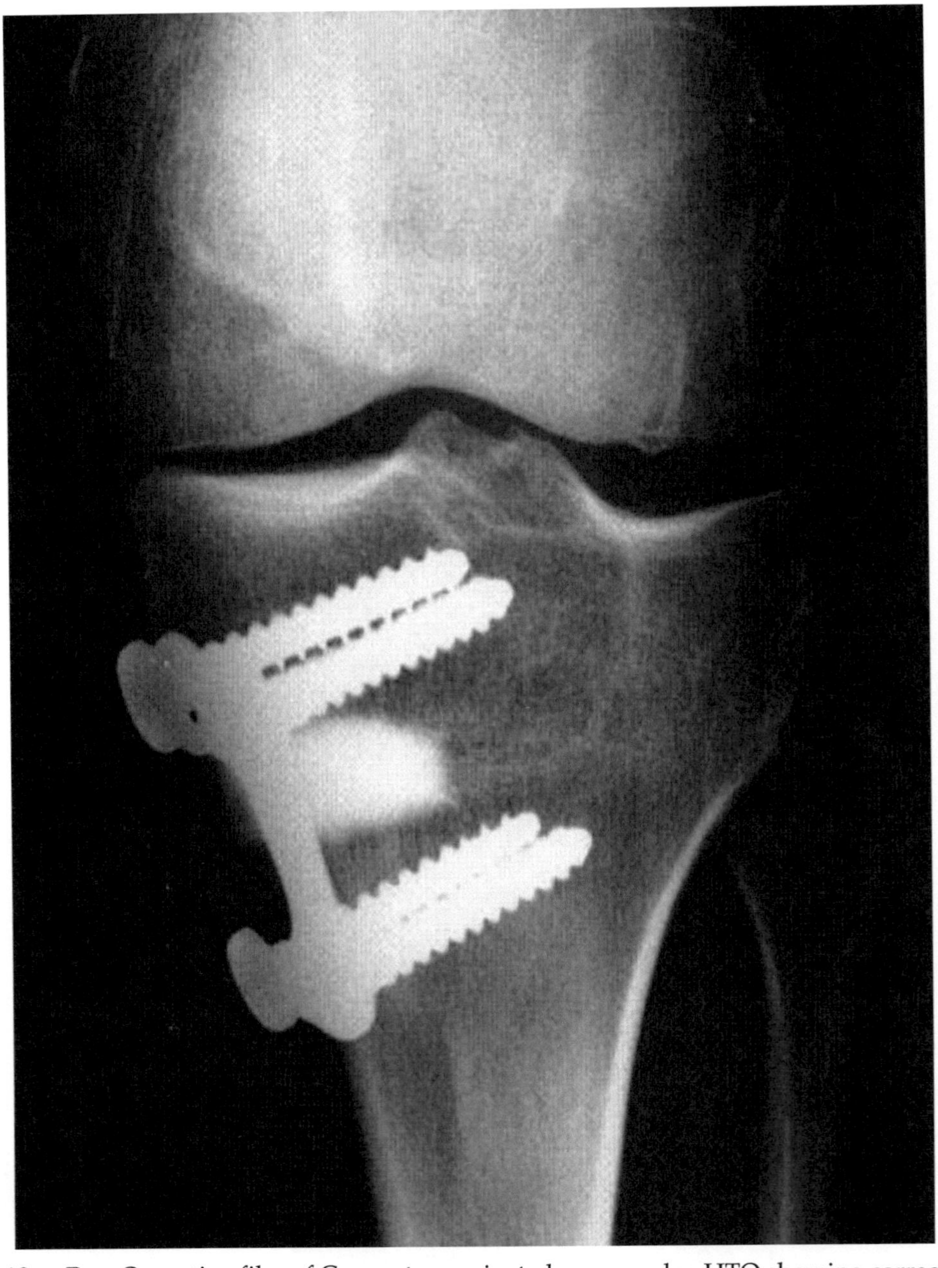

Fig. 10. c: Post Operative film of Computer navigated open wedge HTO showing correction of the varus deformity.

3.2 Computer-assisted double level osteotomy (Fig.11 a,b,c)

The first stage is essentially the same as for an HTO : percutaneous insertion of the rigid body markers (high enough not to hamper the femoral osteotomy and low enough on the other level to avoid interfering with the tibial osteotomy), followed by kinematic acquisition of the hip centre, middle of the knee and tibio-tarsal joints in order to find the mechanical axis of the lower limb.

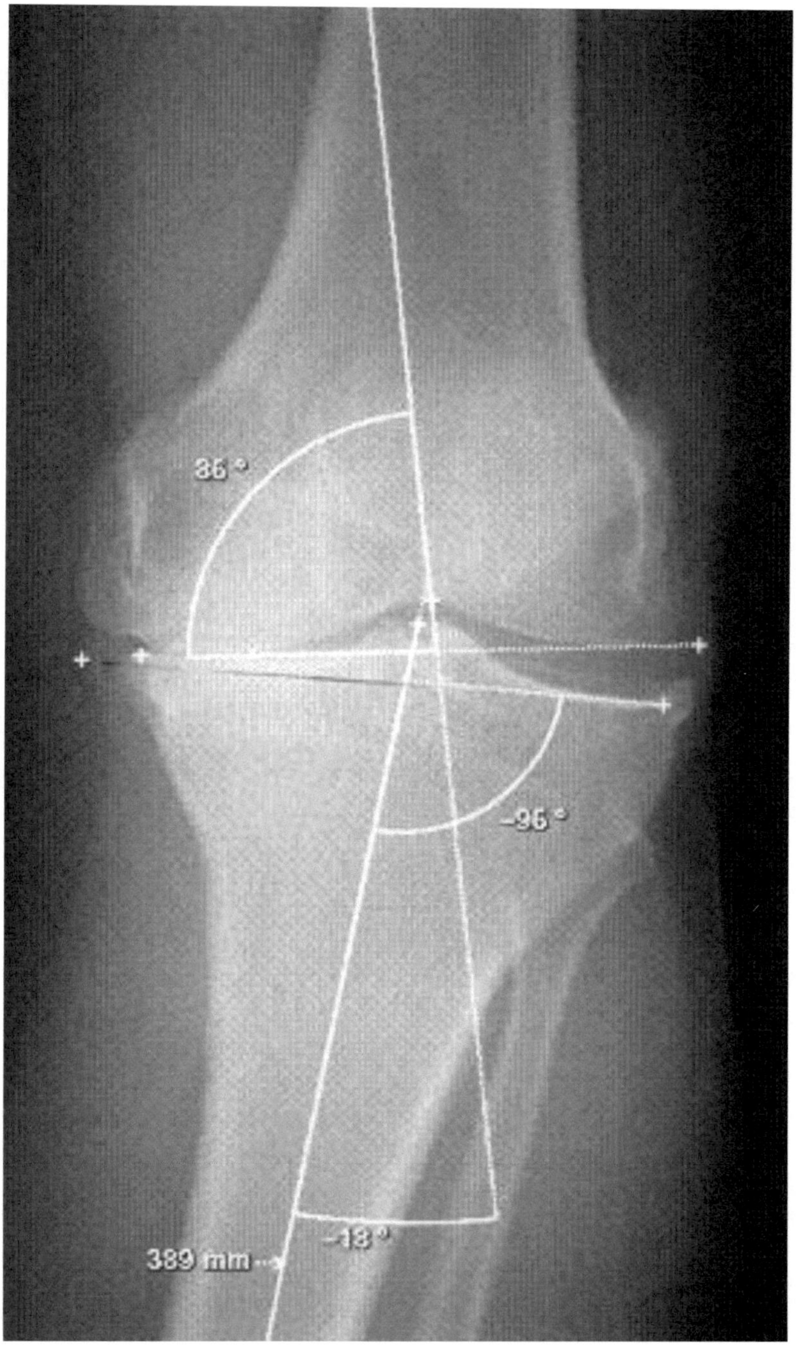

Fig. 11. a: A Pre-operative x-ray film of left knee, femoral and tibia varus deformity. Measurements show the degree of deformity in each bone needing to be corrected.

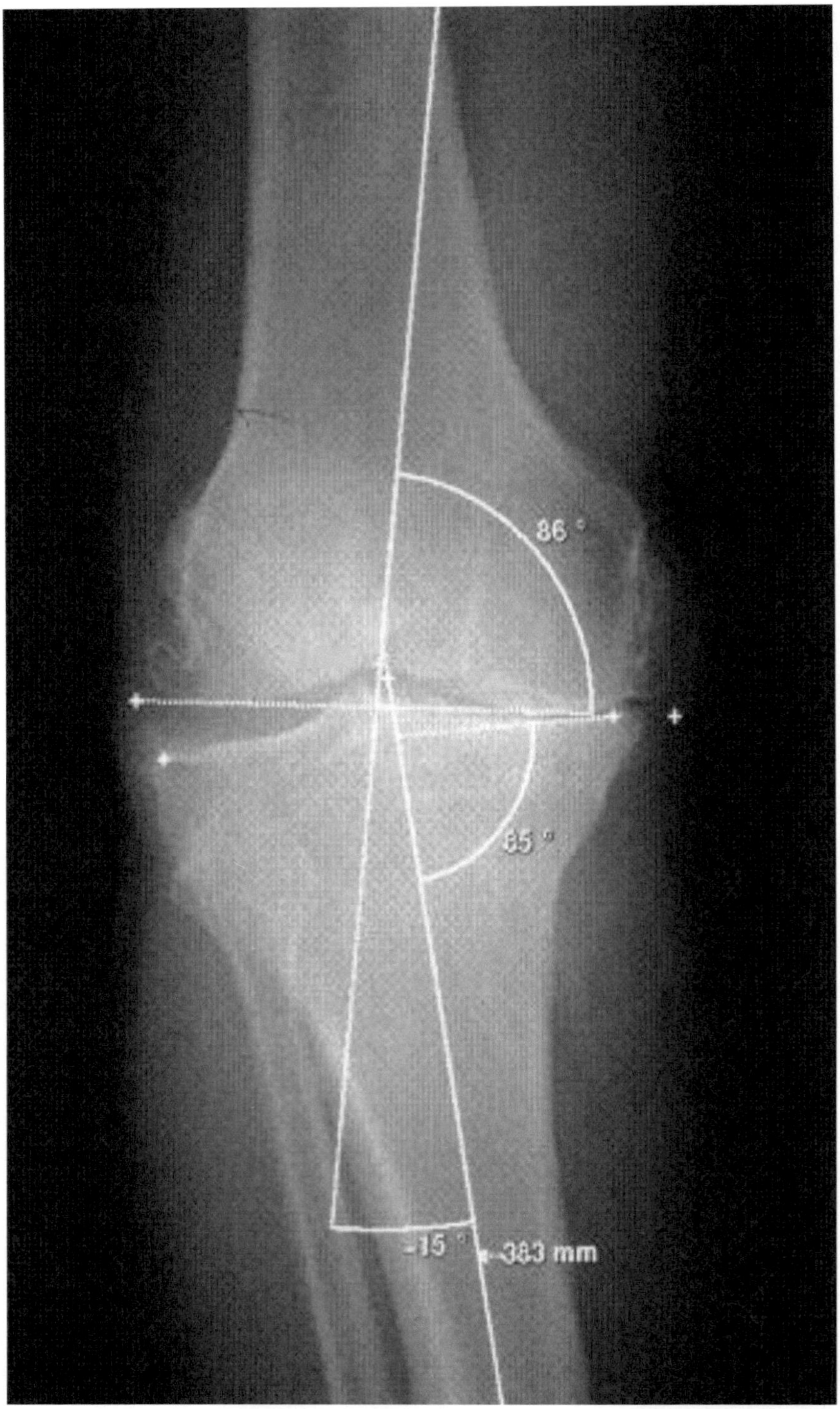

Fig. 11. b: Pre-op x-ray film of the right knee, femoral and tibia varus deformity. Measurements show the degree of deformity in each bone needing to be corrected.

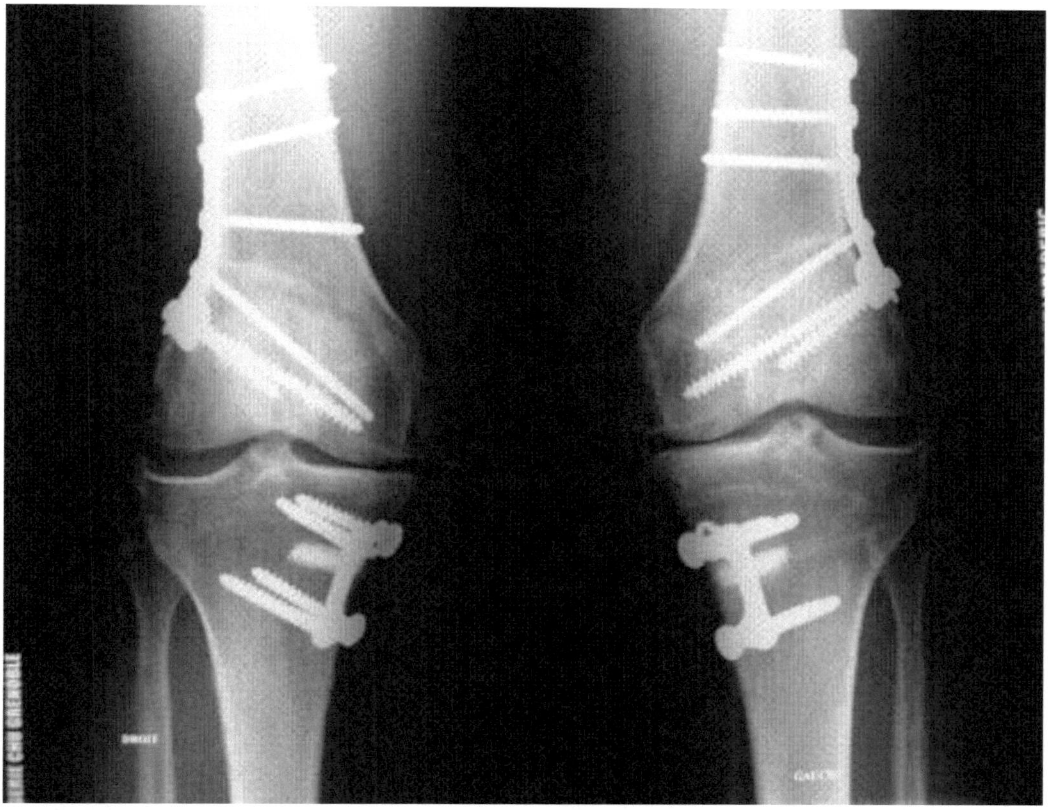

Fig. 11. c: Post operative Film of: Computer navigated double osteotomy for femoral tibia varus deformity. The deformity in both legs were corrected maintaining the joint line.

The second stage consists of making the femoral closing osteotomy in the distal femur (in general a 5-6° alteration is made, although sometimes more in congenital femoral varus) and fixing it in position with a T-plate (AO/ Synthes). A lateral approach with elevation of the vastus lateralis is chosen, to allow the location of the proximal tip of the trochlea. The track of the osteotomy lies proximal to the trochlea and is directed obliquely from proximal lateral to distal medial femoral cortex (Fig.12). A wedge of bone is then excised from the distal femur with a 4-5 mm lateral base, corresponding to a 5-6° correction (Fig.13). The osteotomy is then fixed with the T-plate after placing the femur into valgus manually (Fig. 14). Once this stage is reached the mechanical axis is rechecked so the required correction at the level of the tibia can be calculated in order to achieve the pre-operative objectives. Then the wound is closed on a drain. The last stage is to perform the HTO exactly in the fashion described earlier. The definitive axis is then displayed on the computer screen and the osteosynthesis is checked with the image intensifier.

3.3 Computer-assisted distal femoral osteotomy

The procedure is the same as described previously and we prefer to make a closing wedge osteotomy rather than an opening one because of the difficulty to get good stability after plating the distal femur.

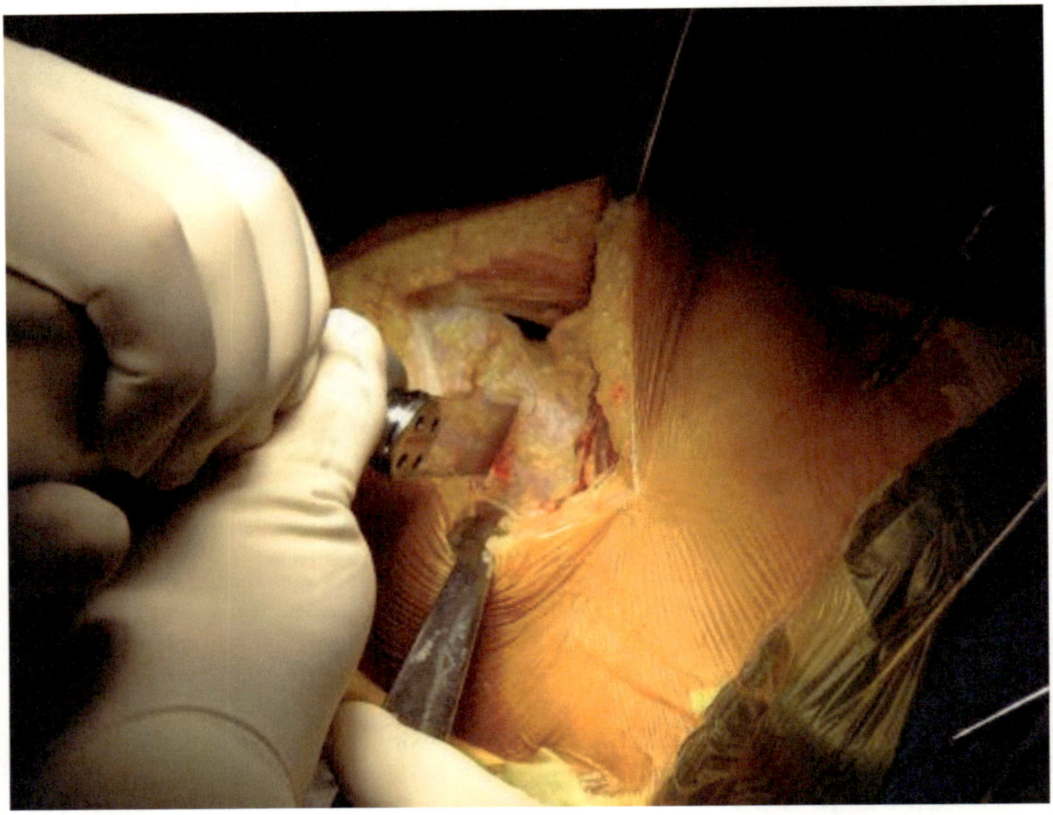

Fig. 12. Intra operation view of the direction of osteotomy proximal to trochlea aiming obliquely to distal medial femoral cortex.

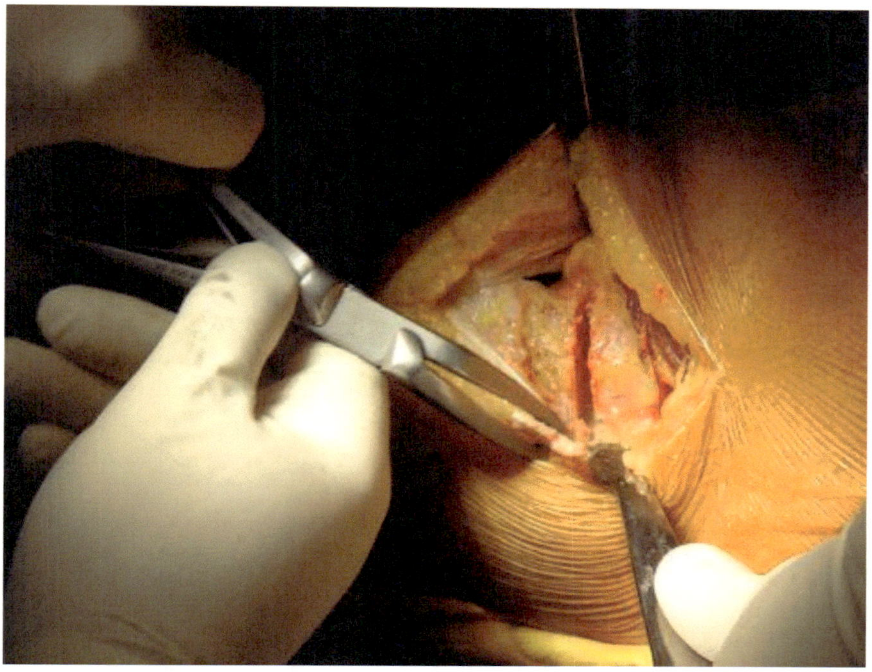

Fig. 13. Excision of 4-5 mm wedge of femur correspond to almost 5° - 6° of deformity correction allowing 1-2 mm of saw play to avoid overcorrection.

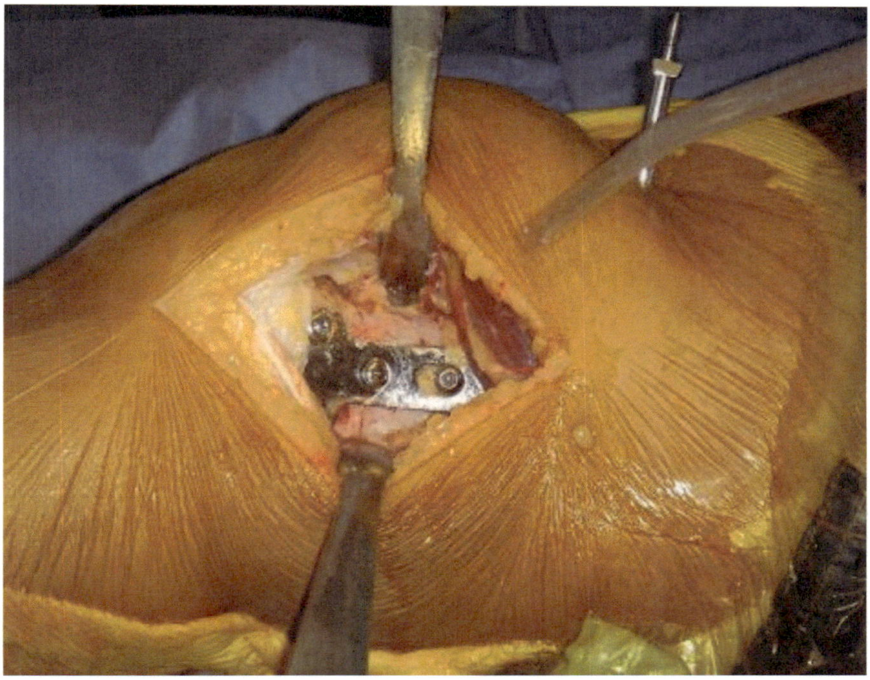

Fig. 14. Intra operation view showing correction of femoral varus deformity and maintaining it with a T-Plate.

4. Postoperative management

The patient can stand up the day after the operation and walk with two crutches. Partial weight bearing is allowed for 4-6 weeks when performing an HTO and 10-12 weeks when performing DLO. Full range of motion is regained quickly after HTO and after 6-8 weeks for DLO, because of the distal femoral osteotomy which slows down rehabilitation. However, being an extra articular procedure, postoperative arthrofibrosis does not occur.

5. Indications

The best indication for osteotomy is a non-sedentary patient with a low arthritis grade (Coventry, MB & Ilstrup, DM & Wallrichs, SL 1993; Yasuda, K & Majima, T & Tsuchida, T et al 1992) and below 60 to 65 years. In some cases (very active patients under the age of 50 years) we have performed double level osteotomy for grade 4 and five with a good result but this is far from being the rule.

6. Discussion

When should double level osteotomy be performed? If we consider the "normal" mechanical axis of the lower limb as described by Kapandji (Kapandji, IA 1974) and later taken up by Hungerford and Krackow (Hungerford, DS & Krackow, KA 1985) it should be 180° with an MDFMA of 93° and an MPTMA of 87° resulting in a joint line perfectly parallel to the ground. However this assumption is not confirmed in case of osteoarthritis with varus deformity because, in unpublished series of senior author (D.S.) of 89 TKR, we found an MDFMA of 93° in only 43.8% of the cases. It was at 90° in 33.7% of the cases, below 90° in 13.5%, and above 93° in 9%.

Thus, before performing high tibial osteotomy, it is crucial to have high quality and reproducible full-length AP radiographs of the lower limb, according to a specific protocol. The HKA angle, the MDFMA and the MPTMA should be determined on this goniometry (Fig.3a and 3b). Lateral instability testing has become less important than it once was, being that since the indications for osteotomy in this setting have become rare. In case of femoral valgus (MDFMA > 90°), it is illogical to perform a femoral osteotomy because we do not want to create in the femur, the error, we are trying to avoid in the tibia. If the femur is in varus or at 90°, we think, we should proceed with a femoral osteotomy to achieve an MDFMA of around 93° (93° +/- 2°), and then complete it with a tibial osteotomy to achieve an HKA angle of 182° +/- 2°. In our experience, to overcorrect more than this, may jeopardize satisfactory results (Fig. 3c). Overcorrection, whether femoral or tibial, can distort the anatomy and lead to a much more complicated revision TKR. However we think a longer follow-up is needed to prove overcorrection by +/-2° is enough for a lasting good result. If the tibia is not in varus (MPTMA over 88°), we should perform a femoral osteotomy specially if the femur is at 90° or in varus or contraindicate any osteotomy if it leads to joint line obliquity of more than 5°. If we strictly adhere to these criteria, indications for double level osteotomy will likely increase with the development of navigation systems, since as mentioned earlier, femurs in varus are not rare, and more so, those at 90°.

Combined distal femoral and proximal tibial osteotomy in the treatment of genu varum is technically difficult. Little has been said about this technique in the literature and we could find only one paper reporting on 24 patients (29 knees) operated on with a conventional technique (two closing wedge osteotomies) (Babis GC, An KN, Chao E. YS, et al, 2002). The mean preoperative HKA angle was 193.3° (which is 13.3° of varus) and they used a computer-aided analysis of the mechanical status of the knee for preoperative planning. This was limited to preoperative evaluation, and the reliability of the preoperative radiographic evaluation was not assessed. The results showed a mean postoperative HKA angle of 176.9° (169.4° to 184.9°). They had a residual varus in 2 cases (4.6° and 4.9°) and an over correction of more than 4° in 10 cases and more than 6° in 5. One knows an under correction may lead to failure of the operative procedure and a too much overcorrection to discomfort.

The difficulty of the technique comes from the fact once the first osteotomy is performed, whether femoral or tibial, landmarks change and the ability to achieve a satisfactory alignment with the second osteotomy becomes challenging in the absence of reliable intra-operative landmarks. Martres et al (Martres, S & Servien, E & Aït Si Selmi, T, et al 2004) suggested performing this operation in two different stages to improve its accuracy and reproducibility. It is also justified to consider complication occurring at both osteotomy sites could lead to disastrous result. On the other hand, every surgeon operating on osteoarthritic knees should be aware of the risk of malunion in the proximal tibia, for a procedure often considered temporary, particularly when performing an isolated HTO. In fact every osteotomy in a young adult is susceptible to lead subsequently to a TKR, and thus it is essential to plan ahead for the iterative surgery called revision.

Computer-assisted surgery allows controlling of the femoro-tibial axis (HKA angle) at every step of the procedure and thus makes it more accurate. Our first results (Saragaglia, D & Pradel, PH & Picard, F 2004) showed in a comparative cohort study of computer-assisted versus conventional HTO, a 96% reproducibility in achieving a mechanical axis of 184°+/-2° in the computer navigated group versus 71% in the conventional osteotomy group ($p< 0.0015$). In another prospective series including 16 cases of DLO (Saragaglia, D & Rubens-Duval, B & Chaussard, C 2007) we showed 87.5% success in reaching our pre-operative goal for HKA angle, and 100% success in reaching the desired MPTMA (90° +/- 2°), which in terms of performance is remarkable. At the femoral level, results were less accurate (75% of MDFMA at 95° +/-2°). This could be related to the closing wedge osteotomy, which is less straight forward. Moreover, with the Orthopilot® device (kinematic model without pre-op imaging), controlling the MDFMA and the MPTMA following the two osteotomies is not possible because a large arthrotomy would be required to identify and palpate specific landmarks similar to the ones used for TKA.

Thus the only navigated parameter is the HKA angle; the others are calculated from pre and post-operative X-Rays using the most rigorous planning. Regarding mid-term clinical and radiological results of DLO we reviewed recently 42 cases operated on between August 2001 and June 2010 that is with a mean follow up of 46+/-27 months (12-108). The mean Lyshölm-Tegner score (Tegner, Y & Lysholm, J & Lysholm, M & Gillquist, J 1986) improved from 41.2 +/- 8.9 points (22-69) to 83.3 +/- 7.5 points (62-91) and the KOOS score (Roos, EM & Roos, HP & Ekdahl, C & Lohmander, LS 1998) was 95.1+/- 3.2 points (89-100). 40 Patients were satisfied (22) or very satisfied (18) of the result. The radiological results showed the preoperative goal was reached in 92.7% of the cases for the HKA angle and in 88.1% for the

MPTMA, with only one case over 93°. The mean HKA angle was 181.83° +/- 1.80° (177°-185°), the mean MPTMA of 89.71° +/- 1.72° (85°-93°) and the mean MDFMA of 92.76° +/- 2.02° (89°-97°). No patient was revised to total knee arthroplasty.

Finally, despite our trust in opening wedge osteotomies, we think, at the femoral level, one should perform a closing wedge osteotomy to avoid excessive lengthening of the limb when performing DLO (double opening) and also to avoid a less stable osteosynthesis.

7. Conclusion

Young patient genu varum deformity can be corrected by high tibial valgus osteotomy, but it is not the sole way to do. The indication is based on an accurate and reproducible radiological protocol including at least standing AP long leg X-ray. One must measure not only the HKA angle but also the medial distal femoral mechanical angle (MDFMA) and the medial proximal tibial mechanical angle (MPTMA). These measures will guide the surgeon to choose the best indication. When the MDFMA is in valgus (93° or more) and the MPTMA in varus (below 88°) the best one is HTO. When the MDFMA is in varus (90° or less) and the MPTMA in varus (below 88°) the best indication is DLO. Finally, when the MDFMA is in varus and the MPTMA above 88° the best indication is DFO. This way of thinking should avoid too much oblique joint line, which is a difficult condition when performing revision to TKA.

8. References

Babis GC, An KN, Chao E.YS, et al (2002) Double level osteotomy of the knee :: a method to retain joint-line obliquity. J Bone J Surg Am 84 ::1380-13881.

Coventry MB, Ilstrup DM, Wallrichs SL (1993) Proximal tibial osteotomy :: a critical long-term study of eighty-seven cases. J Bone Joint Surg Am 75 ::196-201

Hakki S, Saleh K, Bilotta V, et al. (2009) Navigational predictors in determining the necessity for collateral ligament release in total knee replacement. JBJS - Br, Vol 91-B, Issue 9, 1178-1182.

Hernigou Ph, Medevielle D, Debeyre J, et al (1987) Proximal tibial osteotomy for osteoarthritis with varus deformity :: a ten to thirteen-year follow-up study. J Bone Joint Surg Am 69 ::332-354

Hungerford DS, Krackow KA (1985) Total joint arthroplasty of the knee. Clin Orthop 192 ::23-30

Jackson JP, Waugh W (1961) Tibial osteotomy for osteoarthritis of the knee. J Bone Joint Surg Br 43 ::746-751

Jenny JY, Tavan A, Jenny G, et al (1998) Taux de survie à long terme des ostéotomies tibiales de valgisation pour gonarthrose. Rev chir Orthop 84 ::350-357

Judet R, Dupuis JF, Honnard F, et al (1964) Désaxations et arthroses du genou. Le genu varum de l'adulte. Indications thérapeutiques, résultats. Rev Chir Orthop 13 ::1-28

Kapandji IA (1974) Physiologie articulaire . Fascicule II quatrième édition :: membre inférieur. Paris , PA :: Maloine SA ; ::104

Lerat JL (2000) Ostéotomies dans la gonarthrose. Cahiers d'enseignement de la SOFCOT 2000. Paris, PA :: Elsevier ; ::165-201

Lootvoet L, Massinon A, Rossillon R, et al (1993) Ostéotomie tibiale haute de valgisation pour gonarthrose sur genu varum :: à propos d'une série de 193 cas revus après 6 à 10 ans de recul. Rev Chir Orthop 79 ::375-384

Martres S, Servien E, Aït Si Selmi T, et al (2004) Double ostéotomie :: indication dans la gonarthrose. Rev Chir Orthop 90 suppl au n°6 :: 2S137-2S138

Merle d'Aubigné R, Ramadier JO (1961) Arthrose du genou et surcharge articulaire. Acta Orthop Belg 27 ::365-375

Papachristou G, Plessas S, Sourlas J, Levidiotis C, Chronopoulos E, Papachristou C (2006). Deterioration of long-term results following high tibial osteotomy in patients under 60 years of age. Int orthop 30: 406-408

Picard F, Leitner F, Raoult A, et al (1999) Computer assisted knee arthroplasty. In « Reschnergestützte Verfahren in Orthopädie und Unfallchirurgie ». Steinkopff Darmstadt, PA :: Jerosch, Nichol and Peikenkam; :: 461-471.

Ramadier JO, Buard JE, Lortat-Jacob A, et al (1982) Mesure radiologique des déformations frontales du genou. Procédé du profil vrai radiologique. Rev Chir Orthop 68 ::75-78

Rinonapoli E, Mancini GB, Corvaglia A, et al (1998) Tibial osteotomy for varus gonarthrosis. A 0 to 21-year follow-up study. Clin Orthop 353 :: 185-193

Roos EM, Roos HP, Ekdahl C, Lohmander LS (1998) Knee Injury and Osteoarthritis Outcome Score (KOOS): validation of a swedish version. Scand J Med Sci Sports 8: 439-48

Saragaglia D, Blaysat M, Inman D, Mercier N (2010) Outcome of opening wedge High tibial osteotomy augmented with a Biosorb wedge and fixed by a plate with a mean of ten years follow up. Int Orthop. Published on line in August 2010 (DOI 10.1007/s00264-010-1102-9)

Saragaglia D, Pradel Ph, Picard F (2004) L'ostéotomie de valgisation assistée par ordinateur dans le genu varum arthrosique :: résultats radiologiques d'une étude cas-témoin de 56 cas. E-mémoires de l'Académie Nationale de Chirurgie 3 :: 21-25. Available at :: http://www.bium.univ-paris5.fr/acad-chirurgie.

Saragaglia D, Picard F, Chaussard C, et al (2001) Mise en place des prothèses totales du genou assistée par ordinateur :: comparaison avec la technique conventionnelle. Résultats d'une étude prospective randomisée de 50 cas. Rev chir Orthop 87 ::18-28

Saragaglia D, Roberts J (2005) Navigated osteotomies around the knee in 170 patients with osteoarthritis secondary to genu varum. Orthopaedics 28 Suppl n° 10 ::S1269 - S1274

Saragaglia D, Rubens-Duval B, Chaussard C (2007) Double ostéotomie assistée par ordinateur dans les grands genu varum. Résultats préliminaires à propos de 16 cas. Rev Chir Orthop 93::351-356

Tegner Y, Lysholm J, Lysholm M, Gillquist J (1986) A performance test to monitor rehabilitation and evaluate anterior cruciate ligament injuries. Am J Sports Med 14 : 156-159

Yasuda K, Majima T, Tsuchida T, et al (1992) A ten to 15 year follow-up observation of high tibial osteotomy in medial compartment osteoarthrosis. Clin Orthop 282 ::186-195

9

Digital Templating and Correction of a Valgus Post-Traumatic Lower Limb Deformity

Francisco Lajara-Marco, Francisco J. Ricón,
Carlos E. Morales and José E Salinas
Hospital Vega Baja Orihuela (Alicante)
Spain

1. Introduction

The management of post-traumatic deformities of the lower limb, either occurring immediately after failed primary fracture treatment leading to malunion, or developing gradually caused by an injury of the growth mechanism, is an everlasting challenge, the orthopaedic surgeon has to face.

Precise preoperative planning is a key principle of success in orthopaedic surgery. Traditionally, preoperative planning has been performed on standard radiographs with various techniques. Recently, digital templating has been proposed as a method using electronically overlay templates from a digital library on clinical radiographs for arthroplasties.

2. Case report

A 37-years-old man was suffering of mechanical knee pain. He previously had a non-union left diaphyseal tibial fracture and had undergone a reduction and internal fixation at least three times, an anterior cruciate ligament reconstruction with a patellar tendon autograft and a medial collateral ligament reconstruction with hamstring tendon autograft some 15 years ago. Pre-morbility, he was HBV positive. Clinical examination revealed a combined valgus deformity by a medial collateral ligament insufficiency and a tibial shaft deformity in a multioperated lower limb with range of motion (ROM) of 0° to 140°. Radiographs revealed a malunited diaphyseal tibial fracture and degenerative changes in articular cartilage of the lateral compartment of the knee (Fig. 1). The patient, was at a relatively young age to receive a total knee arthroplasty. Additionally, he displayed good range of motion, so the patient was candidate for an osteotomy to correct the supero-lateral tilt to the joint line. (Badhe & Foster, 2002; Goradia and Van Allen, 2002; Phisitkul et al, 2006).

2.1 Deformity analysis

In order to analyze deformity and choose the osteotomy level we used the methods which have been described by Paley 2002. The authors have developed a universal system of geometric deformity planning based on the mechanical or anatomic axes. The place where the axes intersect is the center of rotation angulation (CORA) of a deformity. Osteotomy level and type should be considered relative to the CORA enabling us to avoid creating secondary deformities. This type of planning is applicable to both frontal and sagittal plane deformities.

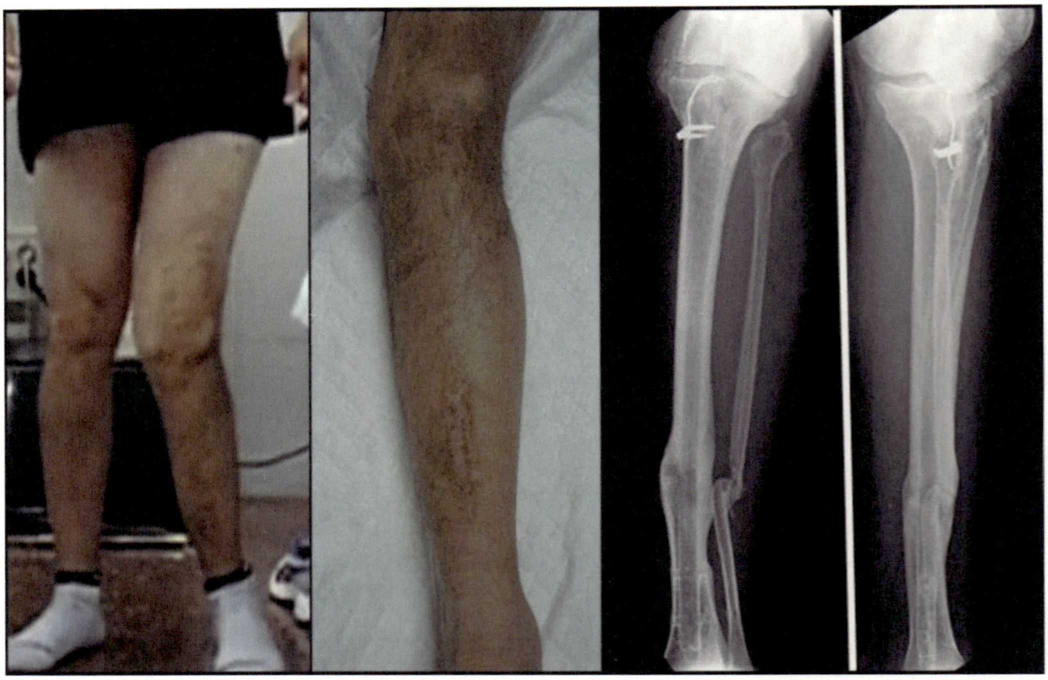

Fig. 1. Initial clinical and radiographs examination

True anteroposterior (AP) and lateral radiographs of the femur and tibia should be obtained with the knee in neutral rotation (patella forward on the AP projection). A full-length standing AP radiograph of both lower extremities including the hip, knee, and ankle on one film with the patella forward allows simultaneous assessment of alignment, length, and knee joint stability.

We have no significative deformity in the axial or sagittal plane and have a valgus knee deformity in the coronal plane that is more evident when the patient is walking because of medial collateral ligament insufficiency. So we have a static deformity due to malunited diaphyseal tibial fracture and a dynamic valgus instability caused by medial ligament injury.

When we apply the Paley´s analysis we realise that we have another static component, the medial distal femoral mechanical angle (MDFMA) has 83° when the normal MDFMA has 87°. And what can we say about the tibial shaft? When we make the tibial mechanical axis planning, we come to the conclusion that this is a multiapical angulation with two CORAs, one proximal to eight centimetres of the knee joint and one distal to 13 centimetres of the ankle joint, this is the site of the old tibial shaft fracture (Fig 2).

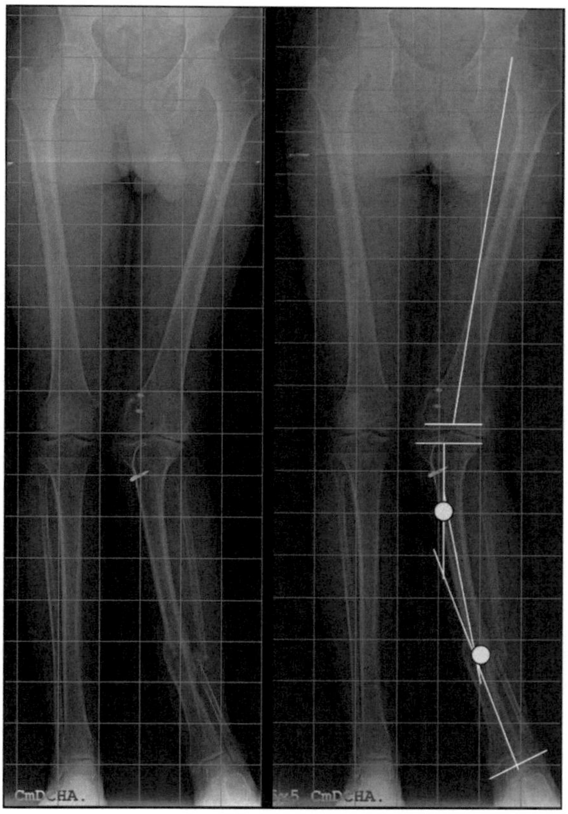

Fig. 2. Full-length standing AP radiograph of both lower extremities including the hip, knee, and ankle. Osteotomy Planning Using the Anatomic Method described by Paley

We have used **digital templating** in a clinical session, with commercially available software (Adobe1 Photoshop1 CS4; Adobe Systems Inc, San Jose, CA) (Jamali, 2009) to quickly and conveniently choose two osteotomies options. The size and shape of an opening wedge and closing wedge can be predicted and planned before surgery with the software. The virtually osteotomized tibia can then be freely transformed and rotated until the desired correction is achieved on the image. The final mechanical axis of the extremity can also be confirmed on this image to run in the desired position.

In order to prepare the two strategies we have used digital templating: (A) **Osteotomy level selection:** The level of the initial transverse osteotomy is drawn on the long, standing radiograph, then, the selection tool is used to select a rectangle around the entire tibia, ankle, and foot. (B) **Osteotomy fragment reorientation:** This image selection is copied and pasted into a new layer using the software. The virtually osteotomized tibia can then be rotated using "rotate canvas arbitrary". This command rotates the image (clockwise or anticlockwise) by an arbitrary angle. However, we decide the value of the rotation angle in degrees, the value of the osteotomy. The final mechanical axis of the extremity can also be confirmed on this image to run in the desired position and the lateral cortical opening can be measured on the pre-operative plan. (Fig 3)

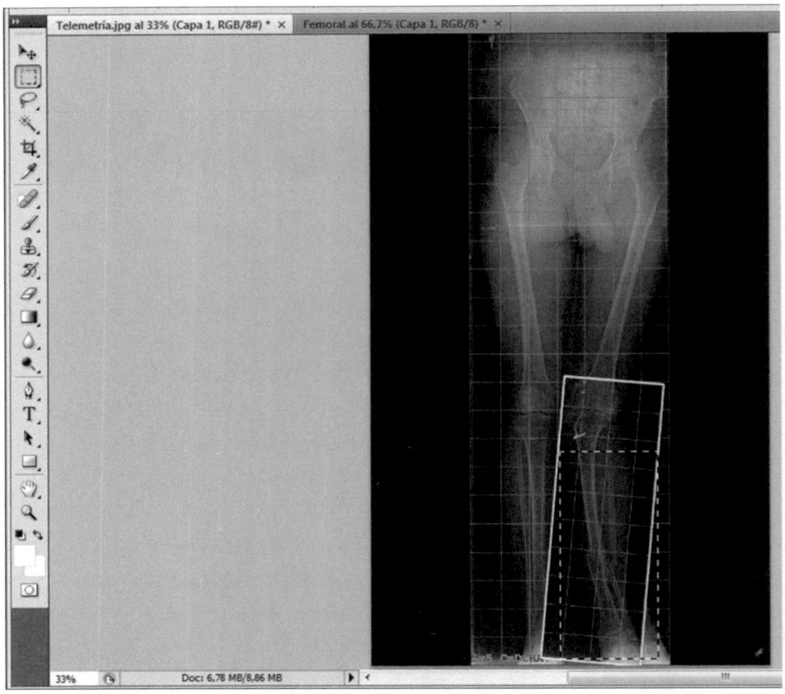

Fig. 3. Osteotomy level selection and osteotomy fragment reorientation with Adobe1 Photoshop1 CS4.

In this case, we plan two strategies. First option (no shown), one osteotomy for each problem, making of a lateral opening wedge femoral osteotomy of 5° and two tibial osteotomies one in each CORA, a proximal medial closing wedge tibial osteotomy of 9° and other distal lateral opening wedge tibial osteotomy of 6°. But we have to be aware that we are going to do last osteotomy on an old fracture focus. Second option (Fig 4) is making a lateral opening wedge femoral osteotomy of 5° and one medial closing wedge tibal osteotomy of 16° upper of the proximal CORA. This option has some advantages; there are places that don't have any previous surgeries, with no skin incisions and allowing fixation with two plates. However we have to accept a slight translational deformity. We opted for the second strategy.

2.2 Surgical technique

Distal femoral opening wedge osteotomy was performed according to Puddu (Arthrex, Naples, FL) at the distal epiphyseal region. The distal femur was approached laterally at the distal epiphyseal region. A 3-mm guide wire is drilled in the lateral condyl 1 cm above the lateral epicondyle, and directed to the origin of the medial collateral ligament (adductor tubercle) under fluoroscopic control. Over this wire a special sleeve is placed to determine the osteotomy plane. The osteotomy is made using an oscillating saw ending approximately 5 mm lateral of the medial cortex. The osteotomy plane is spread using special spreading wedges. The Puddu plate, which is designed with varying spacer blocks, is then placed over the osteotomy gap and secured proximally with traditional bicortical screws and distally with partially threaded cancellous screws. The wedge is filled with bone allografts.

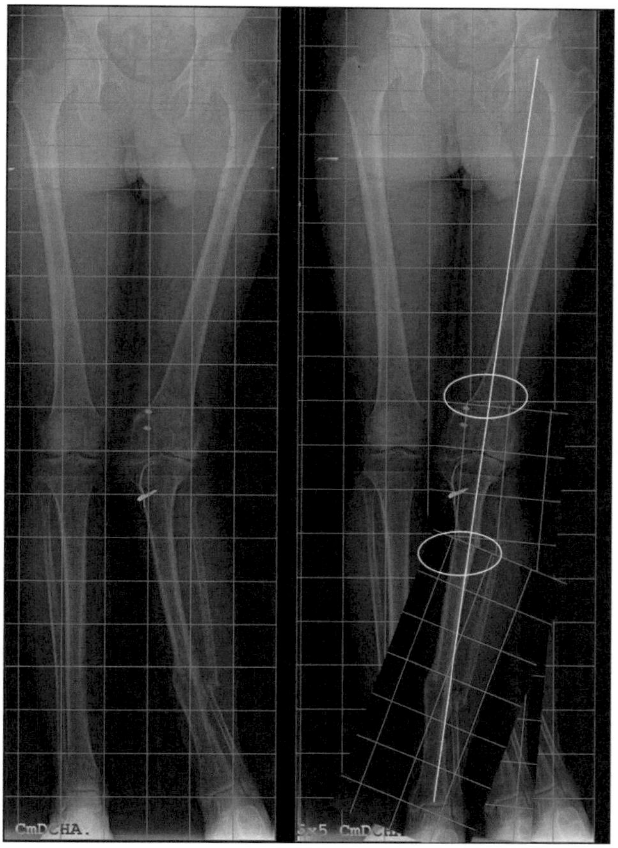

Fig. 4. Option selcted: Lateral opening wedge femoral osteotomy of 5° and one medial closing wedge tibal osteotomy of 16° upper of the proximal CORA

Before medial closing wedge tibial osteotomy (TO) was made, a fibular transection was performed at the junction of the middle and distal thirds through a separate incision and the peroneal nerve was exposed and protected. A five to 6 centimetres long incision is made on the medial side of the tibia just at the level of the osteotomy, which is confirmed by placing a needle under fluoroscopic control, then we performed the TO using an oscillating saw, 8 cm below the medial joint line, bone wedge size was based on the preoperative calculations from the long leg standing radiograph (Fig 5). Finally, fixing it provisionally in position with a medial small locking compression plate (3,5mm LCP plate Synthes, Paoli, PA) and was ultimately fixed with a lateral 4,5mm LCP plate.

The definitive axis and the osteosynthesis are checked with the image intensifier. In order to assess mechanical axis deviation correction intraoperatively, a cautery cord is stretched from the center of the femoral head to the centre of the ankle plafond.

The last stage is to perform the posteromedial ligaments reconstruction with contralateral gracilis autograft, through a curvilinear medial-sided incision from the anteromedial proximal tibia to the medial femoral epicondyle. It is tensioned at 30 degrees and fixed with two bioabsorbable interference screws.

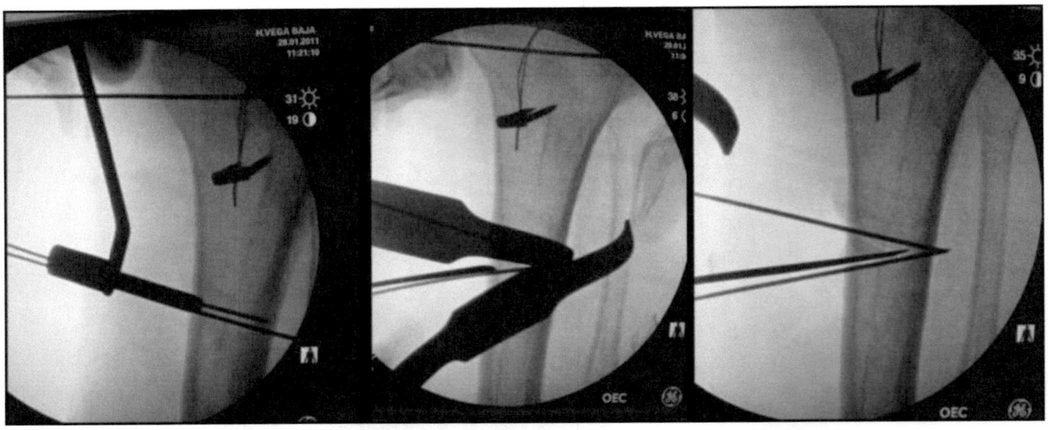

Fig. 5. Medial closing wedge TO fluoroscopic control

2.3 Postoperative management

Postoperatively, the leg was placed in a hinged knee brace locked 30º of flexion (Fig), due to medial ligaments reconstruction. The patient was initially non-weight bearing, with crutches. The patient was allowed to undergo protected range of motion from 0 to 90º at 4 weeks postoperatively. Full range of motion was regained after 8 weeks, because of the distal femoral osteotomy which slowed down rehabilitation. However, even with two extra articular procedures, postoperative arthrofibrosis did not occur. Partial weight bearing was allowed 12 weeks after the operation. The patient returned to full weight bearing 20 weeks after the operation.

2.4 Results

Patient was very satisfied with the result. He kept a full range of motion and he could walk and ride a bike without any significant pain (Fig 6) However, even if improvement in gait pattern was achieved the medial collateral ligament remained slightly lax.

His osteotomy sites appeared healed and the tibiofemoral angle was corrected, the time needed to achieve complete clinical and radiographic bone union was 12 weeks. No complications were encountered, such as delayed union, nonunion, deep infection, skin necrosis, peroneal nerve and vascular injury. There was one case of superficial infection; this was fixed by surgical debridement and antibiotic treatment.

3. Conclusion

Commercially available software can be used with a step-by-step technique for orthopaedic applications with lower cost and increased flexibility than commercial orthopaedic software. We have used this technique of digital templating to discuss all osteotomies options in order to quickly and conveniently choose the best option for this post-traumatic valgus deformity. The size and shape of an opening wedge and closing wedge can be predicted and planned before surgery with the software.

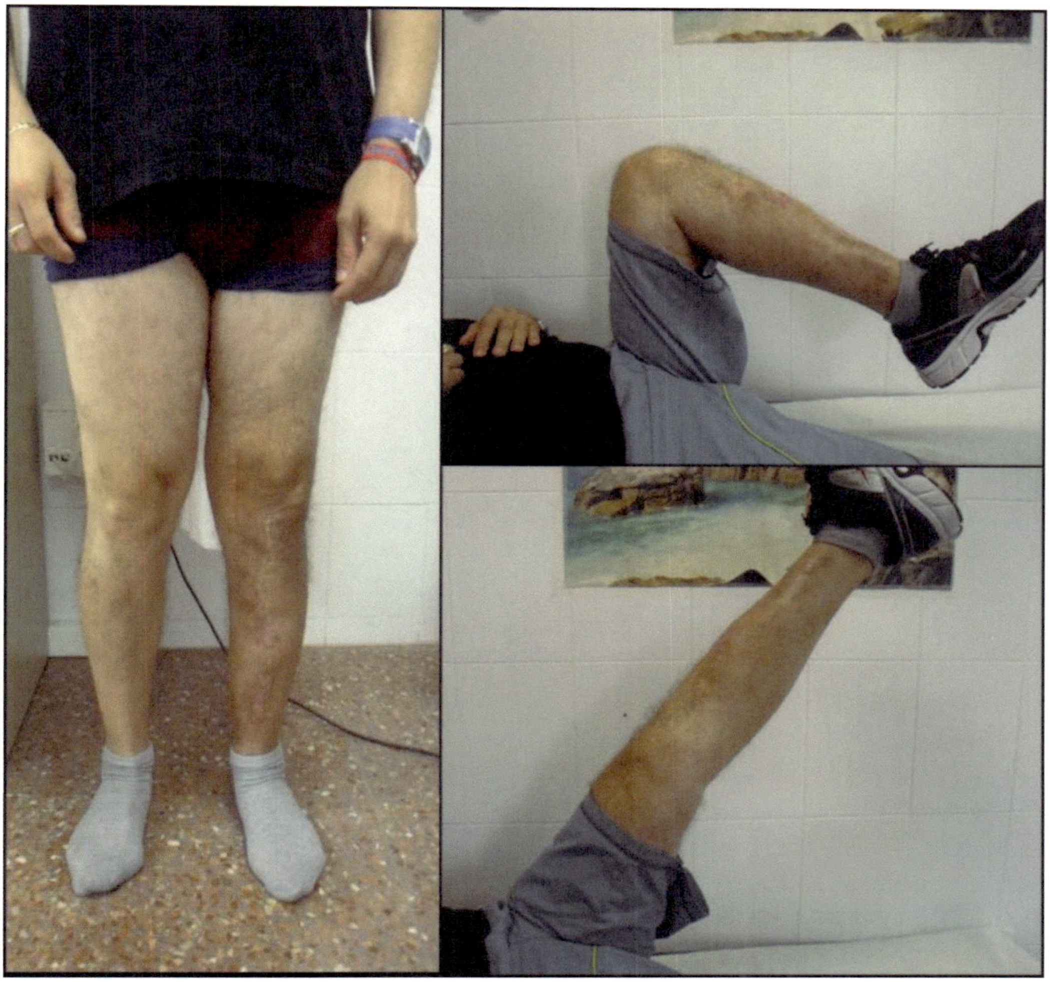

Fig. 6. Clinical view and range of motion at the last follow-up.

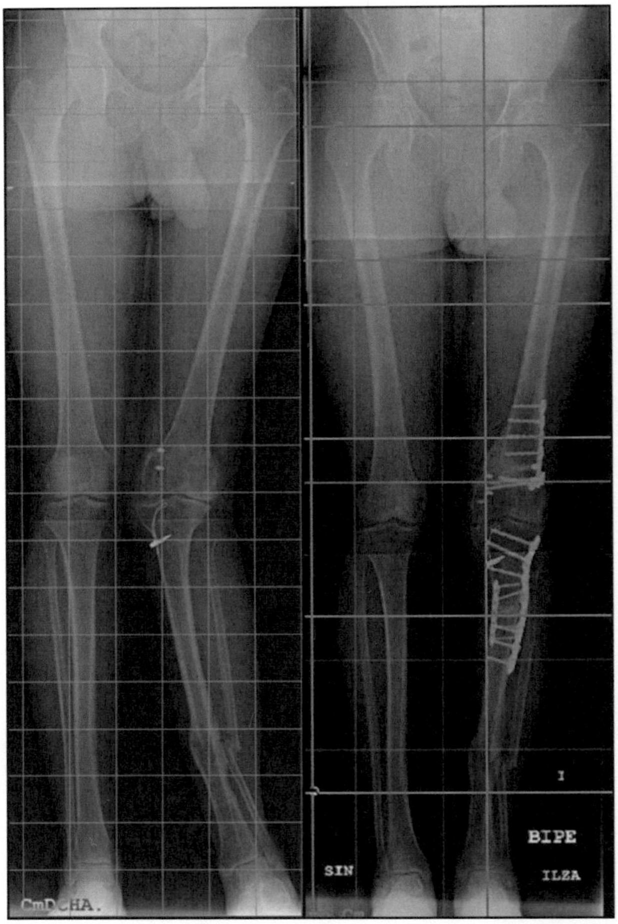

Fig. 7. Full-length standing AP radiograph of both lower extremities. Before (left side) and after (right side) osteotomies.

4. References

Badhe NP, Forster IW. (2002) High tibial osteotomy in knee instability: the rational of treatment and early results. *Knee Surg Sports Traumatol Arthrosc.* Vol 10, No 1, (January 2001), pp 38-43, ISSN. 0942-2056

Goradia VK, Van Allen J. (2002) Chronic lateral knee instability treated with high tibial osteotomy. *Arthroscopy* Vol 18, No7, (September 2001) pp 807-811. ISSN 0749-8063

Jamali AA. (2009) Digital templating and preoperative deformity analysis with standard imaging software. *Clin Orthop Relat Res.* Vol 467, No 10, (May 2009), pp 2695-704. ISSN : 1528-1132

Paley D. (2002). *Principles of Deformity Correction* (1st edition), Springer-Verlag, ISBN : 3-540-41665-X, New York, NY.

Phisitkul P, Wolf BR, Amendola A. (2006) Role of high tibial and distal femoral osteotomies in the treatment of lateral-posterolateral and medial instabilities of the knee. *Sports Med Arthrosc.* Vol.14, No 2, (June 2005), pp 96-104. ISSN 1062-8592

10

Aiming Accuracy and Reliable Opposite Site Cortical Sparing Wedge Ostoetomy Technique – A Surgical Trick

Zoltán Csernátony, Sándor Manó and László Kiss
University of Debrecen, Department of Orthopaedic Surgery, Hungary

1. Introduction

Osteotomy is one of the most ancient orthopaedic procedures still used today (Macewen, 1880). Osteotomy means the severance of a bony structure. It can be made for different purposes, such as ablation of an unneeded or disturbing bony prominence, elimination of an unhealthy bone segment or modification of the axis of a bone among others. When performing an axial correction on a bone, most frequently we make a wedge osteotomy, which is a common procedure in orthopaedics. To perform this we have two options. The first option is to cut across the whole bone with the elimination or addition of a triangular or trapezoidal piece of bone, or the cut section is incomplete, that is the opposite cortex is spared (Toksvig-Larsen 1992).

2. Background and surgical technique

Axial correction is carried out most often on long bones. Human long bones are tubular. Stress analysts distinguish two types of tubes, the thin and the large walled ones because of their different mechanical behaviour. A tube reacts to the bending force depending on its wall thickness. Due to genetical determination and the fact that the long bone is a living structure frequently receiving bending stress, its tubular form is consequently differing from a regular tube. This way the long bones are similar to irregularly shaped thick walled tubes.

However when we are correcting the axis of a long bone by means of preliminary incomplete cut, shear forces rise in the remaining part of the tube wall, which has a short section curved area. Incomplete section means that the bone is only partially cut, this way sparing the cortical on the opposite site. Also there is a difference if the cut end is just next to the inner cortical wall or if it is also biting it a bit (Fig. 1.).

This remaining integral cortical will serve as a hinge when correcting the angle (Fig. 2.). Depending on if we are carrying out an opening or a closing wedge osteotomy the stress rising on this cortical will be inverse. During opening wedge osteotomy in the external half of the cortical a compression stress, while in its internal part a tension stress occurs (Fig. 3.). In case of a closing wedge osteotomy the stress distribution appears inversely.

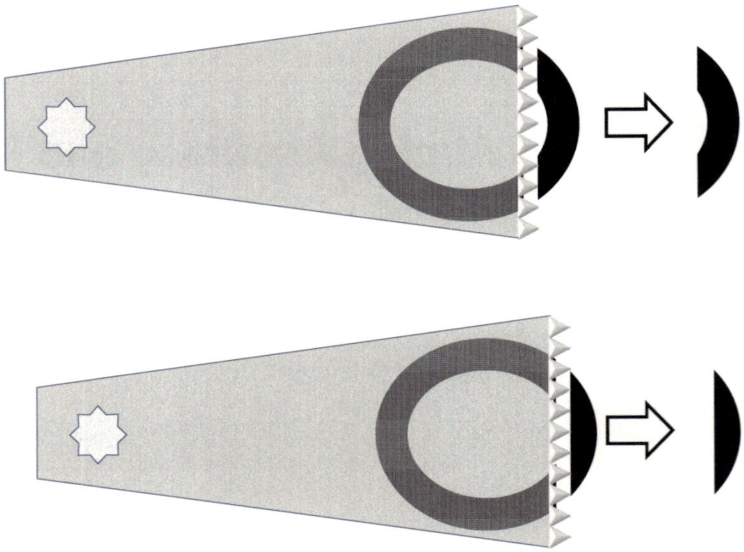

Fig. 1. Schematic drawing of the two types of incomplete cuts. The top figure shows the cut when the inner cortical wall is not reached, and the bottom figure shows the cut where the cut extends to the inner cortical.

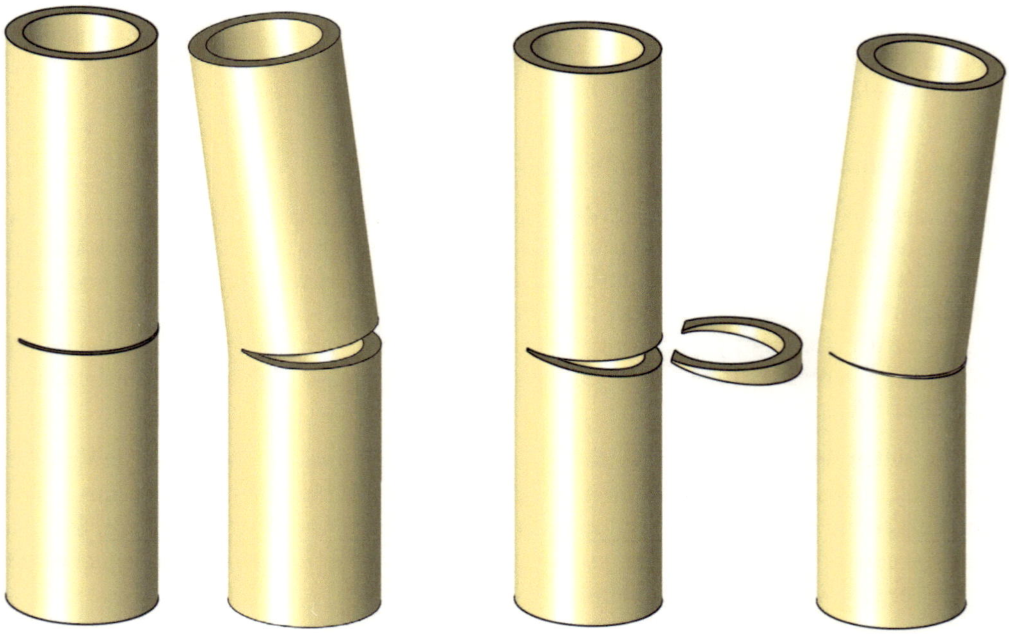

Fig. 2. Schematic drawing demonstrating opening and closing wedge osteotomy on long bones.

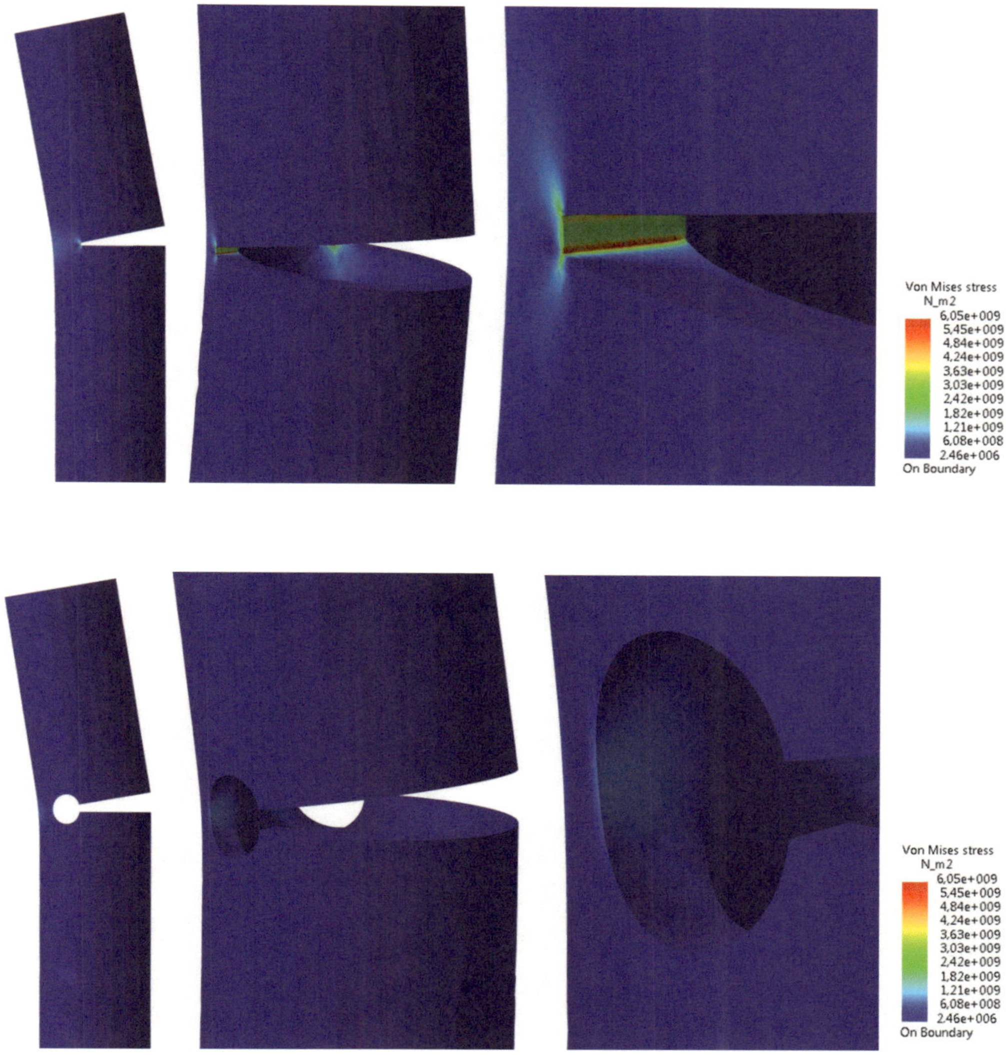

Fig. 3. Finite element model of the stress rise in case of opening wedge osteotomy in case of traditional cut (top) and after a perpendicular drill hole (bottom).

Irrespectively if we are opening or closing, the rising stress risks to surpass the resistance of the remaining cortical bone resulting in its break through, this means the loss of the hinge (Miller et al., 2009). If there is no hinge, the task of osteosynthesis is burdensome. In this case since the nature of the operation changed, the required osteosynthesis hardware and technique is completely different (Fillinger, 2001).

Up to this point we considered bone as a homogeneous material. However we have to keep in mind the importance of the bone's microstructure hierarchy on its mechanical properties. Crack initiation, propagation and finally completion is somehow resisted by the longitudinally oriented osteonal architecture. This way stress concentration itself does not determine the occurrence of material failure.

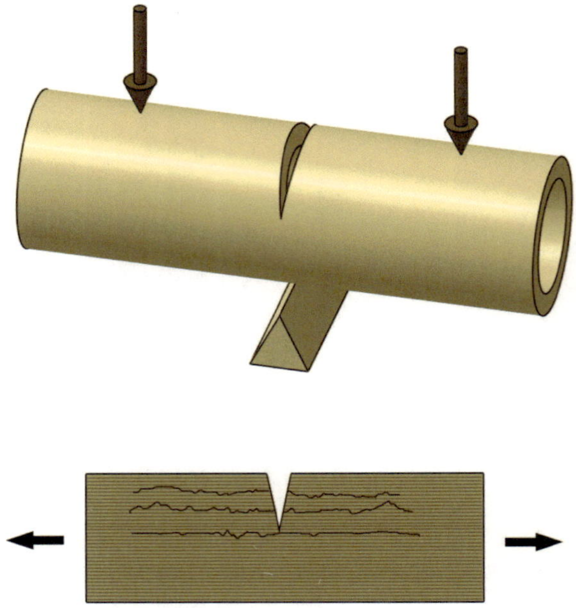

Fig. 4. Crack propagation following incomplete sharply ending cut.

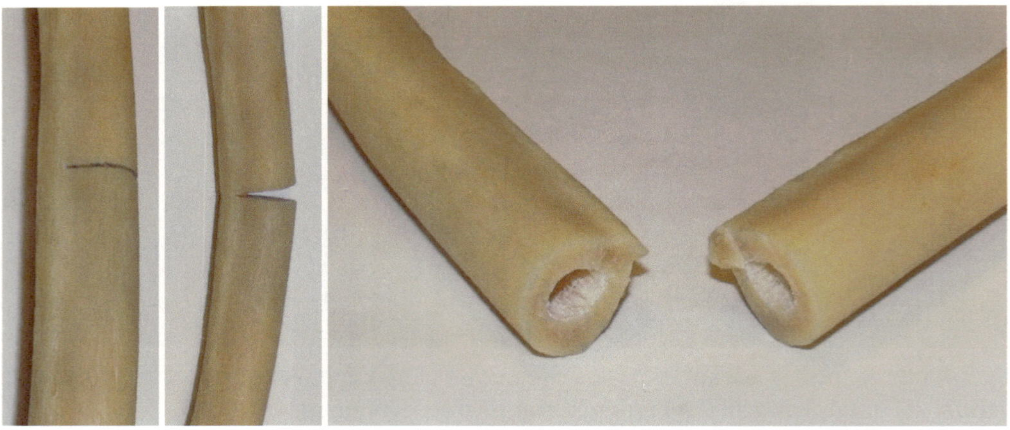

Fig. 5. Incomplete cut on a femoral diaphysis broken through during an opening wedge osteotomy.

If the vitality of the bone is not compromised by excessive devitalisation during the operation and the correcting manoeuvres don't cause immediate failure, the viable bone responds by an expedient remodelling process according to Wolff's law.

We felt that there is a lack of a technique which secures reliable control of sparing opposite site cortical (Fig. 5.), that is why we had recourse to a wide spread craftsman's method. All carpenters and locksmiths know that when performing a partial kerf cut before bending a piece of wood or metal the best way to make it safe, preventing breakage, is to drill a hole receiving the cut slot (Fig. 6.).

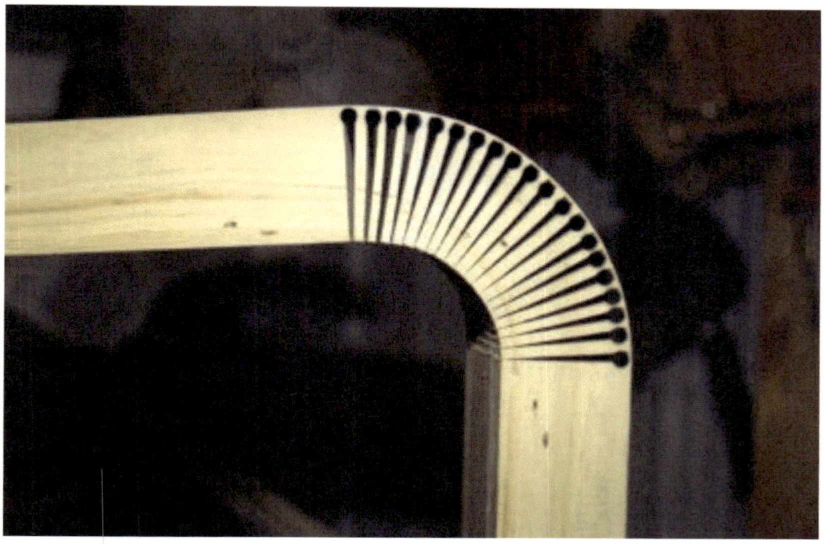

Fig. 6. A safe way to realize a serial incomplete wood cut for bending.

We adapted this technique during opening and closing wedge osteotomies in our clinical practice since 2006 (Csernátony et al., 2008). The method consists of drilling a juxtacortical hole positioned at the desired ending of the osteotomy cut. The diameter of the drill bit depends on the diameter of the bone cut. For instance in case of a proximal tibia osteotomy a 6 to 8 mm diameter is suitable, while in case of the first metatarsal bone a 4.5 mm diameter is sufficient (Fig. 7.). Here too it has an importance if the drilled hole is just against the inner cortical wall, or entering it, or is somehow away from it (Fig. 8.).

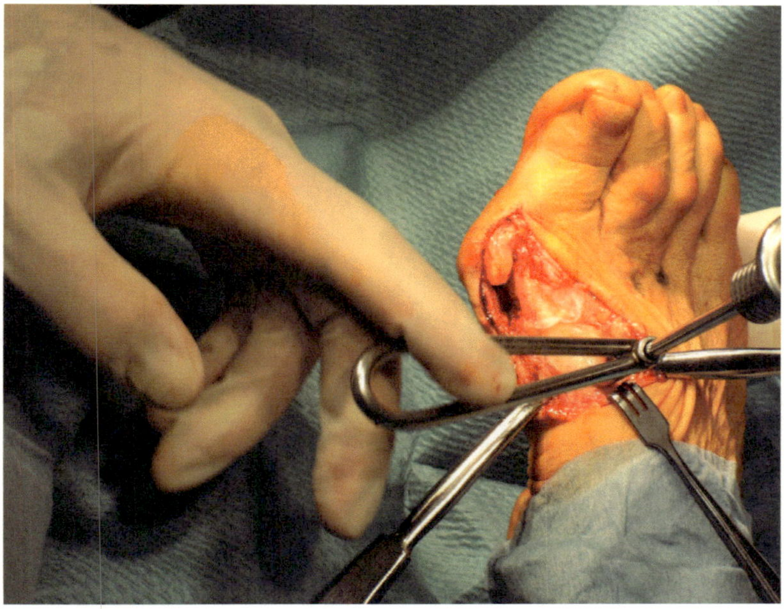

Fig. 7. A 4.5 mm drill hole is made on the opposite cortex in case a proximal osteotomy for metatarsus primus varus.

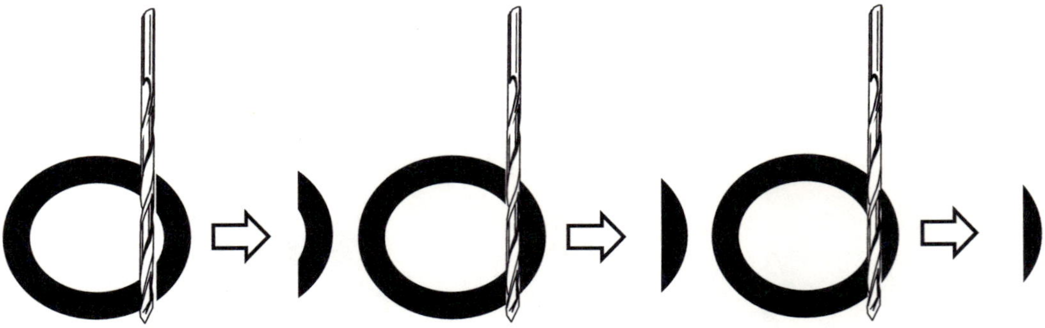

Fig. 8. Schematic drawing showing the three possible drill holes next to the opposite cortex.

Another practical difficulty in case of freehand bone cutting is the accuracy of cut. Preciseness might be easily disturbed by the fact, that only a small part of the leg is exposed during surgery and all remaining part of the body is covered with isolating sheets. One of the often used techniques is direct pencil marking on the bone. However many circumstances may divert during an operation the surgeon's attention, so reliable guide for precise execution is necessary.

Our way of execution adds a solution to the aiming of the osteotomy orientation. If the drill bit is left in place after removing it from the chuck, the drill bit can serve as a tracer guide when performing the osteotomy of the bone (Fig. 9.). Preciseness requires only directing the saw blade onto the midline of the drill-bit. After the osteotomy is performed the drill-bit is removed and the opening or closing wedge osteotomy is performed as usual (Fig. 10.). The drill hole on the opposite cortex decreases the amount of stress on the cortex and this way the chance of fracture is also decreased.

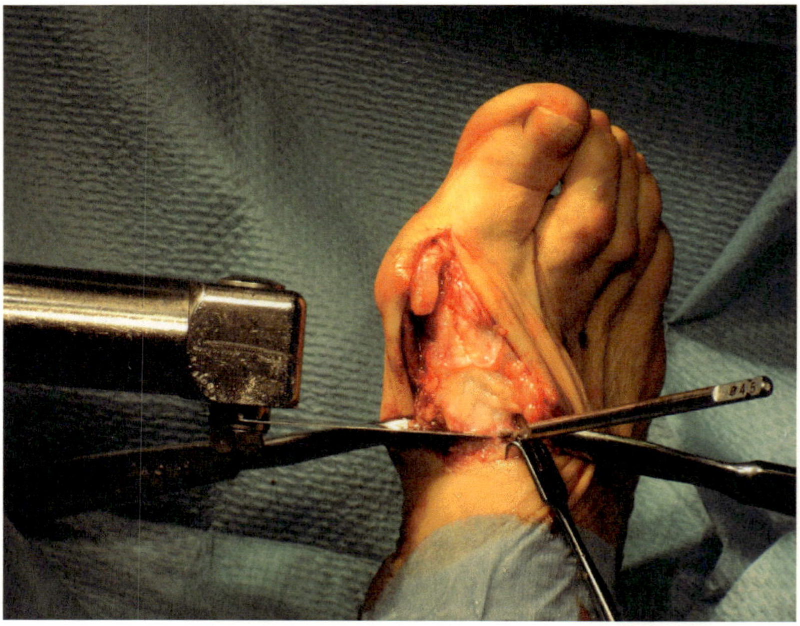

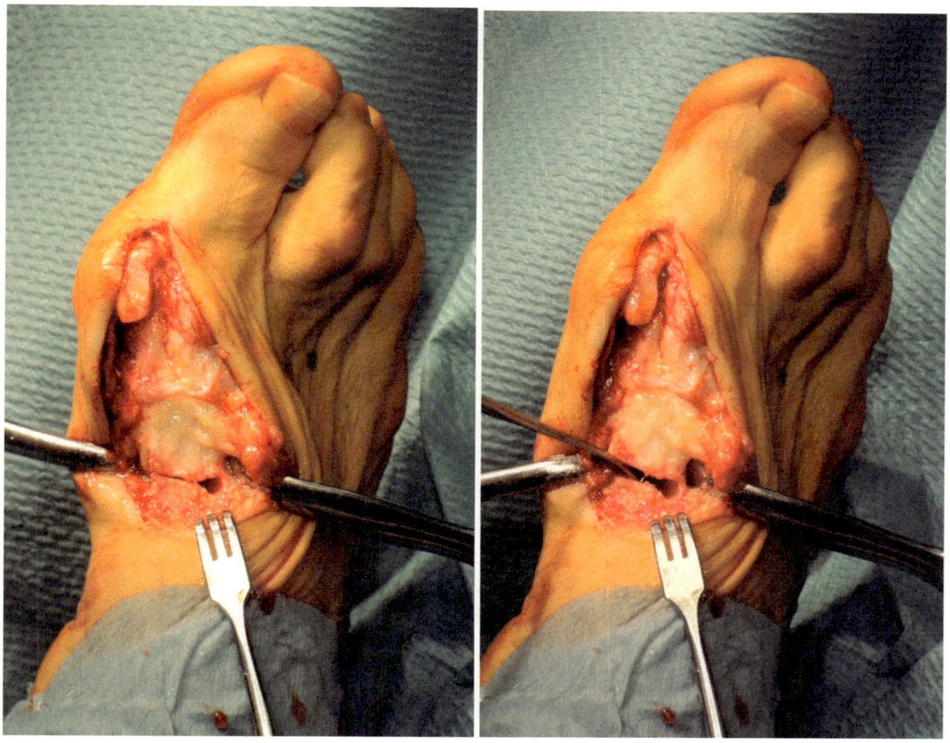

Fig. 9. Performing the osteotomy while using the drill-bit at the opposite cortex as a guide

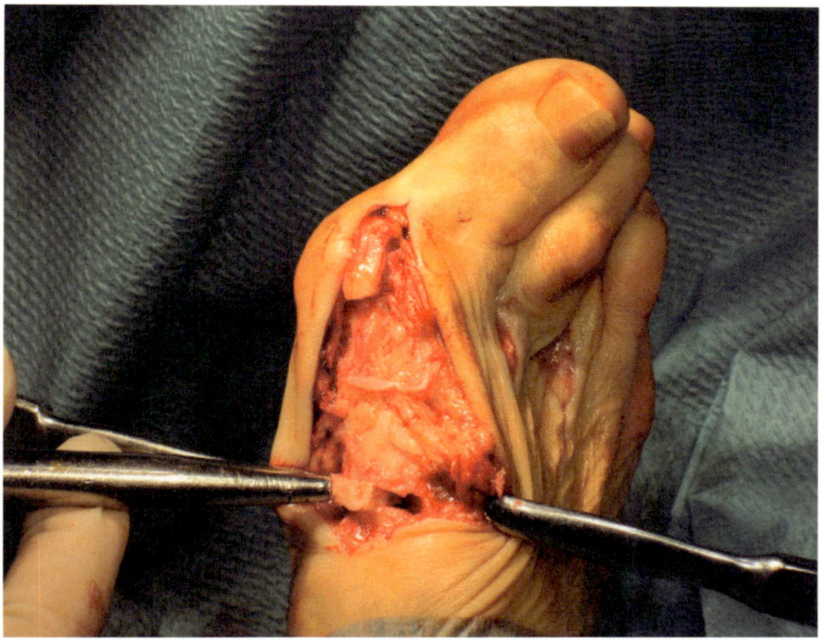

Fig. 10. In this opening wedge osteotomy the bone removed from the bunion is impacted into the osteotomy site.

3. Conclusion

We think that on the one hand nowadays in some fields of surgery we are over assisted by highly sophisticated instruments and navigation systems, however on the other hand there are still frequently used techniques relying simply on good manual skill. Our technique adds to the surgical precision without the invocation of a new dear instrumentation.

4. References

Macewen, W. (Ed.). (1880). *Osteotomy, with an inquiry into aetiology and pathology of knockknee, bow-leg and other osseus deformities of lower limbs.* Vol.16. I and A Churcill, London, UK

Toksvig-Larsen, S. (1992). *On bone cutting*. University Department of Orthopedics, Lund

Csernátony, Z.; Kiss, L. ; Manó, S. (2008). A new technique of wedge osteotomy to diminish undesirable fractures. *Eur J Orthop Surg Traumatol,* Vol.18, No.7, pp. 485-488

Miller, BS.; Downie, B.; McDonough, EB.; Woytys EM. (2009). Complications after medial opening wedge high tibila osteotomy. *Arthroscopy,* Vol.25, No.6, pp. 639-646

Fillinger, EB.; McGuire, JW.; Hesse, DF.; Solomon, MG. (2001). Inherent stability of proximal first metatarsal osteotomies: a comparative analysis. *The Journal of Foot and Ankle Surgery* Vol.40, No.5, pp. 292-302

11

Role of High Tibial Osteotomy in Chronic Posterior Cruciate Ligament and Posterolateral Corner Knee Instability

Salvatore Bisicchia[1] and Eugenio Savarese[2]
[1]*University of Rome "Tor Vergata",*
[2]*"Tor Vergata", San Carlo Hospital, Potenza,*
Italy

1. Introduction

High tibial osteotomy (HTO) has traditionally been performed to correct the mechanical axis of the knee in patients with osteoarthritis (OA) of the medial compartment associated with pain and functional impairment; in these patients the restoration of the alignment was related to the regeneration of the articular cartilage that seemed apparently normal (Fujisawa et al., 1979; Odenbring et al., 1992). Recently, HTO has also become very popular is association with cartilage techniques and meniscal grafts (Noyes et al., 2004). In the past chronic knee instability and varus thrust have been considered a contraindication for HTO (Coventry et al., 1993; Naudie et al., 1999), but nowadays, chronic instability is an indication for HTO, because allows to correct both the coronal and the sagittal alignment, improving the function of an unstable knee. Soft tissue techniques alone, without correction of the alignment, often give poor results because a bone deformity overstresses them (Christel, 2003; Goradia & Van Allen, 2002; Insall et al., 1984; Neyret et al., 1993). Soft tissue destruction causes a decrease in neuromuscular joint control, which in time can worsen the malalignment (Lephart et al., 1998). Reconstruction of the Posterior Cruciate Ligament (PCL), without repair or reconstruction of the Posterolateral Corner (PLC), often gives poor results (Christel, 2003; Krudwig et al., 2002; LaPrade & Wentorf, 2002; Noyes et al., 2005; Strobel et al., 2000. Some Authors (Badhe & Forster, 2002; Coventry et al., 1993; Hernigou et al., 1987; Insall et al., 1984; Nagel et al., 1996; Naudie et al. 1999) have reported satisfying results after HTO in monocompartimental knee OA and varus alignment, whereas there are few studies about the results of HTO in the unstable knee [9,17,18]. Recent papers suggest to perform this procedure before soft tissue reconstruction for the treatment of a PCL/PLC deficient knee associated with varus malalignment, to improve function and stability (Badhe & Forster, 2002; Fowler et al., 1994; Goradia & Van Allen, 2002). HTO is also useful in the treatment of an Anterior Cruciate Ligament (ACL) lesion associated with a varus of the knee (Dejour & Bonnin, 1994; Dejour et al., 1994; Fowler et al., 1994; Lattermann & Jakob, 1996; Lerat et al., 1993; Neuschwander et al., 1993; Noyes et al., 1993, 1996, 2000).

2. Anatomy

The tibia is a large bone transmitting, from the knee to the ankle, most of the stress of walking. It is surrounded by three compartments of muscles: the antero-lateral, the lateral and the posterior. The medial surface of the tibia is not covered by muscles providing an easier access to the bone (Hoppenfeld et al., 2003). The proximal anteromedial tibial cortex, viewed in a cross section, has an oblique or triangular shape, and it forms an angle of 45°±6° with the posterior margin of the tibia; whereas the lateral tibial cortex is nearly perpendicular to the posterior margin of the tibia (Noyes et al, 2005).

The PCL originates from the lateral aspect of the medial condyle and it inserts on the posterior edge of the tibial plateau. It has 2 boundles, the antero-lateral and the postero-medial (Ahmad et al., 2003; Amis et al., 2006; Takahashi et al., 2006).

PLC consists of three layers (Seebacher et al., 1982). The external layer is formed by the biceps femoris and the ileo-tibial tract. The middle layer is formed by the quadriceps retinaculum and the patello-femoral ligaments. The internal layer consists of a superficial lamina, formed by the lateral collateral ligament (LCL) and the fabello-fibular ligament, and a deep lamina, formed by the popliteo-fibular ligament, the arcuate ligament and the popliteus muscle with its tendon. The two laminae of the internal layer are the most important stabilizers of the PLC.

3. Biomechanics

There are three geometric variables to consider in the correction of a deformity (Paley, 1992):

1. Center of Rotation of Angulation (CORA): is the intersection between the proximal mechanical axis (PMA) with the distal mechanical axis (DMA). It is not under surgeon's control because it is related to the morphology of the deformity.
2. Angulation Correction Axis (ACA): is the axis around which the deformity is corrected. It is partially under the control of the surgeon.
3. Level of osteotomy: is totally under surgeon's control.

Given these geometric variables, there are three rules for osteotomies (Paley, 1992):

1. If the level of osteotomy and ACA pass for CORA, the re-alignment takes place without translation.
2. If ACA passes for CORA but the osteotomy is at a different level, the re-alignment takes place with angulation and translation at the osteotomy site.
3. If osteotomy and ACA are above or under CORA, the re-alignment takes place with translation.

ACA and CORA have to be as close as possible to avoid a secondary deformity with translation after the osteotomy is performed. In HTO, ACA and CORA are very close to each other, for this reason only the angular deformity will be corrected after surgery.

Patients with a varus of the knee and posterolateral instability often present the so-called "hyperextension varus thrust gait": during the gait cycle the knee goes into varus and hyperextension, the medial compartment narrows and the lateral compartment enlarges. In chronic lesions, posterolateral structures become overused with a further decrease in function. This phenomenon is increased during gait because all the weight bears on a limb (Chang et al., 2004; Miller et al., 2002; Noyes et al., 2006) (Fig. 1).

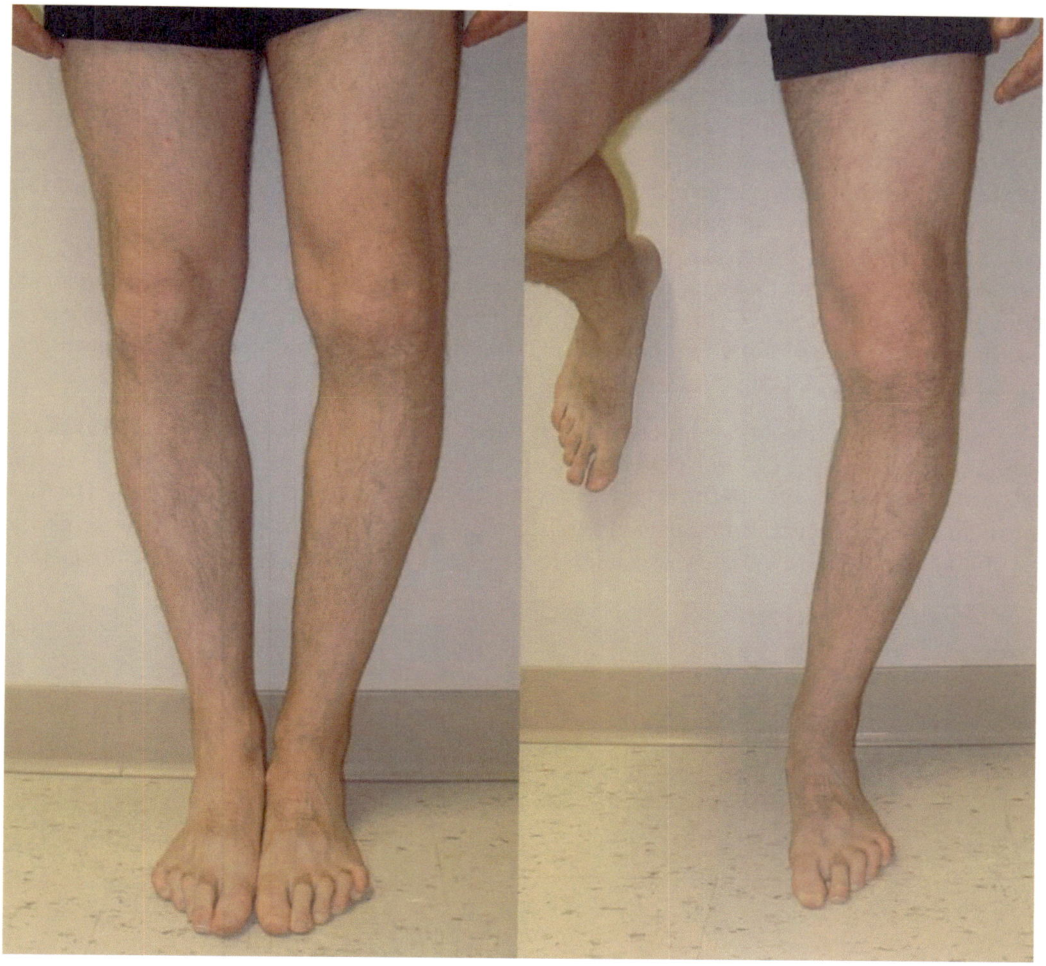

Fig. 1. One foot standing increases hyperextension varus thrust.

3.1 Effects of a chronic PCL/PLC lesion

An isolated chronic PCL lesion causes the tibia to translate posteriorly and to rotate externally about the femur. During all the different phases of the gait cycle the knee with a PCL lesion hyperextends, if compared with a normal knee (Noyes et al., 1996; Miller et al, 2002):

- Heel strike with PCL: 1.3°±1.6° of knee flexion
- Heel strike without PCL -5.6°±2.8 of relative knee flexion (hyperextension)
- Midstance with PCL: 14.9°±5° of knee flexion
- Midstance without PCL: 6.2°±10.9° of knee flexion
- Off Toe with PCL: 6.6°±4° of knee flexion
- Off Toe without PCL: -7.3°±4.4° of relative knee flexion (hyperextension)

A chronic PCL lesion can have effects on osteo-cartilagineous structures and on soft tissues of the knee. An osteoarthritic degeneration of the medial compartment of the knee is possible because of the aforementioned biomechanical changes and a quantitative reduction of PCL mechanoceptors (Safran et al., 1999). After a PCL lesion, the pressure increases of about 30% in the medial compartment of the knee (LaPrade & Wentorf, 2002; Lephart et al., 1998). Osteoarthritic changes take place even in the patello-femoral joint, due to an increase in pressure of about 16% (Ramaniraka et al., 2005; Skyhar et al, 1993), mainly on the lateral facet (because of an internal femoral rotation depending on external tibial rotation), and on the inferior pole (because the posterior tibial translation increases the tension along the patellar tendon: this increases patellar flexion (Kumagai et al., 2002; Li et al., 2002). Soft tissue effects occur mainly on ACL, which presents a decrease in number, diameter and density of collagen fibers (Ochi et al., 1999) and on PLC. Indeed, forces on PLC increase from 34±25N with PCL to 63±24N without PCL at 30° of knee flexion and from 38±46N with PCL to 86±53N without PCL at 90° of knee flexion (Hoher et al., 1998).

The effects of a PCL lesion are more evident when a PLC lesion is also present. This is not rare, in 60% of cases PCL and PLC lesions are associated [46]. The final result is a chronic posterolateral instability, defined as triple varus (Noyes & Simon, 1994) (Fig. 2). The first varus is osseous, lateral compartment enlargement due to LCL deficiency represents the second varus, the third varus is associated to hyperextension and it is due to PLC deficiency.

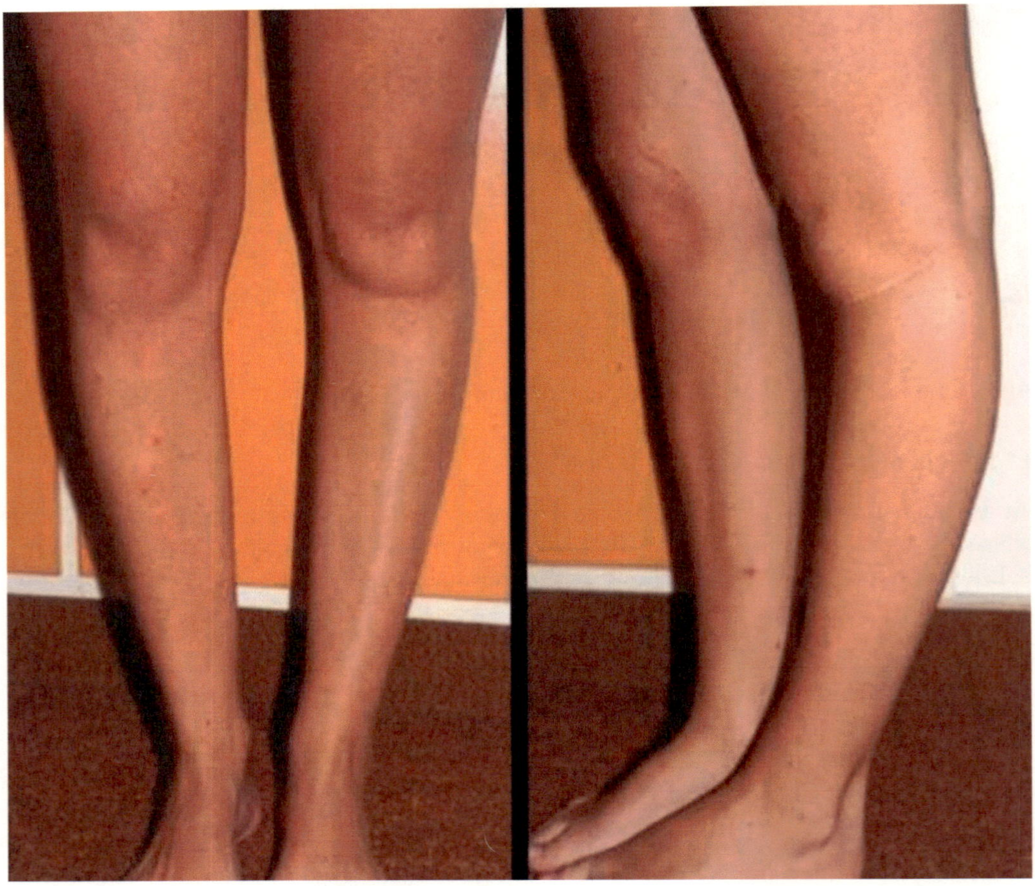

Fig. 2. Posterolateral chronic instability

3.2 Observations about posterior tibial slope

In the normal knee the medial posterior tibial slope is 9°-11° and the lateral posterior tibial slope is 6°-11° however, because there are 5 radiographic techniques described to evaluate its amount (see the Imaging section for more explanations), a wide range of values is reported (Brazier et al., 1996; Chiu et al., 2000; Dejour & Bonnin, 1994; Genin et al., 1993; Insall , 1993; Lecuire et al, 1980; Matsuda et al., 1999; Paley et al., 1994). The sagittal plane of the knee has often been ignored, however its changes affect biomechanics and joint stability. In fact, with an HTO it is possible to modify both the coronal and the sagittal planes, causing an anterior or posterior translation of the tibia about the femur. This has determined a great increase of osteotomies in the last years for the treatment of chronic knee instability. The proximal anteromedial tibial cortex, viewed in a cross section, has an oblique or triangular shape and it forms and angle of 45°±6° with the posterior margin of the tibia; whereas the lateral tibial cortex is nearly perpendicular to the posterior margin of the tibia. Because of these anatomical features a medial opening wedge HTO increases the tibial slope only if the anteromedial gap is equal to the posteromedial gap, whereas the slope does not change if the anteromedial gap is smaller than the posteromedial gap (Noyes et al., 2005). A lateral closing wedge osteotomy causes a small decrease in posterior tibial slope, a posterior translation of the tibia and stabilizes a knee with anterior instability (Amendola et al., 1989; Boileau & Neyret, 1991; Hohmann et al., 2006; Lerat et al., 1993; Levigne & Bonnin, 1991) (Fig. 3). Whereas a medial opening wedge HTO increases the posterior tibial slope, causes an anterior translation of the tibia and stabilizes a knee with posterior instability (Dejour & Bonnin, 1994; Giffin et al., 2007) (Fig. 4). Moreover, HTO preserves the proximal tibio-fibular joint, does not change the length of the posterolateral structures and prevents proximal migration of the fibula that could increase posterolateral instability.

Usually HTO are stabilized with plates: an anteromedial plate increases the slope, a posteromedial plate tends not to modify the posterior tibial slope [60] (Fig. 5). Furthermore, if the anteromedial gap is the half of the posteromedial gap, the tibial slope does not change. For each increase of 1 mm in the anterior gap, there is an increase of 2° in the posterior tibial slope (Noyes et al., 2005), and for every 10° of varus correction, the posterior tibial slope increases on the average of 2.7° and the tibia translates anteriorly of about 6 mm (Bonnin, 1990; Marti et al., 2004). Several authors reported, after HTO, an increase in posterior tibial slope, with an anterior translation of the tibia (Giffin et al., 2004; Naudie et al., 1994) and an decrease of forces on PCL: from 34±14N to 19±15N with the knee flexed at 30° and from 36±29N to 22±11N with the knee flexed at 90° (Giffin et al., 2004). This is a further demonstration that an increase in posterior tibial slope decreases stress forces on posterior structures.

Dome osteotomy (Maquet, 1976) is associated with an increase in posterior tibial slope (Cullù et al., 2005; Nakamura et al., 2001), whereas an opening wedge HTO with emicallotaxis, has little influence on tibial slope (Nakamura et al., 2001). An increase in posterior tibial slope causes a change in the pressure on the articular tibial cartilage: the pressure increases in the anterior portion and decreases in the posterior portion. If the tibia translates anteriorly, the pressure on posterior articular cartilage should increase; however, between 120° of knee flexion and full extension, femoral condyles roll anteriorly on the tibia, shifting anteriorly the contact point (Agneskirchner et al., 2004).

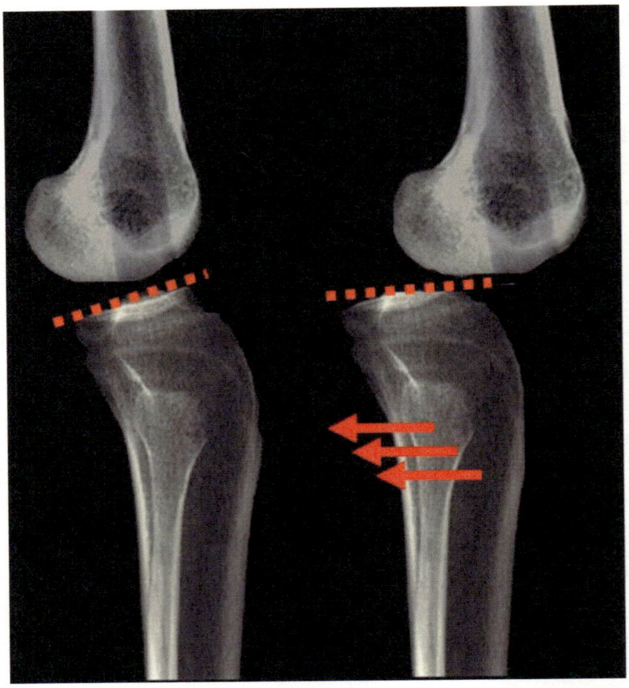

Fig. 3. A closing wedge HTO causes a decrease in posterior tibial slope and a posterior translation of the tibia, it stabilizes a knee with anterior instability.

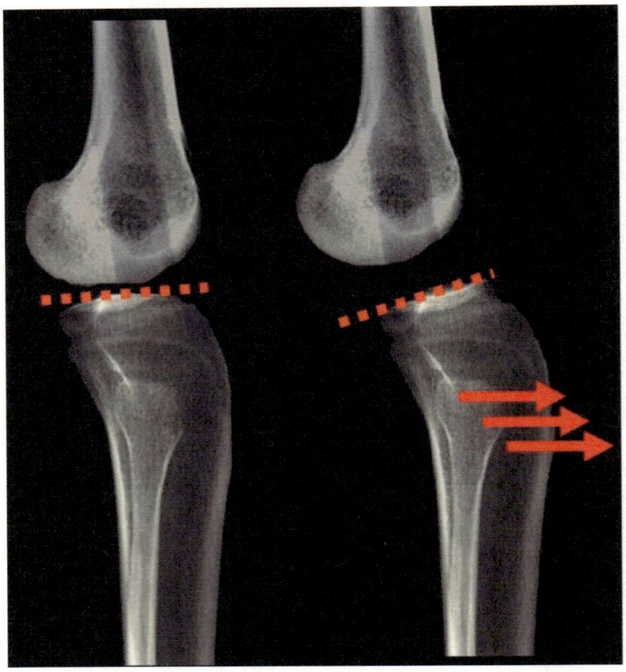

Fig. 4. A opening wedge HTO causes an increase in posterior tibial slope and an anterior translation of the tibia, it stabilizes a knee with posterior instability.

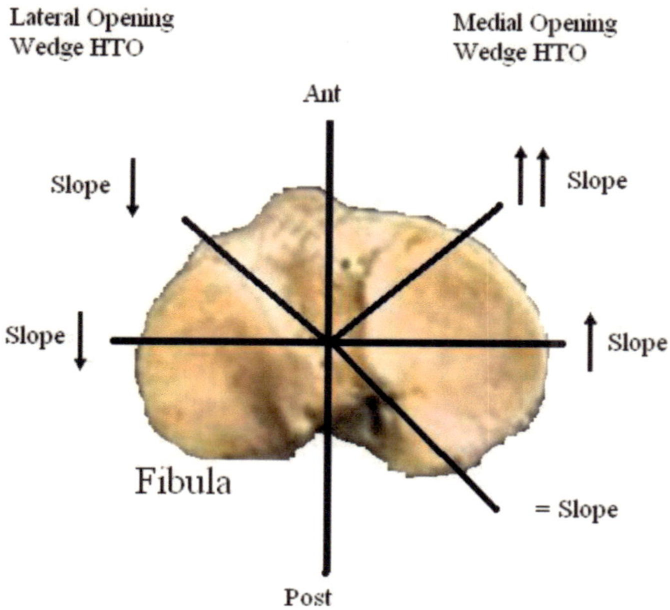

Fig. 5. Relationship between tibial slope and kind and site of osteotomy.

4. History and physical examination

Complete history and physical examination are mandatory in the evaluation of all patients, but in a patient with a PCL/PLC lesion, associated with a varus malalignment, they have a particular value, in fact clinical tests for the diagnosis of PCL and PLC lesions have low sensitivity and, in some cases, also low specificity, for these reasons we advise the clinician to perform all the tests described to rule out such lesions.

Because PCL and PLC lesions are associated in 60% of the cases (Fanelli & Edson, 1995), if a PCL lesion is suspected or detected, the physician should look for a PLC lesion. Patients with a PCL lesion usually complain about non specific symptoms, the mechanism of injury usually reported is a posterior force applied to the tibia with the knee in flexion (football players or a fall on the flexed knee), and hyperextension or hyperflexion with or without a posteriorly directed force applied to the tibia (Petrigliano & McAllister, 2006). After an acute PLC lesion, patients usually refer a blow to the anteromedial aspect of the knee, contact or noncontact hyperextension and a varus noncontact force. About 15% of PLC lesions are associated to a common peroneal nerve injury, it is important to ask the patient about numbness, tingling or muscle weakness, especially in ankle dorsiflexion or great toe extension (LaPrade & Terry, 1997). Because of the biomechanical changes in PLC after a PCL lesion (see the Biomechanics section), patients with a chronic PLC lesion usually do not refer either a specific trauma or a PCL lesion that might have occurred several years before. Chronic lesion should be suspected during physical examination, and gait analysis is useful in detecting them, so we believe that it should be systematically performed.

During physical examination it is important to identify all the factors involved in posterolateral chronic instability, because they are all related to the surgical outcome.

- Gait is the first factor to analyze. Patients with posterolateral instability often present the so-called "hyperextension varus thrust gait" (Fig. 1) (see the Biomechanics section). Gait analysis is important to detect PLC associated lesions because, in some cases, patients with hyperextension varus thrust have poorer results than patients with normal gait (Chang et al., 2004; Miller et al., 2002; Noyes et al., 1996).

Many tests are described for the evaluation of PCL and PLC.

- Posterior Sag Sign (Barton et al., 1984; Mayo Robson, 1903) has 79% sensitivity and 100% specificity (Rubinstein et al., 1994). The patient lies in the supine position with both knees and hip at 90° of flexion while the examiner holds the heels of the patient and compares side by side the posterior translation of the tibia from a lateral view.
- Posterior Drawer Test (Paessler & Michel, 1992; Strobel et al., 1990) has 90% sensitivity and 99% specificity (Rubinstein et al., 1994). The patient lies in the supine position, with the knee at 90° of flexion, the examiner sits on the foot of the patient and applies a posterior force on the anterior tibial shaft comparing side by side the posterior tibial translation.
- Quadriceps contraction (Daniel et al., 1988) has 54% sensitivity and 97% specificity (Rubinstein et al., 1994). The patient lies in the supine position with the knee in the drawer position and is asked to slide the foot down the table, if a PCL lesion is present the tibia translates anteriorly more than 2 mm during quadriceps contraction.
- Dial Test, performed in prone and supine position (Loomer, 1991; Veltri & Warren, 1994). The patient lies in the supine position with both thighs supported by an holder or allowed to hang off the end of the examining table and stabilized by an assistant at 30° of knee flexion. The examiner externally rotates the lower legs and compares the tibial tuberosity external rotation side by side. In the prone position an assistant is not needed and the thigh-foot angle is measured. The test is positive for a PLC lesion if there is an increase of at least 10-15° in comparison to the other knee at 30° of knee flexion. The test is then repeated at 90° of flexion, if a further increase in external rotation is present, a PCL lesion is associated.
- External Rotation Recurvatum Test (Hughston & Norwood, 1980). The patient lies in the supine position with both knees extended. The examiner holds and lifts the great toes of the patient. If a PLC lesion is present, the affected knee hyperextends and goes in varus and in external rotation compared to the contra lateral normal knee.
- Varus Stress test (Hughston et al., 1976; Palmer, 1938). The knee is at 30° of flexion, the examiner grasps the thigh of the patient with one hand and the foot or the lower leg with the other hand and applies a varus force to the knee. The amount of lateral compartment opening indicates the grade of LCL lesion. I grade (0-5 mm), II grade (6-10 mm), III grade (>10 mm).
- Posterolateral drawer test (Hughston & Norwood, 1980). The patient lies in the supine position with the knee at 90° of flexion and the foot 15° in external rotation while the examiner posteriorly translates the tibia. If the affected limb translates posteriorly more than the contra lateral limb, a popliteus tendon or popliteo-fibular ligament injury are suspected.
- Reverse Pivot Shift test (Jakob et al., 1981). The patient lies in the supine position with the knee at 70°-80° of flexion with the foot externally rotated. If a PLC lesion is present the tibia is posteriorly subluxatated. The knee is subsequently extended and at 20° of

flexion this subluxation reduces spontaneously. It is important to consider that the test is positive in 35% of normal knees, especially under anesthesia, so a side to side comparison is mandatory to evaluate the real amount of instability (Cooper, 1991).

Because meniscal injuries are associated to acute PCL lesions in 16% to 28% of cases (Fowler & Messieh, 1987; Hamada M et al., 2000) and to chronic PCL lesions in 36% of cases (Geissler & Whipple, 1993), specific meniscal tests should be systematically performed. Even if neuro-vascular function tests are more important in acute injury, they also should be performed also in patients with chronic lesions.

5. Imaging

Conventional radiology has still an important role in the pre-operative planning of patients with a PCL/PLC lesion, especially if associated to a varus of the knee.

If physical examination reveals any of the following: positive varus stress test, increased varus during thrust, increased tibial external rotation at 30° of knee flexion or varus recurvatum during standing or walking, stress X-rays should be performed. If X-rays are positive, the patient should get supine full length antero-posterior (A-P) X-rays of both legs to evaluate the real alignment. If physical examination reveals none of the aforementioned features, the patient should get full length double-stance A-P X-rays of both legs. If a varus deformity is not present, the patient should undergo a soft tissue reconstruction; if this deformity is present, it is important to evaluate if a lateral joint line opening is associated. If it is the case, the patient should get stress X-rays, if it is not the case there are two methods described to evaluate the amount of correction to perform during surgery (Dugdale et al., 1992; Noyes et al., 2000).

5.1 Standard X-ray

Full length double-stance A-P X-ray is mandatory to evaluate femoro-tibial alignment (Moreland et al., 1987). An A-P. X-ray is taken from the hips to the ankles with the patient standing and the patellae looking forward using a suitable cassette to gradually filter the X-ray beam in order to properly visualize both hips and ankles. There are two methods to quantify the amount of correction to perform if a malalignment is present (Dugdale et al., 1992). In both methods a line along the tibial plateau and its intersection with the desired mechanical axis of the lower extremity are marked, in this section this point is called P for simplicity (see the Indications section for more explanations about the position of P in each patient). Then a line is traced from the centre of the femoral head to P and a line is traced from the centre of the tibio-talar joint to P. In the first method the angle formed at the intersection between these two lines represents the amount of correction required (Fig. 6).

In the second method the radiographic film is cut along the osteotomy line and along a vertical line that converge with the first, leaving a 2 mm hinge at the medial tibial margin, the distal part of the film is rotated until the femoral head, P and the tibio-talar joint are along the same line; the overlapping wedge margin is the amount of correction to perform. If lateral and/or posterolateral soft tissue structures are insufficient, for every increase of 1 mm in the lateral joint line width, there is 1° of added varus. Supine X-rays are important to eliminate the added varus due to deficiency of the lateral and/or posterolateral structures and to evaluate the real amount of correction to perform. After HTO the mechanical axis of the lower extremity is translated laterally of 3-4 mm for each 1° of valgus correction and this value depends on the height of the patient.

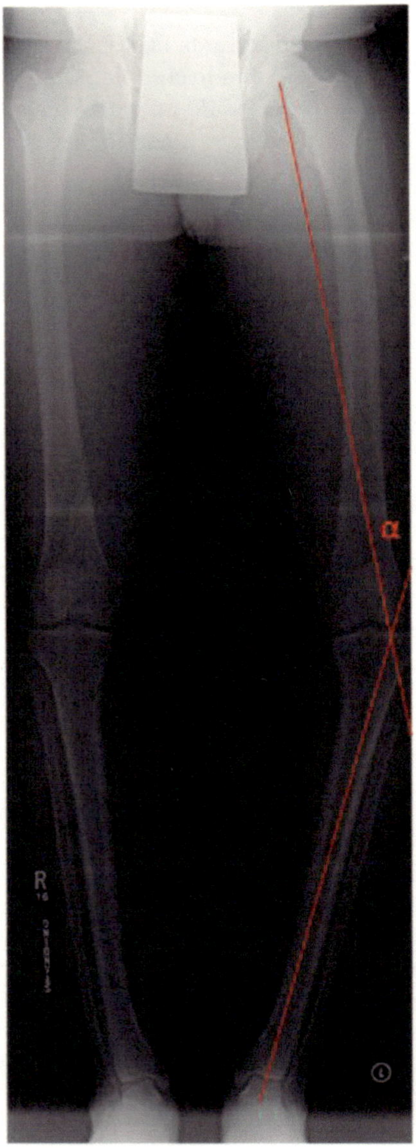

Fig. 6. The angle a represents the correction required

- Real lateral view X-rays are important to evaluate posterior tibial slope. In literature many methods are described to quantify its value (Fig. 7). In all cases a line is traced along the medial tibial plateau, and the angle formed with Proximal Tibial Anatomical Axis (PTAA) (Dejour & Bonnin, 1994), the anterior tibial cortex (ATC) (Moore & Harvey, 1974), the posterior tibial cortex (PTC), the proximal fibular anatomical axis (PFAA) and the fibular shaft axis (FSA) (Brazier et al., 1996) is calculated. Between all these techniques the most reliable are PTAA and PTC (Brazier et al., 1996). Higher values are found using the ATC method and lower values with PFAA method (Cullù et al., 2005).

- Merchant's view (Merchant et al., 1974) is useful to evaluate patello-femoral joint that can undergo degenerative changes. The patient lies in the supine position with the knees at 45° of flexion over the end of the table, the knees are sustained to maintain the femora parallel to the horizontal. The X-Ray collimator is placed above the patient and the beam is directed from proximal to distal forming a 30° angle with the table. The film cassette is placed about 30 cm below the knees, perpendicular to the tibial shaft.
- Rosemberg's view (Rosenberg et al., 1988) is useful to evaluate the lateral compartment of the knee. The patient stands on both legs with thumbs pointing ahead and the patellae touching the film cassette. The knees are at 45° of flexion (25° between the femora and the cassette and 20° between the tibiae and the cassette), the X-Ray beam is directed from posterior to anterior, 10° caudal, so the posterior and the anterior margins of the tibial plateau are superimposed.

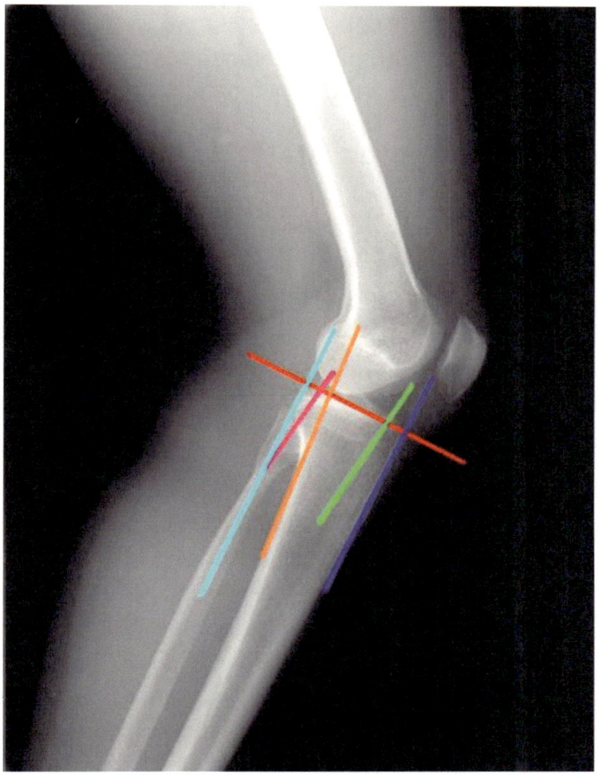

Fig. 7. ATC: Anterior tibial cortex, PTAA: Proximal tibial anatomical axis, PTC: Posterior tibial cortex, PFAA: Proximal fibular anatomical axis, FSA: Fibular shaft axis.

5.2 Stress X-ray

- Lateral stress view according to the Telos method (Jacobsen, 1976). The patient lies in the lateral decubitus with the knee flexed at 90° and is encouraged to relax. The heel is fixed to a stand and the arm of the Telos GA II (Telos, Weterstadt, Germany) applies a posterior force to the tibia. In this position a lateral X-Ray is taken. The test is then performed with the knee at 25° of flexion. This method is very important in chronic PCL deficient knees to evaluate both anterior and posterior tibial translation with regards to the femur and it is useful to detect a fixed posterior tibial subluxation that can be present in 44% of the patients with a PCL lesion (Strobel et al., 2002).

- Lateral stress view according to the Kneeling method (Louisia et al., 2005). The patient knees on a bench with the knee at 90° of flexion, the bench only supports the lower legs up to the tibial tubercle. In this position a lateral X-Ray is taken.
- Lateral stress view with hamstring contraction (Chassaing et al., 1995). The patient lies in the lateral decubitus or in the seated position with the knee at 90° of flexion and the heel fixed to a stand. A lateral X-Ray is taken while the patient contracts his/her hamstring for at least 10 seconds (Chassaing et al., 1995; Jung et al., 2006).
- Lateral stress view according to Gravity method (Staubli & Jakob, 1990). The patient lies in the supine position with the hip and the knee at 90° of flexion supported by an assistant, with the leg in neutral rotation. In this position a lateral X-ray is taken.
- Axial stress view (Puddu et al., 2000). The patient lies in the supine position, with both knees at 70° of flexion, feet plantigrade in moderate plantar flexion and the tibia in neutral rotation. The X-Ray beam is directed parallel to the longitudinal patellar axis, from distal to proximal and the distance between the anterior tibial profile and the centre of the femoral groove is measured. The side to side difference is the amount of posterior instability.

Comparing all these five methods, focusing on posterior translation, side to side difference, condyle rotation, time to perform the test and pain during the test, the most effective methods are Telos at 90° of knee flexion and Kneeling method, even if they are painful and time consuming procedures. Telos is the most expensive but the most reliable in detecting a posterior tibial subluxation (Jung et al., 2006; Margheritini et al., 2003).

5.3 MRI

MRI is useful to evaluate PCL deficient knees, especially associated lesions and subchondral bone (Puddu et al., 2007). Gross et al. (1992) described a classification for PCL lesion that is widely used, however Bellelli et al. (2006) proposed a new MRI classification that considers each PCL bundle independently, emphasizing the importance of SE T2 and STIR sequences. To evaluate PLC, at least 1.5 T MRI scanner is recommended (LaPrade & Wentorf, 2002), because its sensitivity is 66.7%-100% and its specificity is 66.7%-100%, depending on the anatomical structures. Coronal oblique sections (parallel to the popliteus tendon) significantly increases the ability to detect some structures of PLC (i.e. fabello-fibular ligament, arcuate ligament, popliteus tendon and popliteo-fibular ligament) but, also with coronal oblique sections, less than one half of these structures could be imaged (Yu et al., 1996). The use thin slice (2 mm) proton density coronal oblique sequences to evaluate LCL and popliteus tendon is also recommended (LaPrade et al., 2000).

We believe that stress radiographs are mandatory in the evaluation of an unstable knee, but do not help the clinician to identify the injured structures. MRI does not solve this problem, because it cannot fully visualize posterolateral structures in at least 50% of patients (Yu et al., 1996). This is still a problem in the diagnosis of a PLC lesion.

6. Indications and contraindications

A wrong indication is the first cause of failure, so surgery must be preceded by an accurate pre-operative planning. Contraindications to HTO are: inflammatory disease, severe tricompartmental OA, severe medial compartment OA, severe lateral compartment OA, severe osteoporosis, high BMI (relative contraindication), individuals older than 65 years (relative), severe patello-femoral OA (relative). There are three causes of failure of HTO in a varus knee: inability to correct the deformity during surgery, a "tibial teeter-totter effect" (advanced medial tibio-femoral OA and obliquity) and a gradual collapse of the medial compartment over years in which the overall alignment drifts back into varus because of continued medial tibio-femoral OA (Noyes et al., 2000).

PCL and PLC lesion are often associated to malalignment of the knee (Fanelli & Edson, 1995) and they should be corrected 6-8 months after HTO (if the knee is still unstable). In literature poor results for soft tissue procedures alone are reported. This is related to the forces on these structures that do not decrease if the malalignment is not corrected, because a bone deformity overstresses them. Instead HTO reduces these forces and improves the stability and biomechanics of the knee. (See the Biomechanics section for more explanations).

We believe that the evaluation of the deformity in the coronal and the sagittal plane is essential for the treatment of a complex instability of the knee and, before performing any kind of soft tissue surgery, a correct bone alignment should be obtained, both in coronal and in the sagittal plane.

If femoro-tibial OA is present, with narrowing of the medial compartment, the point called P in the Imaging section should be positioned at 62%-66% of the tibial plateau (0% positioned on the medial margin of the tibial plateau and 100% on the lateral margin). This position increases the pressure on the lateral compartment of the knee (most of the weight of the patient bears on the lateral articular cartilage) (Dugdale et al., 1992; Noyes et al., 2000; Viskontas et al., 2006), indeed a small overcorrection prevents progression of medial compartment OA and an early recurrence of the varus deformity (Akizuki et al., 2008; Noyes et al., 2000). If a degenerative narrowing of the medial compartment is not present the new mechanical axis should split the tibial plateau in two halves (Noyes et al., 2000). Medial opening wedge HTO improves symptoms of patello-femoral OA because the anterior translation of the tibia reduces the tension on the patellar tendon, the patella becomes less horizontal and pressure decreases in the lateral facet (Kumagai et al., 2002; Li et al., 2002). So a patello-femoral pain syndrome is not a contraindication for HTO.

Strobel et al (2002) classified fixed posterior tibial subluxation in three grades: I (3-5 mm), II (6-10 mm), III (>10 mm). In first and second grades they recommend a brace in extension with a support under the calf to push the tibia anteriorly (Medi Bayreuth, Bayreuth Germany) because they had good results in 78.4% and 70.1% of the patients respectively. In patients with a third grade lesion conservative treatment has given acceptable result only in 32%, so they recommend surgical treatment. If a fixed tibial subluxation is present, it should be reduced before performing any surgical treatment, to avoid an overstress of the graft and an early failure. HTO modifies the tibial slope, provokes the tibia to translate anteriorly and reduces this subluxation. Subsequently, if the knee is still unstable, PCL could be reconstructed. If meniscal lesions are associated, they should be addressed at the same time of HTO.

Some Authors (Klinger et al., 2001; Ohsawa et al., 2006; Viskontas et al, 2006) suggested that an opening wedge HTO with emicallotaxis and external fixator is the treatment that should be chosen to correct the malalignment, however we prefer to use this technique with a circular external fixator (Taylor Spatial Frame, Smith & Nephew, Memphis, Tennesseee) only in deformities that need a correction greater than 12.5°. In these cases HTO is associated to a greater rate of complications, such as delayed unions, nonunions and an unstable osteotomy, due to a too large osteotomy gap. If an external fixator is applied, the osteotomy is performed distal to the tibial tubercle and it does not change patellar height, instead medial opening wedge HTO is performed proximal to the tibial tubercle and if the gap is too large, patella infera (baja) may occur. This circular external fixator has a computerized program that consents to achieve a triplanar correction of the deformity and to correct also the tibial slope in the sagittal plane (Catagni et al., 1994). An external fixator consents a slow correction of the deformity, improving consolidation even of large osteotomy gaps, the patient can walk earlier, weight bearing X-Rays could be obtained to evaluate the alignment of the lower limbs, the mechanical axis could be corrected at any time during the elongation phase if needed, without a second surgery being performed and a tourniquet is not needed at the time of surgery (Watanabe et al., 2008). But it is uncomfortable for the patient, it is not easy to wear under normal clothes and pin tract infection may occur. Because the external fixator is not rigid, 5° of overcorrection reduces the failure rate in case of loss of correction (Catagni et al., 1994).

A preoperative rehabilitation protocol (strengthening of the muscles of the lower limbs and gait retraining) is needed to avoid the recurrence of hyperextension varus trust gait after surgery (Noyes et al., 2000).

HTO and ACL reconstruction are often associated and good results are reported even in knees with double varus. If triple varus is present, HTO should be performed before soft tissue reconstruction, in order to avoid a long surgery and increased risk of postoperative complications (Noyes et al., 2000). We do not have enough patients for a statistical analysis, but in our clinical experience, in a patient with a chronic PCL deficient knee associated with double or triple varus, HTO should be performed before soft tissue procedures. The patient should be evaluated 6-8 months later and, if the knee is still unstable, soft tissue reconstruction should be performed.

7. Treatment

A closing wedge lateral HTO and a Dome osteotomy according to Maquet slightly decrease the tibial slope and are not useful in the treatment of a PCL/PLC deficient knee. Because an opening wedge medial HTO and HTO with external fixator consent the surgeon to modify the tibial slope, they are the only osteotomies that can be performed in patients with a PCL/PLC deficient knee, and only these osteotomies are discussed in this section. For the description of lateral HTO, Dome osteotomy and soft tissue procedures the reader is advised to consult the specific literature.

All patients should receive a prophylactic pre-operative dose of intravenous antibiotics; general endotracheal anaesthesia should be preferred because it allows the surgeon to get a bone block from the iliac crest, if needed. With the patient lying in a supine position, the leg is draped in a sterile fashion; if a bone block is needed, the omolateral iliac crest is draped in the same fashion. Arthroscopy is performed in all patients to evaluate articular cartilage and menisci and to confirm the indication for HTO (Hernigou et al., 1987; Noyes & Simon, 1994; Noyes et al., 2000).

If a plate is used to stabilize the osteotomy, the leg is raised and tourniquet is inflated. A vertical incision is performed just behind the pes anserine, between the medial border of the patellar tendon and the posterior border of the tibia. Sartorius fascia is cut to visualize hamstring tendons. Under fluoroscopic control a guide wire is positioned from medial to lateral. The wire is placed at the level of the superior aspect of the tibial tubercle, anteromedially, and it arrives about 1 cm below the lateral articular margin of the tibia (Fig. 8). A cortical osteotomy is performed with an oscillating saw, inferiorly to the guide wire, and it will be continued with an osteotome under fluoroscopic control (Fig. 9). When the osteotomy is completed, the medial tibia is opened with a wedge of a suitable width (Fig. 10). Wedges have a graduated scale to quantify the angular correction achieved (Hernigou et al., 1987; Noyes & Simon, 1994; Noyes et al., 2000). The position of the wedge is very

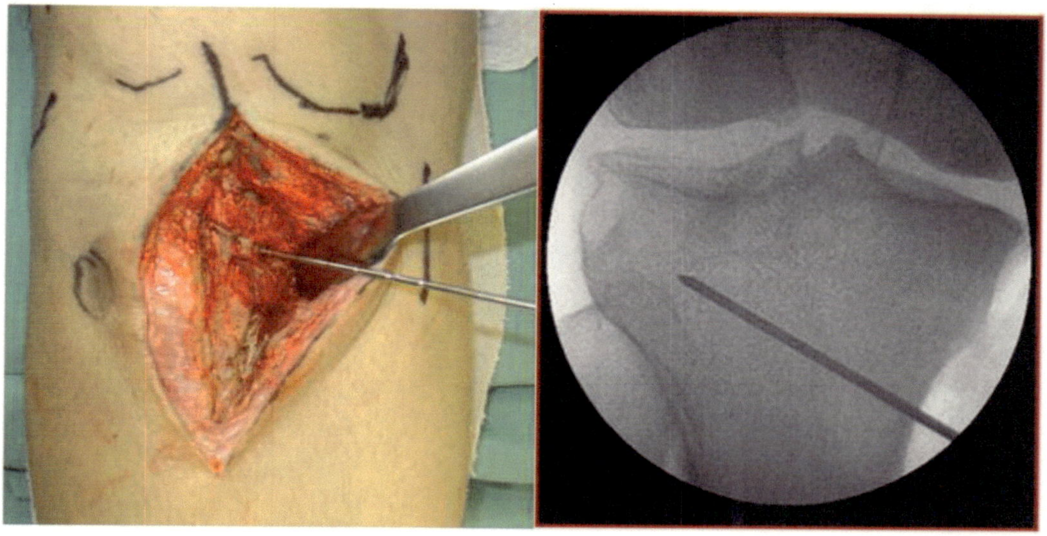

Fig. 8. A guide wire is placed from the superior aspect of the tibial tubercle to about 1 cm below the lateral articular margin of the tibia.

important in order to correct the deformity on the sagittal plane: a wedge placed anteriorly causes an increase in posterior tibial slope, whereas a posterior wedge tends to slightly decrease the posterior tibial slope (Rodner et al., 2006). Anterior and posterior gaps of the osteotomy are then measured with a ruler, this is important to calculate the amount of increase in posterior tibial slope after surgery (Hohmann et al., 2006). If the anteromedial gap is the half of the postermedial gap, the slope will not change; for each millimetre of increase of the anterior gap, the posterior tibial slope will increase of 2°. An image intensifier and an alignment rod are used to control coronal and sagittal alignment during axial loading of the joint (Noyes et al., 2000) (Fig. 11). If the anterior gap is greater than 1 cm, it is better to perform an osteotomy to lift up the tibial tubercle of the same amount in order to avoid patella infera (baja). Generally to fill the osteotomy gap a carefully shaped bone block from a donor is used. Under fluoroscopic control the final result is checked before the tourniquet is deflated, hemostatis and skin suture are then performed (Hernigou et al., 1987; Noyes & Simon, 1994; Noyes et al., 2000) (Fig. 12). When the correction in the two planes is achieved, the osteotomy is stabilized with a plate with four holes (Arthex, Naples, Florida, USA) with two 6.5 mm proximal cancellous screws and two 4.5 mm distal cortical screws (Fig. 13).

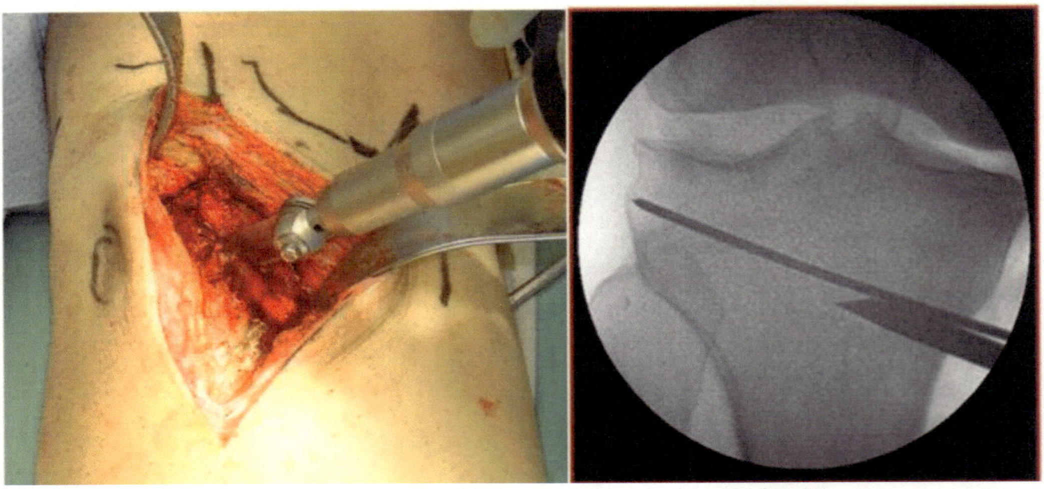

Fig. 9. Cortical osteotomy is performed with an oscillating saw, inferior to the guide wire, and it will be continued with an osteotome.

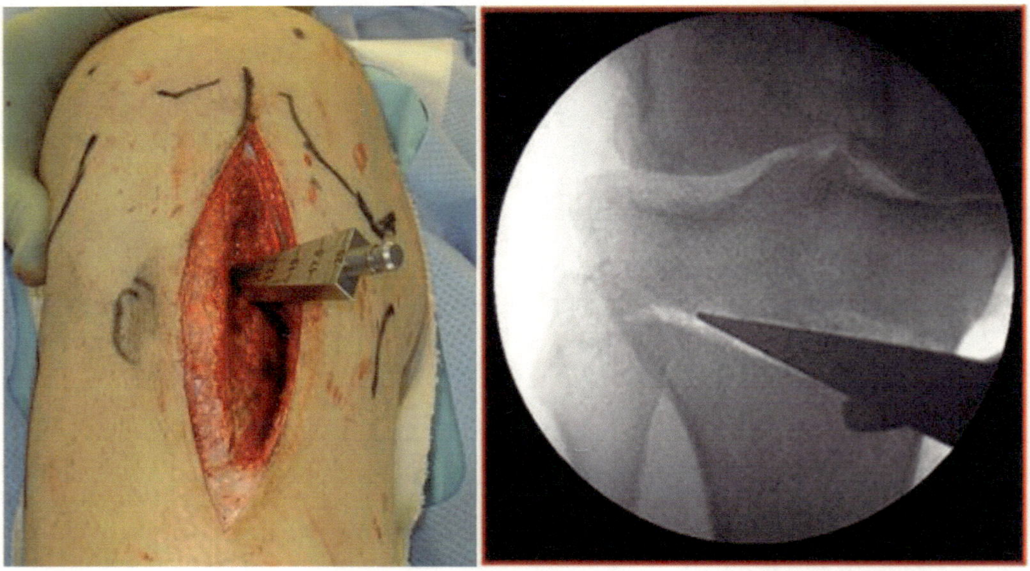

Fig. 10. When the osteotomy is completed, the medial tibia is opened with a wedge of suitable width.

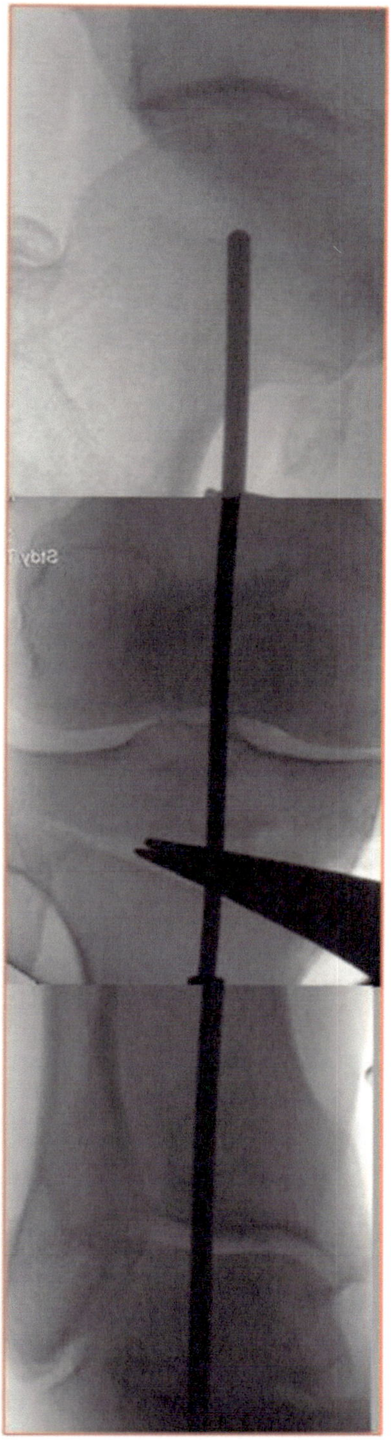

Fig. 11. An image intensifier and an alignment rod are used to control coronal and sagittal alignment during axial loading of the joint.

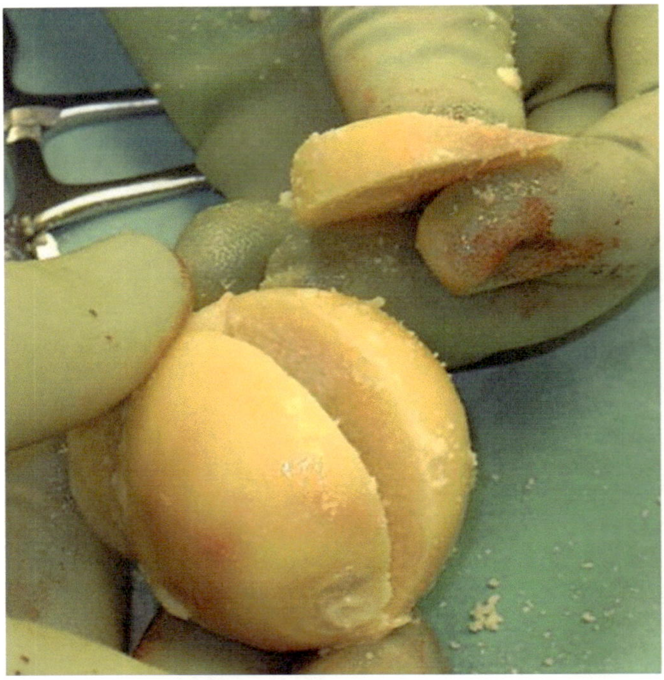

Fig. 12. To fill the osteotomy gap, a carefully shaped bone block from a donor is used.

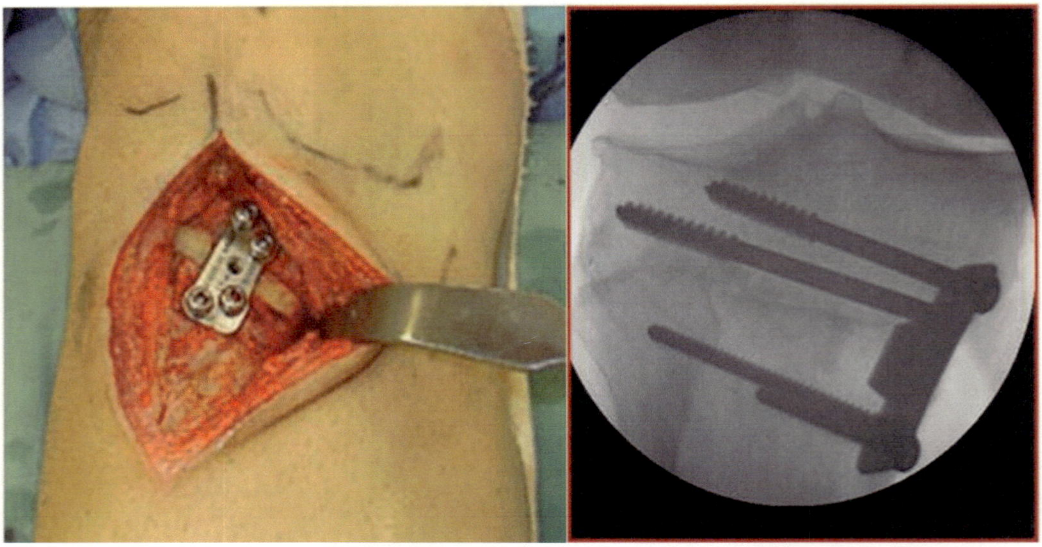

Fig. 13. When correction in the two planes is achieved, the osteotomy is stabilized using a plate with four screws.

Medial opening wedge HTO has some disadvantages like an unstable construct, implant failure, delayed union and nonunions. During surgery it is impossible to exactly predict the position of the mechanical axis during weight bearing, and an overcorrection may occur, requiring a revision surgery (Noyes et al., 2000).

If an external fixator is used, it is assembled preoperatively on the leg of the patient. Three rings, 4 cm larger than the diameter of the tibia, are used. The first is positioned at the level of the fibular head, the second 5 cm below the tibial tubercle, the third 3 cm proximal to the ankle joint. The first and the second ring are joined with 2 tethered rods and the second and the third rings are joined with 4 tethered rods. The proximal ring is held at an angle equal to the correction needed plus 5° (to give some overcorrection). The apparatus is then sterilized (Catagni et al., 1994). During surgery a tourniquet in not needed. A 3 cm incision is made 10 cm below the fibular head posterolaterally, the plane between soleus and peronei is developed and an oblique fibular osteotomy is performed with an oscillating saw. The external fixator is then applied to the leg of the patient and the first ring is stabilized with two wires and one half pin across the tibia. The second ring is stabilized with one wire and one half pin across the tibia, it is important to avoid to transfix the branches of the superficial peroneal nerve, so the wire should be placed slightly more laterally than the medial aspect of the tibia. The third ring is stabilized with two wires that pass across the tibia and the fibula in order to avoid a distal tibio-fibular subluxation. Then a 1.5 cm incision is performed anteriorly just distal to the tibial tuberosity, periosteum is elevated on both sides and a tibial osteotomy is performed with an oscillating saw, a drill, a Gigli saw or an osteotome. The required correction can be achieved acutely during surgery by rotating the first two rings until they are parallel to each other. Otherwise, if the osteotomy gap is too large, the correction can be performed gradually, beginning on the 7th-10th post-operative day, with emicallotaxis technique. The result is verified under image intensifier, a small amount of compression is performed, the rods are tightened and the skin is closed (Catagni et al., 1994; Klinger et al., 2001; Ohsawa et al., 2006; Viskontas et al., 2006).

8. Post-operative protocol

The patient should be encouraged not drinking alcohol or smoking. If a plate is used to stabilize the osteotomy, the knee is protected for six weeks in an articulated brace. During this period the patient makes exercises aimed to completely regain the Range Of Motion and reinforce the "Core stability" (Kibler et al., 2006). Only toe-touch gait with crutches is allowed. After six weeks, an X-Ray is performed and the patients is encouraged to increase progressively weight bearing until twelfth week, at that time a second X-Ray is recommended (Christel, 2003). If a circular external fixator is applied, partial weight bearing is allowed immediately without any brace (Catagni et al., 1994)

9. Conclusion

HTO is an effective and reliable procedure in the treatment of a PCL/PLC deficient knee associated to varus malalignment. If the knee is still unstable, soft tissue procedures should be performed 6-8 months after the correction of the malalignment. HTO allows the surgeon to modify both the coronal and the sagittal plane of the knee; an increased posterior tibial slope stabilizes the joint, reduces forces of posterolateral structures and on the posterior articular cartilage. However more biomechanical and clinical studies are needed in the future.

10. References

Agneskirchner, J.D.; Hurschler, C.; Stukenborg-Colsman, C.; Imhoff, A.B. & Lobenhoffer, P. (2004) Effect of high tibial flexion osteotomy on cartilage pressure and joint kinematics: a biomechanical study in human cadaveric knees. *Arch Orthop Trauma Surg*, Vol. 124, No. 9, (November), pp. 575-584, ISSN 0936-8051

Ahmad, C.S.; Cohen, Z.A.; Levine, W.N.; Gardner, T.R.; Ateshian, G.A. & Mow, V.C. (2003) Codominance of the individual posterior cruciate ligament bundles. An analysis of bundle lengths and orientation. *Am J Sports Med*, Vol. 31, No. 2, (March-April), pp. 221-225, ISSN 0363-5465

Amendola, A.; Rorabeck, C.H.; Bourne, R.B. & Apyan, P.M. (1989) Total knee arthroplasty following high tibial osteotomy for osteoarthritis. *J Arthroplasty, Vol. 4,* Suppl., pp. S11-S17, ISSN 0883-5403

Amis, A.A.; Gupte, C.M.; Bull, A.M. & Edwards, A. (2006) Anatomy of the posterior cruciate ligament and the meniscofemoral ligaments. *Knee Surg Sports Traumatol Arthrosc,*Vol. 14, No. 3 (March), pp. 257-263. Review, ISSN 0942-2056.

Akizuki, S.; Shibakawa, A.; Takizawa, T.; Yamazaki, I. & Horiuchi, H. (2008) The long-term outcome of high tibial osteotomy: a ten- to 20-year follow-up. *J Bone Joint Surg Br*, Vol. 90, No. 5 (May), pp. 592-596, ISSN 0301-620X

Badhe, N.P. & Forster, I.W. (2002) High tibial osteotomy in knee instability: the rationale of treatment and early results. *Knee Surg Sports Traumtol Arthros*, Vol. 10, No. 1 (January), pp. 38-43, ISSN 0942-2056

Barton, T.M.; Torg, J.S. & Das, M. (1984) Posterior cruciate ligament insufficiency. A review of the literature. *Sports Med*, Vol. 1, No. 6, (November-December), pp. 419-430. Review, ISSN 0112-1642

Bellelli, A.; Mancini, P.; Polito, M.; David, V. & Mariani, P.P. (2006) Magnetic resonance imaging of posterior cruciate ligament injuries: a new classification of traumatic tears. *Radiol Med*, Vol. 111, No. 6, (September), pp. 828-35, ISSN: 0033-8362.

Boileau, P. & Neyret P.H. (1991) Resultats des osteotomies tibialis de valgisation assoiees aux plasties du ligament croise' anterieur dans le traitment des laxites anterieures chronique evoluees. In: *7èmes journèes lyonnaises de chirurgie du genu*, Lyon, pp 232-249, ISBN 2853341550 9782853341554

Bonnin, M. (1990) La subluxation tibiale anterieure en appui monopodal dans les ruptures du ligament croise anterieur. Etude clinic et biomechanique (thesis). Lyon, France: Université Claude Bernard.

Brazier, J.; Migaud, H.; Gougeon, F.; Cotten, A.; Fontaine, C. & Duquennoy A. (1996) Evaluation of methods for radiographic measurement of the tibial slope. A study of 83 healthy knee. *Rev Chir Orthop Reparatrice Appar Mot*, Vol. 82, No. 3, pp. 195-200, ISSN 0035-1040

Catagni, M.A.; Guerreschi, F.; Ahmad, T.S. & Cattaneo, R. (1994) Treatment of genu varum in medial compartment osteoarthritis of the knee using the Ilizarov method. *Orthop Clin North Am*. Vol. 25, No. 3, (July), pp. 509-514, ISSN 0030-5898

Chang, A.; Hayes, K.; Dunlop, D.; Hurwitz, D.; Song, J.; Cahue, S.; Genge, R.; & Sharma L. (2004) Thrust during ambulation and the progression of knee osteoarthritis. *Arthritis Rheum*, Vol. 50, No. 12, (December), pp. 3897-3903, ISSN: 1529-0131

Chassaing, V.; Deltour, F.; Touzard, R.; Ceccaldi, J.P. & Miremad, C. (1995) Etude radiologique du L.C.P.'a 90 de flexion. *Rev Chir Orthop*, Vol. 81, pp. 35–38, ISSN 0035-1040

Chiu, K.Y.; Zhang, S.D. & Zhang, G.H. (2000) Posterior slope of tibial plateau in Chinese. *J Arthroplasty*, Vol. 15, No. 2 (February), pp. 224-227, ISSN 0883-5403

Christel P. (2003) Basic principles for surgical reconstruction of the PCL in chronic posterior knee instability. *Knee Surg Sports Traumatol Arthrosc,* Vol. 11, No. 5, (September), pp. 289-296. Review, ISSN 0942-2056

Cooper DE. (1991) Tests for posterolateral instability of the knee in normal subjects. *J Bone Joint Surg Am,* Vol. 73, No. 1, (January), pp 30–36, ISSN 1535-1386

Coventry, M.B.; Ilstrup, D.M. & Wallrichs, S.L. (1993) Proximal tibial osteotomy: A critical long-term study of eighty-seven cases. *J Bone Joint Surg Am,* Vol. 75, No. 2, (February), pp 196-201, ISSN 1535-1386

Cullù, E.; Aydogdu, S.; Alparslan, B. & Sur, H. (2005) Tibial slope changes following dome-type high tibial osteotomy. *Knee Surg Sports Traumatol Arthrosc,* Vol. 13, No. 1 (January), pp. 38-43, ISSN 0942-2056

Daniel, D.M.; Stone, M.L.; Barnett, P. & Sachs, R. (1988) Use of the quadriceps active test to diagnose posterior cruciate-ligament disruption and measure posterior laxity of the knee. *J Bone Joint Surg Am,* Vol. 70, No. 3, (March), pp. 386-391, ISSN 1535-1386

Dejour, H. & Bonnin, M. (1994) Tibial translation after anterior cruciate ligament rupture. Two radiological tests compared. *J Bone Joint Surg Br,* Vol. 76, No. 5, (September), pp. 745-749, ISSN 0301-620X

Dejour, H.; Neyret, P. & Bonnin, M. (1994) Instability and Osteoarthritis, in: *Knee Surgery.* Fu FH, Harner CD, Vince KG (eds), pp . 859-875, Williams & Wilkins, ISBN: 0683033891, Baltimore,

Dugdale, T.W.; Noyes, F.R. & Styer, D. (1992) Preoperative planning for high tibial osteotomy. The effect of lateral tibiofemoral separation and tibiofemoral length. *Clin Orthop Relat Res,* Vol. 274 (January), pp. 248-264. Review, ISSN 0009-921X

Fanelli, G.C. & Edson, C.J. (1995) Posterior cruciate ligament injuries in trauma patients: Part II. *Arthroscopy,* Vol. 11, No. 5, (October), pp. 526-529, ISSN 0749-8063

Fowler, P.J. & Messieh, S.S. (1987) Isolated posterior cruciate ligament injuries in athletes. *Am J Sports Med,* Vol. 15, No. 6, (November-December), pp. 553-557, ISSN 0363-5465

Fowler, P.J.; Kirkley, A. & Roe, J. (1994) Osteotomy of the proximal tibia in the treatment of chronic anterior cruciate ligament insufficiency. *J Bone Joint Surg Br,* Vol. 76, Supp 26, ISSN 0301-620X

Fujisawa, Y.; Masuhara, K.; Shiomi, S. (1979) The effect of high tibial osteotomy on osteoarthritis of the knee. An arthroscopic study of 54 knee joints. *Orthop Clin North Am,* Vol. 10, No. 3, (July), pp. 585-608, ISSN 0030-5898

Geissler, W.B. & Whipple, T.L. (1993) Intraarticular abnormalities in association with posterior cruciate ligament injuries. *Am J SportsMed,* Vol. 21, No. 6, (November-December), pp. 846-849, ISSN 0363-5465

Genin, P.; Weill, G. & Julliard, R. (1993) The tibial slope. Proposal for a measurement method. *J Radiol.* Vol. 74, No. 1, (January), pp. 27-33. Review.

Giffin, J.R.; Vogrin, T.M.; Zantop, T.; Woo, S.L. & Harner, C.D. (2004) Effects of increasing tibial slope on the biomechanics of the knee. *Am J Sports Med.* Vol. 32, No. 2, (March), pp. 376-382, ISSN 0363-5465

Giffin, J.R.; Stabile, K.J.; Zantop, T.; Vogrin, T.M.; Woo, S.L. & Harner, C.D. (2007) Importance of Tibial Slope for Stability of the Posterior Cruciate Ligament-Deficient Knee. *Am J Sports Med,* Vol. 35, No. 9,)September), pp. 1443-1449, ISSN 0363-5465

Goradia, V.K. & Van Allen, J. (2002) Chronic lateral knee instability treated with a high tibial osteotomy. *Arthroscopy,* Vol. 18, No. 7, (September), pp. 807-811, ISSN 0749-8063

Gross, M.L.; Grover, J.S.; Bassett, L.W.; Seeger, L.L. & Finerman, G.A. (1992) Magnetic resonance imaging of the posterior cruciate ligament. Clinical use to improve diagnostic accuracy. *Am J Sports Med,* Vol. 20, No. 6, (November-December), pp. 732-737, ISSN 0363-5465

Hamada, M.; Shino, K.; Mitsuoka, T.; Toritsuka, Y.; Natsu-Ume, T. & Horibe, S. (2000) Chondral injury associated with acute isolated posterior cruciate ligament injury. *Arthroscopy,* Vol. 16, No. 1, (January-February), pp. 59-63, ISSN 0749-8063

Hernigou, P.; Medevielle, D.; Debeyre, J. & Goutallier, D. (1987) Proximal tibial osteotomy for osteoarthritis with varus deformity. A ten to thirteen-year follow-up study. *J Bone Joint Surg Am,* Vol. 69, No. 3, (March), pp. 332-354, ISSN 1535-1386

Hoher, J.; Harner, C.D.; Vogrin, T.M.; Baek, G.H.; Carlin, G.J. & Woo, S.L. (1998) In situ forces in the posterolateral structures of the knee under posterior tibial loading in the intact and posterior cruciate ligament-deficient knee. *J Orthop Res,* Vol. 16, No. 6, (November), pp. 675-681, ISSN 1554-527X

Hohmann, E.; Bryant, A. & Imhoff, A.B. (2006) The effect of closed wedge high tibial osteotomy on tibial slope: a radiographic study. *Knee Surg Sports Traumatol Arthrosc,* Vol. 14, No. 5, (May), pp. 454-459, ISSN 0942-2056

Hoppenfeld, S.; deBoer, P. (2003) The Tibia and Fibula. In: *Surgical Exposures in Orthopaedics: The Anatomic Approach, 3rd Edition,* Lippincott Williams & Wilkins, ISBN-10: 0781742285

Hughston, J.C.; Andrews, J.R.; Cross, M.J. & Moschi, A. (1976) Classification of knee ligament instabilities: Part II. The lateral compartment. *J Bone Joint Surg Am,* Vol. 58, No. 2, (March), pp.173-179, ISSN 1535-1386

Hughston, J.C. & Norwood, L.A. Jr. (1980) The posterolateral drawer test and external rotational recurvatum test for posterolateral rotatory instability of the knee. *Clin Orthop Relat Res,* Vol. 147, (March-April), pp. 82-87, ISSN 0009-921X

Insall, J.N.; Joseph, D.M. & Msika, C. (1984) High tibial osteotomy for varus gonarthrosis. A long-term follow-up study. *J Bone Joint Surg Am,* Vol. 66, No. 7, (September), pp. 1040-1048, ISSN 1535-1386

Insall, J.N. (1993) Total knee arthroplasty in rheumatoid arthritis. *Ryumachi,* Vol. 33, No. 6, (December), pp. 472, ISSN 0300-9157

Jakob, R.P.; Hassler, H. & Staubli, H.U. (1981) Observations on rotator instability of the lateral compartment of the knee. Experimental studies of the functional anatomy and pathomechanism of the true and reverse pivot shift sign. *Acta Orthop Scand Suppl,* Vol. 191, pp. 1–32, ISSN 0001-6470

Jacobsen, K. (1976) Stress radiographical measurement of the anteroposterior, medial and lateral stability of the knee joint. *Acta Orthop Scand,* Vol. 47, No, 3, (June), pp. 335-4, ISSN 0001-6470

Jung, T.M.; Reinhardt, C.; Scheffler, S.U. & Weiler, A. (2006) Stress radiography to measure posterior cruciate ligament insufficiency: a comparison of five different techniques. *Knee Surg Sports Traumatol Arthrosc,* Vol. 14, No. 11, (November), pp. 1116-1121, ISSN 0942-2056

Kibler, W.B.; Press, J. & Sciascia A. (2006) The role of core stability in athletic function. *Sports Med,* Vol. 36, No. 3, pp. 189-198, ISSN 0112-1642

Klinger, H.M.; Lorenz, F.; Harer, T. (2001) Open wedge tibial osteotomy by hemicallotasis for medial compartment osteoarthritis. *Arch Orthop Trauma Surg,* Vol. 121, No. 5, (May), pp. 245-247, ISSN 0936-8051

Kumagai, M.; Mizuno, Y.; Mattessich, S.M.; Elias, J.J.; Cosgarea, A.J. & Chao, E.Y. (2002) Posterior cruciate ligament rupture alters in vitro knee kinematics. *Clin Orthop Relat Res,* Vol. 395, pp. 241-248, ISSN 0009-921X

Krudwig, W.K.; Witzel, U. & Ullrich, K. (2002) Posterolateral aspect and stability of the knee joint. II. Posterolateral instability and effect of isolated and combined posterolateral reconstruction on knee stability: a biomechanical study. *Knee Surg Sports Traumatol Arthrosc,* Vol. 10, No. 2, (March), pp. 91-95, ISSN 0942-2056

LaPrade, R.F. & Terry, G.C. (1997) Injuries to the posterolateral aspect of the knee: association of anatomic injury patterns with clinical instability. *Am J Sports Med,* Vol. 25, No. 4, (July-August), pp. 433–438, ISSN 0363-5465

LaPrade, R.F.; Gilbert, T.J.; Bollom, T.S.; Wentorf, F. & Chaljub, G. (2000) The magnetic resonance imaging appearance of individual structures of the posterolateral knee. A prospective study of normal knees and knees with surgically verified grade III injuries. *Am J Sports Med,* Vol. 28, No. 2, (March-April), pp. 191–199, ISSN 0363-5465

LaPrade, R.F. & Wentorf, F. (2002) Diagnosis and treatment of posterolateral knee injuries. *Clin Orthop Relat Res,* Vol. 402, (September), pp. 110-121. Review, ISSN 0009-921X

Lattermann, C. & Jakob, R.P. (1996) High tibial osteotomy alone or combined with ligament reconstruction in anterior cruciate ligament-deficient knees. *Knee Surg Sports Traumatol Arthrosc,* Vol. 4, No. 1, pp. 32-38, ISSN 0942-2056

Lecuire, F.; Lerat, J.L.; Bousquet, G.; Dejour, H. & Trillat, A. (1980) The treatment of genu recurvatum. *Rev Chir Orthop Reparatrice Appar Mot,* Vol. 66, No. 2, (March), pp. 95-103, ISSN 0035-1040

Lephart, S.M.; Pincivero, D.M. & Rozzi, S.L. (1998) Proprioception of the ankle and knee. *Sports Med,* Vol. 25, No. 3, (March), pp. 149-155. Review, ISSN 0112-1642

Lerat, J.L.; Moyen, B.; Garin, C.; Mandrino, A.; Besse, J.L. & Brunet-Guedj, E. (1993) Anterior laxity and internal arthritis of the knee. Results of the reconstruction of the anterior cruciate ligament associated with tibial osteotomy. *Rev Chir Orthop Reparatrice Appar Mot,* Vol. 79, No. 5, pp. 365-374, ISSN 0035-1040

Levigne, C.H. & Bonnin, M. (1991) Osteotomie tibiale de valgisation pour arthrose femoro-tibale interne. In: *7èmes journees lyonnaise de chirurgie du genu,* Lyon, pp 142-168, ISBN 2853341550 9782853341554

Li, G.; Gill, T.J.; DeFrate, L.E.; Zayontz, S.; Glatt, V. & Zarins, B. (2002) Biomechanical consequences of PCL deficiency in the knee under simulated muscle loads-an in vitro experimental study. *J Orthop Res,* Vol. 20, No. 4, (July), pp. 887-892, ISSN 1554-527X

Loomer, R.L. (1991) A test for knee posterolateral rotatory instability. *Clin Orthop Relat Res,* Vol. 264, (March), pp. 235-238, ISSN 0009-921X

Louisia, S.; Siebold, R.; Canty, J. & Bartlett, R.J. (2005) Assessment of posterior stability in total knee replacement by stress radiographs: prospective comparison of two different types of mobile bearing implants. *Knee Surg Sports Traumatol Arthrosc,* Vol. *13, No.* 6, (September), pp. 476–48, ISSN 0942-2056

Maquet, P. Valgus osteotomy for osteoarthritis of the knee. (1976) *Clin Orthop Relat Res,* Vol. 120, (October), pp. 143-148, ISSN 0009-921X

Margheritini, F.; Mancini, L.; Mauro, C.S.; Mariani, P.P. (2003) Stress radiography for quantifying posterior cruciate ligament deficiency. *Arthroscopy,* Vol. 19, No. 7, (September), pp. 706-711, ISSN 0749-8063

Marti, C.B.; Gautier, E.; Wachtl, S.W. & Jakob, R.P. (2004) Accuracy of frontal and sagittal plane correction in open-wedge high tibial osteotomy. *Arthroscopy,* Vol. 20, No. 4, (April), pp. 366-372. Review, ISSN 0749-8063

Matsuda, S.; Miura, H.; Nagamine, R.; Urabe, K.; Ikenoue, T.; Okazaki, K. & Iwamoto, Y. (1999) Posterior tibial slope in the normal and varus knee. *Am J Knee Surg,* Vol. 12, No. 3, pp. 165-168, ISSN 0899-7403

Mayo Robson, A.W. (1903) Ruptured cruciate ligament and their repair by operation. *Ann Surg Engl.* Vol. 37, No. 5, (May), pp.716-718, ISSN 0003-4932

Merchant, A.C.; Mercer, R.L.; Jacobsen, R.H. & Cool, C.R. (1974) Roentgenographic analysis of patellofemoral congruence. *J Bone Joint Surg Am,* Vol. 56, No. 7, (October), pp. 1391-1396, ISSN 1535-1386

Miller, M.D.; Cooper, D.E.; Fanelli, G.C.; Harner, C.D. & LaPrade, R.F. (2002) Posterior cruciate ligament: current concepts. *Instr Course Lect,* Vol. 51, pp. 347-351. Review, ISSN 0065-6895

Moore, T.M. & Harvey, J.P. Jr. (1974) Roentgenographic measurement of tibial-plateau depression due to fracture. *J Bone Joint Surg Am,* Vol. 56, No. 1, (January), pp. 155-160, ISSN 1535-1386

Moreland, J.R.; Bassett, L.W. & Hanker, G.J. (1987) Radiographic analysis of the axial alignment of the lower extremity. *J Bone Joint Surg Am,* Vol. 69, No. 5, (June), pp. 745-749, ISSN 1535-1386

Nagel, A.; Insall, J.N. & Scuderi, G.R. (1996) Proximal tibial osteotomy: A subjective outcome study. *J Bone Joint Surg Am,* Vol. 78, No. 9, (September), pp. 1353-1358, ISSN 1535-1386

Nakamura, E.; Mizuta, H.; Kudo, S.; Takagi, K. & Sakamoto, K. (2001) Open-wedge osteotomy of the proximal tibia hemicallotasis. *J Bone Joint Surg Br,* Vol. 83, No. 8, (November), pp. 1111-1115, ISSN 0301-620X

Naudie, D.D.; Amendola, A. & Fowler, P.J. (1994) Opening wedge high tibial osteotomy for symptomatic hyperextension-varus thrust. *Am J Sports Med,* Vol. 32, No.1, (January-February), pp. 60-70, ISSN 0363-5465

Naudie, D.D.; Bourne, R.B.; Rorabeck, C.H. & Bourne, T.J. (1999) The Install Award. Survivorship of the high tibial valgus osteotomy. A 10- to -22-year followup study. *Clin Orthop Relat Res,* Vol. 367, (October), pp.18-27, ISSN 0009-921X

Neuschwander, D.C.; Drez, D. Jr. & Paine, R.M. (1993) Simultaneous high tibial osteotomy and ACL reconstruction for combined genu varum and symptomatic ACL tear. *Orthopedics,* Vol. 16, No. 6, (June), pp. 679-684, ISSN 0147-7447

Neyret, P.; Donell, S.T. & Dejour, H. (1993) Results of partial meniscectomy related to the state of the anterior cruciate ligament. Review at 20 to 35 years. *J Bone Joint Surg Br,* Vol. 75, No. 1, (January), pp. 36-40, ISSN 0301-620X

Noyes, F.R.; Barber-Westin, S.D. & Simon, R. (1993) High tibial osteotomy and ligament reconstruction in varus angulated, anterior cruciate ligament-deficient knees. A two-to-seven year follow-up study. *Am J Sports Med,* Vol. 21, No. 1, (January-February), pp. 2-12, ISSN 0363-5465

Noyes, F.R. & Simon, R. (1994) The role of high tibial osteotomy in the anterior cruciate ligament-deficient knee with varus alignment, In: *Orthopaedic Sports Medicine. Principles and Practice,* DeLee J.C. & Drez D, pp 1401-1443, WB Saunders, ISBN-10: 0721688454, Philadelphia,

Noyes, F.R.; Dunworth, L.A.; Andriacchi, T.P.; Andrews, M. & Hewett, T.E. (1996) Knee hyperextension gait abnormalities in unstable knees. Recognition and preoperative gait retraining. *Am J Sports Med,* Vol. 24, No. 1, (January-February), pp. 35-45, ISSN 0363-5465

Noyes, F.R.; Barber-Westin, S.D. & Hewett, T.E. (2000) High tibial osteotomy and ligament reconstruction for varus angulated anterior cruciate ligament-deficient knees. *Am J Sports Med,* Vol. 28, No. 3, (May-June), pp. 282-296, ISSN 0363-5465

Noyes, F.R.; Barber-Westin, S.D. & Rankin, M. (2004) Meniscal transplantation in symptomatic patients less than fifty years old. *J Bone Joint Surg Am,* Vol. 86, No. 7, (July), pp. 1392-1404, ISSN 1535-1386

Noyes, F.R.; Goebel, S.X. & West, J. (2005) Opening wedge tibial osteotomy: the 3-triangle method to correct axial alignment and tibial slope. *Am J Sports Med,* Vol. 33, No. 3, (March), pp. 378-387, ISSN 0363-5465

Ochi, M.; Murao, T.; Sumen, Y.; Kobayashi, K. & Adachi, N. (1999) Isolated posterior cruciate ligament insufficiency induces morphological changes of anterior cruciate ligament collagen fibrils. *Arthroscopy,* Vol. 15, No. 3, (April), pp. 292-296, ISSN 0749-8063

Odenbring, S.; Egund, N.; Lindstrand, A.; Lohmander, L.S. & Willen, H. (1992) Cartilage regeneration after proximal tibial osteotomy for medial gonarthrosis. An arthroscopic, roentgenographic, and histologic study. *Clin Orthop Relat Res,* Vol. 277, (April), pp. 210-216, ISSN 0009-921X

Ohsawa, S.; Hukuda, K.; Inamori, Y. & Yasui, N. (2006) High tibial osteotomy for osteoarthritis of the knee with varus deformity utilizing the hemicallotasis method. *Arch Orthop Trauma Surg,* Vol. 126, No. 9, (November), pp. 588-593, ISSN 0936-8051

Paessler, H.H. & Michel, D. (1992) How new is the Lachman test? *Am J Sports Med,* Vol. 20, No. 1, (January-February), pp. 95-98, ISSN 0363-5465

Paley, D.R. (2002) *Principles of Deformity Correction,* Springer-Verlag, ISBN 3-540-41665-X, Berlin.

Paley, D.R.; Herzenberg, J.E.; Tetsworth, K.; McKie, J. & Bhave, A. (1994) Deformity planning for frontal and sagittal plane corrective osteotomies. *Orthop Clin North Am,* Vol. 25, No 3, (July), pp. 425-465. Review, ISSN 0030-5898

Palmer, I. (1938) On injuries the ligaments of the knee joint. A clinical study. *Acta Chir Scand* Suppl, Vol. 53, pp. 282, ISSN 0301-1860

Petrigliano, F.A.; McAllister, D.R. (2006) Isolated Posterior Cruciate Ligament Injuries of the Knee. *Sports Med Arthrosc Rev,* Vol. 14, No. 4, (December), pp. 206–212, ISSN 1062-8592

Puddu, G.; Gianni, E.; Chambat, P. & De Paulis, F. (2000) The axial view in evaluating tibial translation in cases of insufficiency of the posterior cruciate ligament. *Arthroscopy,* Vol. 16, No. 2, (March), pp. 217-220, ISSN 0749-8063

Puddu, G.; Cipolla, M.; Cerullo, G.; Franco, V. & Gianni E. (2007) Osteotomies: the surgical treatment of the valgus knee. *Sports Med Arthrosc,* Vol. 15, No. 1, (March), pp. 15-22. Review, ISSN 1062-8592

Ramaniraka, N.A.; Terrier, A.; Theumann, N. & Siegrist, O. (2005) Effects of the posterior cruciate ligament reconstruction on the biomechanics of the knee joint: a finite element analysis. *Clin Biomech (Bristol, Avon),* Vol. 20, No. 4, (May), pp. 434-442, ISBN/ISSN 02680033

Rodner, C.M.; Adams, D.J.; Diaz-Doran, V.; Tate, J.P.; Santangelo, S.A.; Mazzocca, A.D. & Arciero, R.A. (2006) Medial opening wedge tibial osteotomy and the sagittal plane:

the effect of increasing tibial slope on tibiofemoral contact pressure. *Am J Sports Med,* Vol. 34, No. 9, (September), pp. 1431-1441, ISSN 0363-5465

Rosenberg, T.D.; Paulos, L.E.; Parker, R.D.; Coward, D.B. & Scott, S.M. (1988) The forty-five-degree posteroanterior flexion weight-bearing radiograph of the knee. *J Bone Joint Surg Am,* Vol. 70, No. 10, (December), pp. 1479-1483, ISSN 1535-1386

Rubinstein, R.A. Jr.; Shelbourne, K.D.; McCarroll, J.R.; VanMeter, C.D. & Rettig, A.C. (1994) The accuracy of the clinical examination in the setting of posterior cruciate ligament injuries. *Am J Sports Med,* Vol. 22, No. 4, (July-August), pp. 550-557, ISSN 0363-5465

Safran, M.R.; Allen, A.A.; Lephart, S.M.; Borsa, P.A.; Fu, F.H. & Harner, CD. (1999) Proprioception in the posterior cruciate ligament deficient knee. *Knee Surg Sports Traumatol Arthrosc,* Vol. 7, No. 5, pp. 310-317, ISSN 0942-2056

Seebacher, J.R.; Inglis, A.E.; Marshall, J.L. & Warren, R.F. (1982) The structure of the posterolateral aspect of the knee. *J Bone Joint Surg Am,* Vol. 64, No. 4, (April), pp. 536-541, ISSN 1535-1386

Skyhar, M.J.; Warren, R.F.; Ortiz, G.J.; Schwartz, E. & Otis, J.C. (1993) The effects of sectioning of the posterior cruciate ligament and the posterolateral complex on the articular contact pressures within the knee. *J Bone Joint Surg Am,* Vol. 75, No. 5, (May), pp. 694-699, ISSN 1535-1386

Staubli, H.U. & Jakob, R.P. (1990) Posterior instability of the knee extension. A clinical and stress radiographic analysis of acute injuries of the posterior cruciate ligament. *J Bone Joint Surg Br,* Vol. 72, No. 2, (March), pp. 225-230, ISSN 0301-620X

Strobel, M.; Stedtfeld, H.W.; Feagia, J.A. & Telger, T.C. (1990) *Diagnostic evaluation of the knee,* Springer-Verlag, ISBN-10: 3540507108, New York

Strobel, M.J.; Weiler, A. & Eichhorn HJ. (2000) Diagnosis and therapy of fresh and chronic posterior cruciate ligament lesions: *Chirurg,* Vol. 71, No. 9, (September), pp. 1066-1081. Review, ISSN 0009-4722

Strobel, M.J.; Weiler, A.; Schulz, M.S.; Russe, K. & Eichhorn, H.J. (2002) Fixed posterior subluxation in posterior cruciate ligament-deficient knees: diagnosis and treatment of a new clinical sign. *Am J Sports Med,* Vol. 30, No. 1, (January-February), pp. 32-38, ISSN 0363-5465

Takahashi, M.; Matsubara, T.; Doi, M.; Suzuki, D. & Nagano A. (2006) Anatomical study of the femoral and tibial insertions of the anterolateral and posteromedial bundles of human posterior cruciate ligament. *Knee Surg Sports Traumatol Arthrosc,* Vol. 14, No. 11, (November), pp. 1055-1059, ISSN 0942-2056

Veltri, D.M. & Warren, R.F. (1994) Anatomy, biomechanics, and physical findings in posterolateral knee instability. *Clin Sports Med,* Vol. 13, No. 3, (July), pp. 599-614. Review, ISSN 0112-1642

Viskontas, D.G.; MacLeod, M.D. & Sanders, D.W. (2006) High tibial osteotomy with use of the Taylor Spatial Frame external fixator for osteoarthritis of the knee. *Can J Surg,* Vol. 49, No. 4, (August), pp. 245-250, ISSN 0008-428X

Watanabe, K.; Tsuchiya, H.; Matsubara, H.; Kitano, S. & Tomita, K. (2008) Revision high tibial osteotomy with the Taylor spatial frame for failed opening-wedge high tibial osteotomy. *J Orthop Sci,* Vol. 13, No. 2, (March), pp. 145-149, ISSN 0949-2658

Yu, J.S.; Salonen, D.C.; Hodler, J.; Haghighi, P.; Trudell, D. & Resnick, D. (1996) Posterolateral aspect of the knee: improved MR imaging with a coronal oblique technique. *Radiology,* Vol. 198, No. 1, pp. 199-204, ISSN 0033-8419

Part 5

Wrist

12

Three-Dimensional Computer-Assisted Corrective Osteotomy Techniques for the Malunited Distal Radius

Joy C. Vroemen and Simon D. Strackee
Department of Plastic, Reconstructive and Hand Surgery,
Academic Medical Center,
University of Amsterdam,
The Netherlands

1. Introduction

A corrective osteotomy is a frequently required procedure for symptomatic malunions of the distal radius. A multitude of different methods have been proposed for correction of distal radius malunions. However, precise correction of a severe malunion that requires simultaneous adjustment of displacement and rotation in multiple planes remains a challenge. Technological advancements have resulted in improved techniques to perform radial corrective osteotomy. In the last few decades a number of computer-assisted techniques have been proposed. Computer-assisted surgery with the use of three-dimensional (3D) pre-operative planning offers multiple advantages. 3D imaging and reconstructions are more intuitive and show details that cannot be observed from two-dimensional (2D) radiographs. This chapter describes and discusses current techniques in computer-assisted corrective osteotomy techniques of the malunited distal radius.

1.1 Malunion of the distal radius

A small number of distal radius fractures results in a symptomatic malunion of the bone. However, because the fracture of the distal radius is the most common fracture in the upper limb, the absolute number of symptomatic malunited distal radii is considerably large. (Cooney et al, 1980; Menon et al, 2008; Solgaard & Petersen, 1985) Symptoms of a malunited radius may include pain, reduced range of motion, reduced grip strength, carpal instability and eventually osteoarthritis. (Cheng et al, 2008; Crisco et al, 2007) Pain and other symptoms have various causes.

Malalignment of the distal radius segment after trauma contributes in most of the cases to a loss of the normal palmar tilt and radial inclination. This leads to a wrong position of the sigmoid notch, which can result in pain and limited forearm rotation, whereby the patient is less able to perform pronation or supination. The mismatch between sigmoid notch and the ulna also causes an adaptive position of the carpus. Carpal malalignment following the malunited distal radial fracture is described to develop as an adaptation to realign the position of the hand to the malunion (Gupta et al., 2002) and may contribute to carpal instability. Changes in the sigmoid notch and thus the DRU joint mechanics are involved in the dysfunction associated with malunion of the distal radius. (Crisco et al., 2007) Clinical studies have shown that poor clinical outcomes are associated with malunited distal radius fractures that heal with more than 20° of dorsal tilt or loss of more than 10° of radial inclination (Kihara et al, 1996), especially in young, manually active patients.

Another problem in malunions of the radius is the shortening of the radial bone, which leads to a positive ulnar variance. This may cause ulnar abutment. In the treatment of the malunited distal radius, it is important to take the relationship between the lengths of the radius and ulna into account.

If the patient has severe complaints that seem to belong to the malunion of the distal radius, a corrective osteotomy can be performed to reduce the pain and improve the function. The goal of a corrective osteotomy is to restore the original position of the distal radius segment and thus the original anatomical relationships in the wrist.

It is shown that there is a correlation between the accuracy of the anatomical reconstruction of the wrist and its function. (Brogren et al., 2011; Pogue et al., 1990) To increase accuracy in the corrective osteotomy of the radius, accurate pre-operative planning is important.

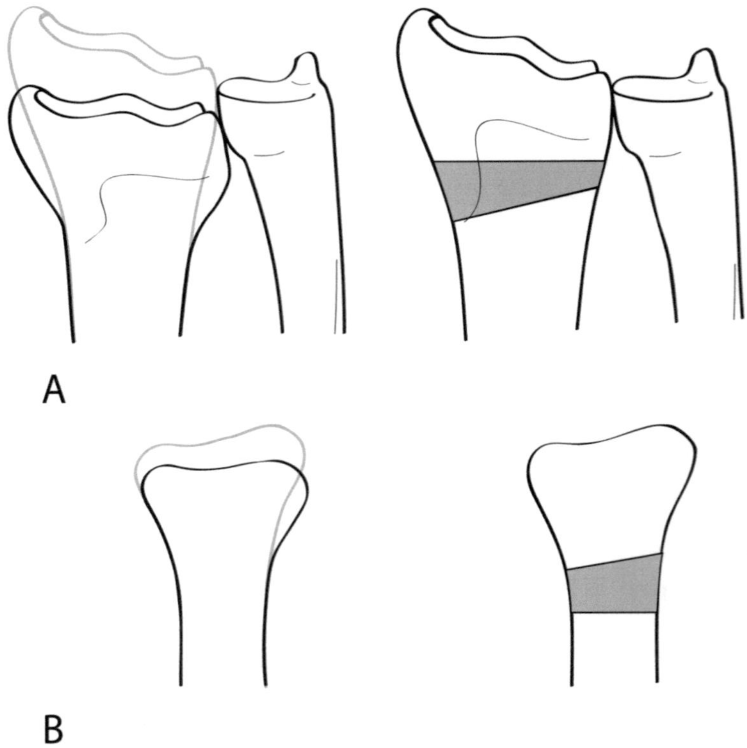

Fig. 1. Schematic representation of the corrective osteotomy procedure of the malunited distal radius. Fig. 1A shows the posterior-anterior view and Fig. 1B the lateral view of the wrist. The left side represents the malunited situation and on the right side the corrected situation is displayed.

1.2 Conventional techniques for radial corrective osteotomy

In the conventional technique, the pre-operative planning of a corrective osteotomy of the radius is done on plain 2D radiographs of the malunited radius. The planning is based on three radiographically obtained parameters: the radial inclination, palmar tilt and ulnar variance. These parameters are used to assess the shape of the supporting bone graft pre-operatively. In early surgery, average values of population data of these parameters were used for surgical planning, and subsequent techniques use the radiograph of the contralateral arm as a reference for planning and restoring the malunited distal radius.

The procedure involves cutting the malunited distal radius near its original fracture site and restoring the original position of the distal radius segment (Fig. 1). The new situation is often supported by a wedge-shaped bone graft or bone substitute, followed by fixation of the osseous structures with a fracture-fixation plate. Sometimes no supporting structures are used, and the fixation is by a fixed-angle fracture-fixation plate alone.

1.3 Computer-assisted radial corrective osteotomy

Since there is a correlation between the accuracy of the reconstruction of the radius and the eventual wrist function, it is important to restore the original position of the distal radius segment as accurate as possible. Lately, the reliability of measurements on 2D radiographs is frequently questioned in the literature. The radiographic parameters are hampered by inter- en intra-observer variations and overprojection, which hides rotations around the longitudinal axis of the bone. (Capo et al., 2009; Pennock et al., 2005) When planning a corrective osteotomy, these limitations of 2D imaging may cause a misinterpretation of the correction parameters. Six parameters are required for optimal planning of repositioning the radial distal segment: three displacements and three rotations around three axes. Therefore 3D planning should be used in performing a corrective osteotomy. This allows correction of all six repositioning parameters, not only the shortening and the angulations seen on 2D radiographs.

In the last few decades a number of 3D computer-assisted techniques have been proposed for corrective surgery. In these new techniques the malunited radius is restored with the help of the unaffected mirrored contralateral radius, which serves as a reference. Because the surgeon has no information about the former position of the radius and does not want to differ too much from the original anatomy, the only reference is currently the contralateral healthy radius. In that way there is an objective goal for the computer-assisted pre-operative planning.

The procedure of a corrective osteotomy for the malunited distal radius experienced major technological advancements in the last decade. This chapter gives a chronological overview of the different computer-assisted techniques for the planning and treatment of radial corrective osteotomy that are described in the literature so far.

2. Current computer-assisted techniques

Most computer-assisted corrective osteotomy techniques use the mirrored image of the unaffected contralateral radius as a template for the affected side. A computer-assisted planning procedure is divided into different phases. The first phase is data collection through imaging, the second phase is creation of virtual 3D models and performing a virtual osteotomy on the affected radius. By matching a proximal and distal segment of the virtual affected radius with the virtual healthy radius, the required position of the distal segment of the affected radius after the osteotomy is calculated. This is the preoperative plan. The third and last phase is the translation of the preoperative plan to the operating room. Computer-assisted techniques have different ways to perform each phase but every technique will have to go through these three phases.

2.1 The BIZCAD method

In 1988 Bilic and Zdravkovic presented a computer-aided planning method for preoperative planning of corrective osteotomy of malunited fractures of the radius. (Bilic & Zdravkovic, 1988a, 1988b) Conventional orthogonal radiographs are used and the goal of the whole procedure is to make the entire procedure as simple as possible, and to make preoperative planning decisions easy and objective. Bizcad is a computer-aided preoperative planning method which provides 3D wire models of bones. From these models the dimensions of the required bone graft and the amount and direction of angulation and translation at the osteotomy can be calculated.

Two plain radiographs are taken from both the affected and the unaffected wrist. From these radiographs, wire models of the distal end of the radius of both hands are constructed and presented in a Cartesian coordinate system with a one-millimeter raster. A null coordinate system point is defined on both projection radiographs of both hands. In this way the lateral and the posterior-anterior view can be linked. Fourteen points are recognized on both views and used as vertex points for a model reconstruction. These points were typical landmarks such as the top of the styloid process, the volar edge of the ulnar notch, and points along the osteotomy line. (Fig. 2A) These reference points of the distal end of the radius were used to generate a computer wire model. (Fig. 2B) After determination of axis lines, vertex points and an osteotomy line, the coordinates were measured and data was processed with a computer. Models of both wrists are constructed and the model of the unaffected radius is mirrored to serve as a reference for the affected side. The model of the part of the radius where the osteotomy is to be made can now be interactively translated and rotated by the surgeon until the point of best fit to the healthy radius model is reached. After this, the shape and measurements of the bone graft needed are calculated and displayed.

This method seems more precise than the conventional planning method of two radiographs and three radiographic parameters. In the conventional corrective osteotomy, when planning a surgical procedure, the surgeon passes from one radiographic view to the other and no allowance is made for the fact that changes in the lateral view imply changes in the anterior-posterior view. The Bizcad method solves this problem. Disadvantages are a complicated planning procedure and an incomplete solution for problems concerning rotational deviations of the distal radius fragment. The system is unable to provide intraoperative guidance and represents details poorly. An advantage of this method is that plain radiographs keep the procedure cheap and simple.

2.2 Computer generated solid plastic bone models

In 1992 Jupiter et al. reported on computer-assisted design and a manufacturing technology to create solid plastic models of complex, multidirectional malunions of the distal radius.

(Jupiter et al., 1992) By the ability to perform the surgical procedure on these models preoperatively, the intention is to enhance the preoperative planning. In this method patients underwent CT scans of both wrists. CT image data are reformatted and transferred to a computer numerically controlled milling machine, which creates a master model that is used to produce plastic models of the malunion and also of the opposite uninjured side. The distal ulna and carpal bones are included in these models. (Fig. 3) The surgical procedure can be readily performed on these solid models. In addition to provide a hands-on exercise for the surgical team, the dimensions of the required bone graft, the size and shape of the internal fixation, and the potential for articular realignment can be visually appreciated. The preoperative solid models make it possible to have a better understanding of the 3D nature of the malunion, especially if there is a malrotation present. Rotational correction can be judged by comparison with the model of the unaffected radius.

An advantage is the availability of a true-to-life 3D appreciation of the deformity. A disadvantage is the extra cost due to the CT scan and producing the solid models. The authors recommend that this method should only be used in cases of unusually complex, multidirectional deformities in which it proves difficult to gain a 3D understanding from plain radiographs.

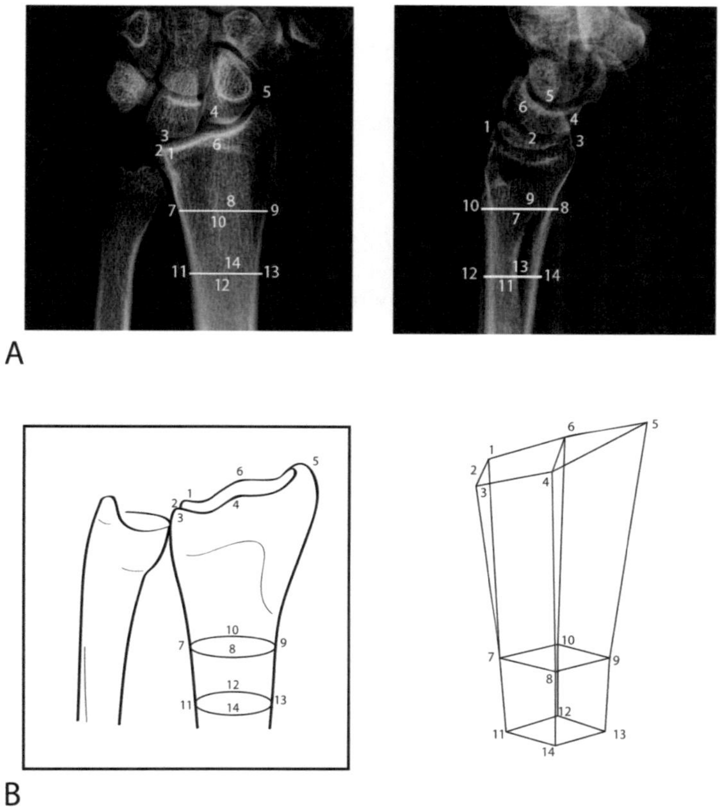

Fig. 2. Reference points of the distal radius segment on two projections for the computer wire model generation are shown on Fig. 2A. Fig. 2B represents the creation of the wire model. This image represents a healthy left wrist. (Method described by Bilic & Zdravkovic et al.)

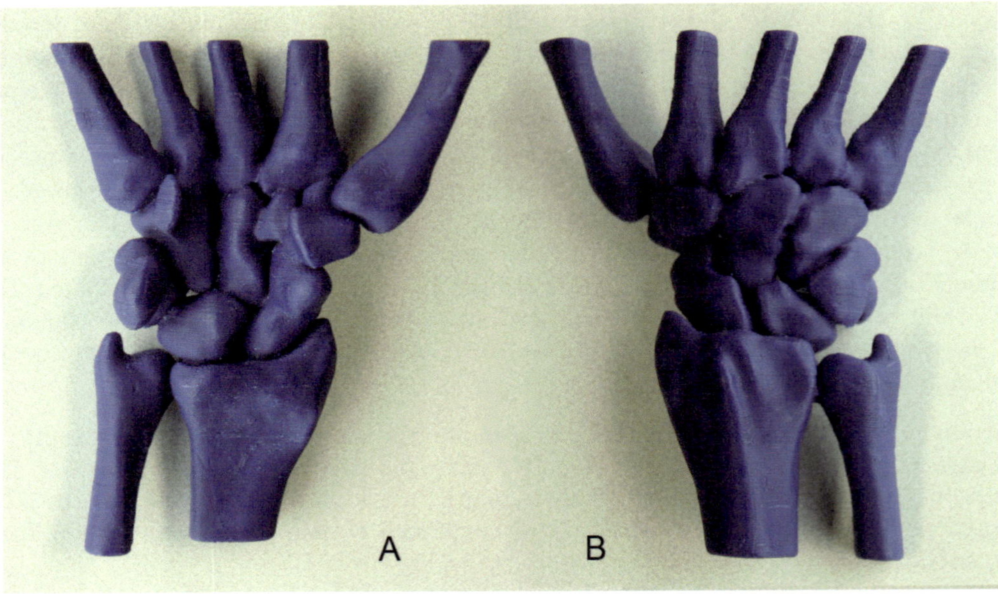

Fig. 3. An example of a computer generated solid plastic bone model of a healthy wrist joint. Fig. 3A is the view of the volar side and Fig. 3B of the dorsal side.

2.3 Computer-assisted fixation-based surgery

In 2001 and 2003 a fixation-based 3D preoperative planner and an intraoperative guidance system for distal radius osteotomy was introduced. (Croitoru et al., 2001; Athwal et al., 2003) Fixation-based surgery is a technique using a fixation device, such as a fracture-fixation plate, during the alignment and distraction phases of an osteotomy. In this technique patient-specific measurements are used, in which the malunited wrist is realigned to match the unaffected wrist.

The computer-assisted system described by Croitoru et al. and Athwal et al. is a two-step process. The first step is the preoperative plan, which contains a 3D reconstructed virtual model of both forearms from CT images and a digitized model of a fracture-fixation plate. A virtual osteotomy is conducted with the preoperative planner and the malunited distal radius segment is realigned to best fit the virtual model of the unaffected radius. Then the digitized fracture-fixation plate is virtually fit to the corrected radius. In this way the positions of the proximal and distal screw holes are known onto the original malunion model. These coordinates, along with the coordinates for the osteotomy plane, are saved and imported into the guidance software.

The second step is the intraoperative guidance system, which is used to translate the preoperative plan towards the operation room. Registration is obtained by matching the patient-specific preoperative plan with landmarks on the patient's in vivo distal radius. This is done by attachment of infrared emitting diodes (IRED) to the radius, which are monitored by an optical tracking device. An IRED target is also attached to the drill. That way the location and orientation of the drill in space is known and can be referenced to the preoperative plan and to precise locations on the patient's exposed distal radius. During the operation, the surgeon sees virtual images of the radius with the planned locations of the screw holes and in this same image the real-time position of the surgical drill. The user-computer interface guides the surgical tools to the location of the planned osteotomy and to the locations of the screw holes in the fracture-fixation plate. Pilot holes are drilled into the bone as indicated by the plan. (Fig. 4B) The osteotomy cut is made, and the distal fragment is shaved to fit the plate. (Fig. 4C) The plate is then fixed to the distal fragment. When the holes through the plate align with the pilot holes in the bone, the surgeon knows that the correct alignment has been achieved and the plate is in the correct position for fixation. (Fig. 4D) The osteotomy gap is filled with a bone graft or bone substitute, and the plate then acts as fixation for the reconstructed radius.

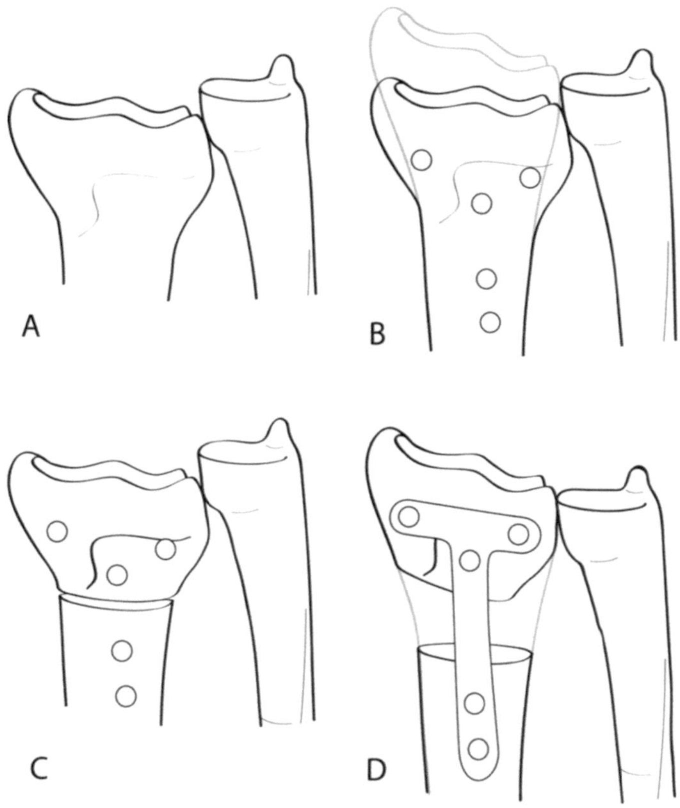

Fig. 4. Schematic view of the computer-assisted fixation-based surgery technique for corrective osteotomy of the distal radius. (Method described by Croitoru et al. and Athwal et al.) Fig. 4A is the malunited radius, Fig. 4B is the malunited radius with pilot holes drilled into the bone as indicated by the preoperative plan. On Fig. 4C the osteotomy is made and in Fig. 4D the plate is fixed to the bone and correct alignment is achieved.

Advantages of computer-assisted fixation-based surgery include that the computer system is simple to use and that the technique takes the required six degrees of freedom of correction into account. The procedure reduces X-ray radiation by eliminating the use of fluoroscopy for achieving the alignment. Furthermore, it is possible to perform multiple simulations of the surgical procedure preoperatively, which can optimize the plan and makes it easy to identify potential problems during realignment. Also exceptionally large defects can be corrected. A disadvantage is the additional preoperative time needed for the planning process. Also, registration of the patient to the surgical planner and guidance system is critical; poor registration may lead to poor outcomes.

2.4 Computer-assisted creation of a repositioning device

In 2004 Rieger et al described a computer-assisted technique with the use of a patient-specific repositioning device. (Rieger et al., 2004) In this method, 3D virtual models of both radii are again created from CT images. The ulna, and a proximal and distal part of the malunited radius, are digitally matched with the ulna and radius of the contralateral healthy forearm, which is mirrored and used as a reference. The planning software of this technique allows the exact calculation of the geometry of the gap in the radius after the virtual osteotomy and positioning. A 3D model that resembles the gap is then created. This model is used to manufacture a synthetic template (i.e. the repositioning device) of stereolithographic material. This repositioning device is placed at the surgical osteotomy site to reposition objectively the distal radius segment before fixation of the osseous structures. The level of osteotomy is determined preoperatively in the virtual planning procedure. After the fixation with the fracture-fixation plate, the repositioning device is replaced with a bone graft or bone subtitute. (Fig. 5)

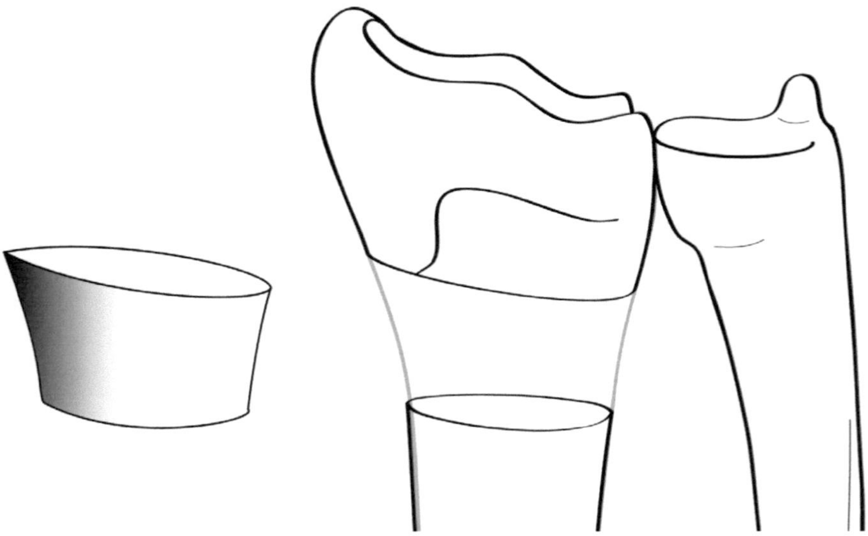

Fig. 5. Schematic view of the computer-assisted technique for corrective osteotomy of the malunited radius using a patient-specific repositioning device. (Method described by Rieger et al.)

This method provides a preoperative insight of the individual operative field and shows, virtually, possible limitations in advance. Also, objective details of the appropriate position of the distal radius segment and the measurements of the required bone graft are known. An advantage of this computer-assisted technique is the fast operative procedure. Disadvantages are the costs and the difficulty to correct rotational misalignment, which is difficult to assess despite the repositioning device.

2.5 Computer-assisted stereolithographic surgical guide

Several studies have been published on computer-assisted corrective osteotomy techniques using patient-specific surgical guides. (Miyake et al., 2010; Oka et al., 2010) These described methods have the same principle.

The corrective osteotomy is simulated and planned with the help of 3D virtual radii models created using CT images of both forearms. Then appropriate screw holes are simulated in the affected radius using computer-assisted design data of a fracture-fixation plate. The location and direction of the screw holes are calculated by the computer to automatically correct the malunion after osteotomy and fixation with a volar fracture-fixation plate.

To translate the preoperative plan to the actual surgery, a patient-specific custom-made osteotomy template with drilling guide holes and an osteotomy slit were designed to exactly fit the surface of the distal radius. The surgical guide is a plastic model made by rapid prototyping technology. With this guide the simulated screw holes can be drilled in the right place. Only then the osteotomy is made through the osteotomy slit. (Fig. 6) The predrilled holes are used to fixate the plate, resulting in automatic reduction of the distal radius segment into the planned position.

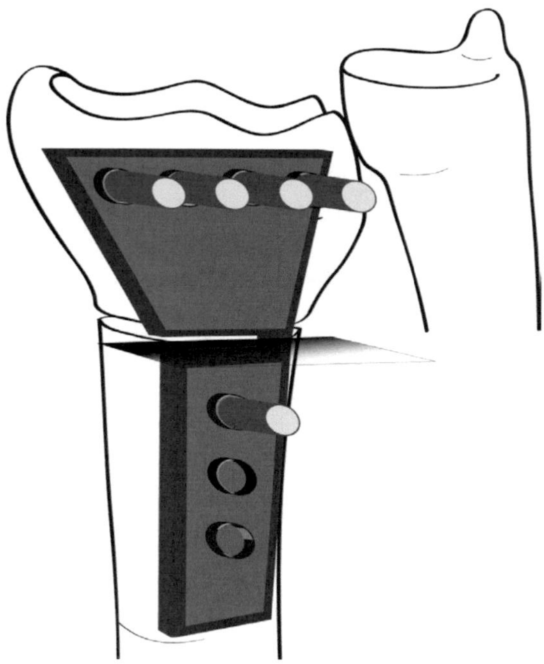

Fig. 6. Schematic view of the computer-assisted corrective osteotomy technique using a patient-specific stereolithographic surgical guide with drilling guide holes and an osteotomy slit. (Method described by Miyake et al. and Oka et al.)

The final step is filling the osteotomy gap with a bone graft or bone substitute. Another option is to combine this method with the creation of a patient-specific repositioning device (see paragraph 2.4) made of biocompatible material. In the latter case no additional surgery is needed at the bone graft site.

One of the advantages of this technique using a custom-made surgical guide is that the intraoperative procedure is simple and undemanding to accomplish. A disadvantage is the rather invasive operation technique. To fit the surgical guide to the bony surface of the radius, the incision must be rather large.

2.6 Computer-assisted correction with manipulator-fixator system

The paper of Dobbe et al. in 2011 introduces a new technique that uses preoperative planning based on 3D CT images in combination with intraoperative 3D imaging. (Dobbe et al., 2011) In this method the first step is again the preoperative planning based on 3D virtual models created from CT images of both the affected and the contralateral healthy radius. Intraoperatively, the distal bone segment needs to be aligned and fixated in the correct position that is determined in the preoperative plan. This is accomplished using Kirschner wires (K-wires) and a positioning tool, called a manipulator-fixator system. The positioning tool is very similar to existing external fixators, the difference is that it is already in the right configuration.

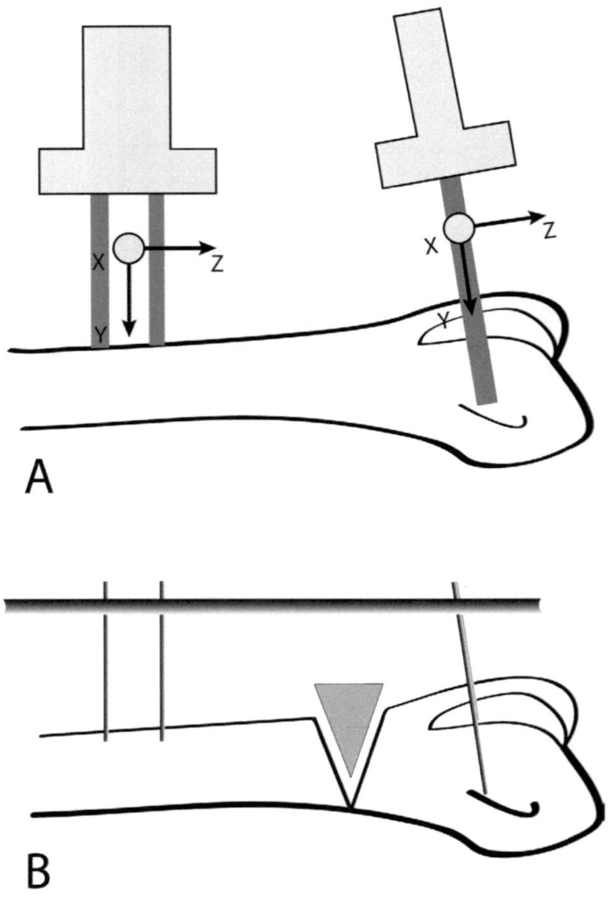

Fig. 7. The manipulator-fixator system that is used in the computer-assisted radial corrective osteotomy technique. (Method by Dobbe et al.)

During the operation, two parallel K-wires are drilled into the proximal part of the radius and a second pair of K-wires into the distal radius segment. Then marker tools are slid over the K-wire pairs and an intraoperative 3D scan is made with a 3DRX scanner. (Fig. 7A) The marker tools allow detection of the K-wires. The preoperative plan and the intraoperative imaging are matched and in this way the positions of the k-wires are known in the preoperative plan. With this information the positioning tool (i.e. the fixator) is adjusted into the right configuration. This is done according to the results of the image analysis software by using a computer-controlled manipulator. The fixator, in the adjusted configuration is attached to the K-wires and in this way the distal radius segment is navigated to the correct position. (Fig. 7B) The osseous structures can now be fixated in this position.

The major advantages of this method are the ease of applicability in the operating room and a high accuracy of repositioning and evaluation using all six degrees of freedom. This method is the first that aims at a minimally invasive technique by making it possible to perform the osteotomy and the bone segment positioning through only small incisions. This could result in less wound problems and less muscle, tendon and nerve complications. Unfortunately, a limitation is that there is currently no minimally invasive fixation method available instead of the fracture-fixation plate and screws.

3. Conclusion

In this chapter the focus is on computer-assisted techniques for corrective osteotomy of the distal radius. However, conclusions in this paragraph also cover other corrective osteotomy procedures, such as osteotomies of the ulna, humerus, clavicula or bones of the lower extremity.

3.1 Advantages of computer-assisted techniques for corrective osteotomies

The greatest advantage of computer-assisted corrective osteotomy that is already described in the introduction is the fact that the preoperative planning is done in 3D instead of the conventional 2D methods. 3D imaging has several potential advantages over 2D radiographs and CT scans. (Guitton & Ring, 2010) Three-dimensional imaging is more intuitive and shows details that cannot be observed on 2D imaging. This allows better preoperative planning and makes the surgeon's mental and psycho-motor preparation easier. Also, 3D physical models can add the sense of touch and immediate 3D manipulations. There is also the possibility for practicing procedures on models preoperatively. Models can be used in the communication with the patient, educational settings, research and development.

3.2 Disadvantages of computer-assisted techniques for corrective osteotomies

Disadvantages of current computer-assisted techniques are radiation exposure for the CT images and the time and effort required for the preoperative planning procedures. The major disadvantage of computer-assisted techniques is the often high manufacturing costs. Of course the new techniques described above are only applied small-scale so far, and cheaper options will be presented. Besides, research has shown that 3D reconstructions may outweigh this latter disadvantage, as both the surgeon and the patient will benefit significantly.

Regarding the disadvantages of the individual current techniques described in this chapter: the use of an intraoperative guidance system like IRED and optical tracking devices requires many touching landmarks at the surface of the bone. This is only possible if the incision for the operative procedure is large and thus invasive. This also applies for the current techniques using a patient-specific stereolithographic surgical guide. To fit the often bulky guide to the bony surface of the radius, the bone must be completely dissected.

Also, another important disadvantage of computer-assisted corrective osteotomy is the requirement of a healthy unaffected contralateral radius, which serves as a reference for the affected radius. There are often cases where a patient has a radius fracture or malunion in both forearms, and this would limit the preoperative planning considerably.

3.3 Perspectives

The perspectives of the newly introduced computer-assisted techniques are promising and it seems that these techniques will have many further applications. The pre-operative 3D planning described in this chapter could also be applied in corrective osteotomies of other long bones, such as the ulna, humerus, clavicula and bones of the lower extremity.

What can be concluded from the advantages and disadvantages of the current computer-assisted techniques is that there are still a few important points that need to be improved. For example, to make computer-assisted corrective osteotomies also minimal invasive, new fixation methods have to be developed, since the bone fixation with a fracture-fixation plate and screws always requires a relatively large incision. Furthermore, the issue of a possible absence of a healthy contralateral radius needs to be addressed. It would be an important development if there would be a statistical model of the wrist joint. In this way relationships between the different bones in the wrist could be calculated and analyzed without the need of an extra CT scan of the contralateral wrist. Of course, this applies to multiple joints which also undergo corrective surgery. Finally, a perspective is that not only the preoperative planning, but also the intraoperative and postoperative evaluation will be in 3D instead of the current postoperative evaluation on 2D radiographs.

Our recommendation for future computer-assisted techniques is a mechanism that resembles the method described by Dobbe et al. (see paragraph 2.6). This technique aims at a system that is minimal invasive and also reusable. By avoiding the need for the manufacturing of patient-specific surgical guides for each individual patient, there will be a significant reduction in cost, and it will be time-saving. More importantly, it will be a technique that is universally applicable and it allows a 3D assessment during the operative procedure.

4. Acknowledgment

The authors would like to thank R.T. Bosscha for the illustrations in this chapter.

5. References

Athwal, GS; Ellis, RE; Small, CF & Pichora, DR. (2003). Computer-assisted distal radius osteotomy. American Journal of Hand Surgery, Vol.28A, No.6, (November 2003), pp. 951-958

Bilic, R & Zdravkovic, V. (1988a). Planning corrective osteotomy of the distal end of the radius. 1. Improved method. *Unfallchirurg*, Vol.91, No.12, (December 1988), pp. 571-574

Bilic, R & Zdravkovic, V. (1988b). Planning corrective osteotomy of the distal end of the radius. 2. Computer-aided planning and postoperative follow-up. *Unfallchirurg*, Vol.91, No.12, (December 1988), pp. 575-580

Brogren, E; Hofer, M; Petranek, M; Wagner, P; Dahlin, LB & Atroshi, I. (2011) Relationships between distal radius fracture malunion and arm-related disability: a prospective population-based cohort study with 1-year follow-up. *BMC Musculoskeletal Disorders*, Vol.12, No.9, (January 2011), pp. 1-9, ISSN 1471-2474

Capo, JT; Accousti, K; Jacob, G & Tan, V. (2009). The effect of rotational malalignment on X-rays of the wrist. *Journal of Hand Surgery European Volume*, Vol.34, No.2, (April 2009), pp. 166-172

Cheng, HS; Hung, LK; Ho, PC & Wong, J. (2008). An analysis of causes and treatment outcome of chronic wrist pain after distal radial fractures. *Hand Surgery*, Vol.13, No.1, (Feburary 2008), pp. 1-10

Cooney, WP; Dobyns, JH; & Linscheid, RL. (1980). Complications of Colles fractures. *American Journal of Bone and Joint Surgery*, Vol.62, No.4, (June 1980), pp. 613-619

Crisco, JJ; Moore, DC; Maral, GE; Laidlaw, DH; Akelman, E; Weiss, AP & Wolfe, SW. (2007). Effects of distal radius malunion on distal radioulnar joint mechanics, an in vivo study. *Journal of Orthopaedic Research*, Vol.25, No.4, (April 2007), pp. 547-555

Croitoru, H; Ellis, RE; Prihar, R; Small, CF & Pichora, DR. (2001). Fixation-based surgery: a new technique for distal radius osteotomy. Computer Aided Surgery, Vol.6, No.3, (March 2001), pp. 160-169

Dobbe, JGG; Strackee, SD; Schreurs, AW; Jonges, R; Carelsen, B; Vroemen, JC; Grimbergen, CA & Streekstra, GJ. (2011). *IEEE Transactions on Biomedical Engineering*, Vol.58, No.1, (January 2011), pp. 182-190

Guitton, TG & Ring, D. (2010). Three-dimensional computer tomographic imaging and modeling in the upper extremity. *Hand Clinics*, Vol.26, No.3, (August 2010), pp. 447-453

Gupta, A; Batra, S; Jain, P & Sharma, SK. (2002). Carpal alignment in distal radial fractures. *BMC Musculoskeletal Disorders*, Vol.24, No.3, (May 2002), pp. 14-20

Jupiter, JB; Ruder, J & Roth, DA. (1992). Computer-generated bone models in the planning of osteotomy of multidirectional distal radius malunions. *American Journal of Hand Surgery*, Vol.17, No.3, (May 1992), pp. 406-415

Kihara, H; Palmer, AK; Werner, FW; Short, WH & Fortino, MD. (1996). The effect of dorsally angulated distal radius fractures on distal radioulnar joint congruency and forearm rotation. *American Journal of Hand Surgery*, Vol.21, No.1, (January 1996), pp. 40-47

Menon, MRG; Walker, JL & Court-Brown, CM. (2008). The epidemiology of fractures in adolescents with reference to social deprivation. *British Journal of Bone and Joint Surgery*, Vol.90, No.11, (November 2008), pp. 1482-1486

Miyake, J; Murase, T; Moritomo, H; Sugamoto, K & Yoshikawa, H. (2011). Distal radius osteotomy with volar locking plates based on computer simulation. *Clinical Orthopaedics and Related Research*, Vol.469, No.6, (June 2011), pp. 1766-1773

Oka, K; Murase, T; Moritomo, H; Goto, A; Sugamoto, K & Yoshikawa, H. (2010). Corrective osteotomy using customized hydroxyapatite implants prepared by preoperative computer simulation. *International Journal of Medical Robotics and Computer Assisted Surgery*, Vol.6, No.2, (June 2010), pp. 186-193

Pennock, AT; Phillips, CS; Matzon, JL & Daley, E. (2005). The effects of forearm rotation on three wrist measurements: radial inclination, radial height and palmar tilt. *Hand Surgery*, Vol.10, No.1, (July 2005), pp. 17-22

Pogue, DJ; Viegas, SF; Patterson, RM; Peterson, PD; Jenkins, DK; Sweo, TD & Hokanson, JA. (1990). Effects of distal radius fracture malunion on wrist joint mechanics. *American Journal of Hand Surgery*, Vol.15, No.5, (September 1990), pp. 721-727

Rieger, M; Gabl, M; Gruber, H; Jaschke, WR & Mallouhi, A. (2005). CT virtual reality in the preoperative workup of malunited distal radius fractures: preliminary results. *European Radiology*, Vol.15, No.4, (April 2005), pp. 792-797

Solgaard, S & Petersen, VS. (1985). Epidemiology of distal radius fractures. *Acta Orthopedica*, Vol.56, No.5, (October 1985) pp. 391-393

Part 6

Foot and Ankle

13

Hallux Valgus Correction in Young Patients with Minimally Invasive Technique

Salvatore Moscadini[1] and Giuseppe Moscadini[2]
[1]*Division of Orthopaedics and Traumatology, University of Palermo,*
[2]*Pediatric Orthopaedic Division,*
"Ospedali Riuniti Villa Sofia-Cervello" Hospital, Palermo,
Italy

1. Introduction

Hallux valgus is a common foot problem which in its early stages will affect just the first metatarsophalangeal joint.

Although hallux valgus has been described for over 100 years (Hueter, 1871, as cited in Kelikian, 1965), the etiology and the definitive treatment remain uncertain.

The term hallux valgus was introduced into the literature in 1871 when Hueter (Hueter, 1871, as cited in Kelikian, 1965) defined the deformity as an abduction contracture in which the great toe is turned away from the mid-line of the body(fig. 1). The adjective valgus implies a static deformity and should not be used interchangeably with abductus which refers to movement caused by muscle function.

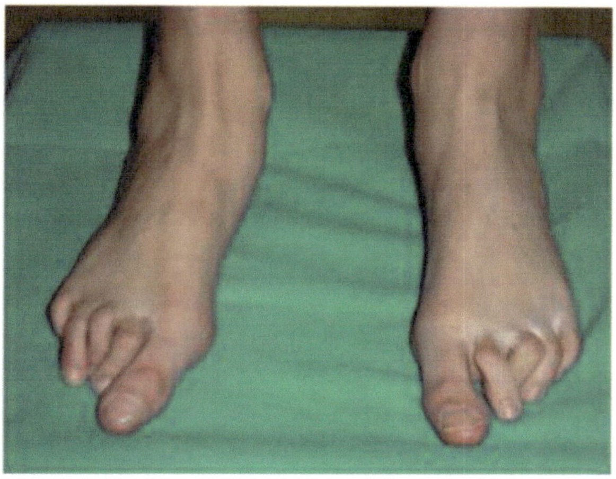

Fig. 1. Bilateral hallux valgus deformity

It is now recognized, particularly in juvenile patients, that a hallux valgus deformity can originate due to lateral deviation of the articular surface of the metatarsal head without subluxation of the first MTP joint.

Bunion is another term, derived from the Latin word bunio (meaning turnip), which is commonly used to describe the hallux valgus deformity and it can refers both to the inflammation of the bursa overlying the MTP joint and to the bony medial eminence which becomes apparent at quite an early stage in the development of hallux valgus.

The dividing line between a normal and a hallux valgus foot is contentious.

It is likely that hallux valgus is not a yes or no phenomenon but rather represents a continuum of variable severity. It can also be associated with abnormal foot mechanics, such us a contracted Achiles tendon, severe pes planus, generalized neuromuscular disease such us cerebral palsy or a cerebrovascular accident, or an acquired deformity of the hindfoot secondary to rupture of the posterior tibial tendon. It can likewise be associated with various inflammatory arthritic conditions, such as rheumatoid arthritis.

2. Anatomy

The articulation of the first MTP joint of the great toe differs from that of the lesser toes in that it has sesamoid mechanism. The head of the first metatarsal articulates with the somewhat smaller, concave elliptical base of the proximal phalanx. A fan-shaped ligamentous band originates from the medial and lateral metatarsal epicondyles and constitutes the collateral ligaments of the MTP joint, that interdigitate with ligaments of the sesamoids.

The two tendons of the flexor hallucis brevis, the abductor and adduttor hallucis, the plantar aponeurosis, and the joint capsule condense on the plantar aspect of the MTP joint to form the plantar plate.

A sesamoid bone is contained in each tendon of the flexor hallucis brevis and articulates by means of cartilage-covered convex facets on its superior surface, with the corresponding longitudinal grooves on the inferior surface of the first metatarsal head. Distally, the two sesamoids are attached by the sesamoid-phalangeal ligament to the base of the proximal phalanx.

The tendons and muscles that move the great toe are arranged around the MTP joint in four groups. Dorsal group: long and short extensor tendons; plantar group: long and short flexor tendons; the last two groups are composed of abductor (medially) and adductor (laterally) hallucis, both pass much nearer the plantar surface than the dorsal surface.

The adductor hallucis, arising from the lesser metatarsal shafts, is made up of two segments, the transverse and the oblique heads, which insert on the plantar lateral aspect of the base of the proximal phalanx and also blend with the plantar plate and the sesamoid complex. The adductor hallucis balances the abductor forces of the abductor hallucis. Acting in the line parallel to this bone and using the head of the first metatarsal as a fulcrum, the abductor hallucis pushes the first metatarsal toward the second metatarsal.

The base of the first metatarsal has a mildly sinusoidal articular surface that articulates with the distal articular surface of the first cuneiform. The orientation of the MTC joint may determinate the amount of the metatarsus primus varus, and the shape of the articulation may affect metatarsal mobility. A medial inclination of up to 8 degrees at the MTC joint is normal. The axis of motion of the tarsometatarsal articulation is quite stable in the central portion because of interlocking of the central metatarsals and cuneiforms. Stability of first and fifth metatarsal, instead, is determined also by the surrounding capsular structures. Therefore, when ligamentous laxity is present, the first metatarsal may deviate medially and the fifth metatarsal laterally in the development of a splay foot deformity.

3. Pathophisiology

The target of a proper treatment of the hallux valgus must include the identification and control of its causes, especially in cases of juvenile hallux valgus. For this reason, it is important understanding which biomechanical dynamics are responsible of the deformity. First of all, we can indentify two foot morphotypes, according to the relationship on the transverse plane between the different sections in which foot can be split (rear tarsus, front tarsus, metatarsus and toes): rectus foot type and adductus foot type. (Root et al.,1977)

In the first one, longitudinal axes of metatarsus and hindfoot tend to be parallel, instead in the adducted forefoot, the metatarsus is angled in adduction respect to the hindfoot.

Regardless of the type of foot, the longitudinal axis of fingers tend to be parallel to the axis of the hindfoot. This allows, in fact, a greater efficiency to the fingers in walking. So, larger is the angle of adduction of the forefoot over the heel, greater is the angle of abduction of the fingers over the metatarsals. This is due to a potential imbalance between the adductors and abductors forces that are exerted on the fingers, with a prevalence of second ones on first ones.

The hallux and the first MTP joint play a significant role in the transfer of weight-bearing forces during locomotion and certain pathologic conditions diminish this ability of the first MTP joint.

Several pathogenetic factors have an important role in the establishment of the deformity.

The excessive pronation of the foot is recognized since long time as a cause of hallux valgus.

In 1965 Kelikian suggested that collapse of the inner border of the midfoot, depressed the base of the first metatarsal downwards, while tilting the metatarsal head upwards. The medial capsule of the first metatarsophalangeal joint offered less resistance than the base of the proximal phalanx and the metatarsal head then subluxed medially.

Pronation of the subtalar joint, in fact, during the push-off phase of gait results in eversion of the foot; it increases the contact area to the ground of the first metatarsal head and causes dorsiflexion of the first metatarsal ray; it, also, hinders the stabilization of the forefoot on the hindfoot and also the stabilization of the cuboid, reflection point of the peroneus longus. Under these conditions, the contraction of the peroneus longus causes lifting of the lateral border of the foot and thus accentuates the pronation of the subtalar joint, instead of inducing plantarflexion and stabilization of the first metatarsal ray (Fig. 2). It determines, then, the unfolding of the long peroneal tendon in its plantar portion, resulting in loss of stabilizing and plantarflexion function on the 1st metatarsal ray (Root et al.,1977).

Once the first MTP become destabilized, it doesn't permit anymore a correct carrying of the weight from the first metatarsus to the great toe.

The loss of stability of the hallux does not allow to the transverse head of the Adductor hallucis to perform its normal function. It stabilizes the foot to the ground, acting on the great toe. Its contraction is necessary to prevent the fan shaped enlargement of metatarsals. If there is a loss of stability of the hallux, the transverse head of the Adductor hallucis acts as an abductor, causing a progressive increase in the MTP angle (hallux abductus), representing a decisive factor in launching the deformity on the transverse plane. The contraction of flexor muscles, longus and brevis, makes the great toe adhering to the ground, trying ineffectually to stabilize the finger even in the case of a first ray hypermobility.

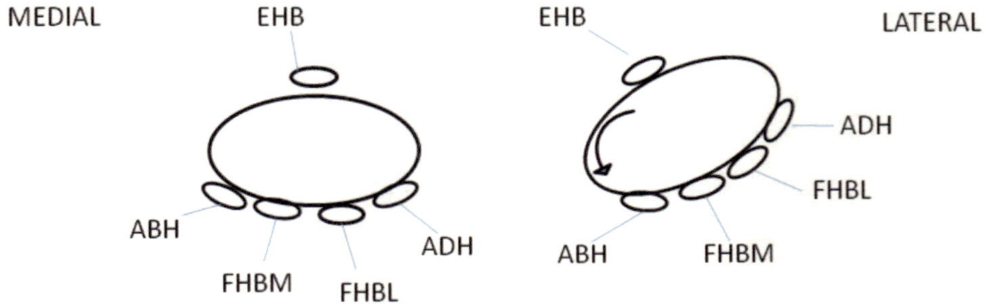

Fig. 2. Representation of tendons around the first metatarsal head. Left: articulation in a balanced state; right: position of the tendons in hallux valgus deformity. ABH, abductor hallucis; ADH, adductor hallucis; EHB, extensor hallucis brevis; FHBL, flexor hallucis brevis lateral head; FHBM, flexor hallucis brevis medial head.

In addition to dorsiflexion, pronation of the foot imposes a longitudinal rotation of the first ray (metatarsal and phalanges), enhanced by weight bearing, that places the axis of the MTP joint in an oblique plane relative to the floor. As under normal conditions, the first MTP joint has not range of motion along the frontal plane, it results in a deformity of the first metatarsal to the lateral direction, and an alteration in valgus of the great toe (Fig. 3). This is the mechanism that initiates the deformity along the frontal plane.

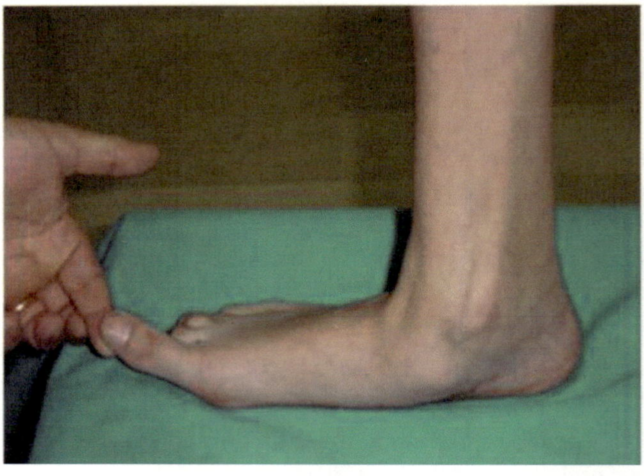

Fig. 3. Pronated foot associated with hallux valgus deformity. Pronation imposes a longitudinal rotation of the first ray that results in a lateral deformity of the first metatarsal, and a valgus great toe.

As the hallux valgus deformity progresses, the soft tissues on the lateral aspect of the MTP joint become contracted, and those on the medial aspect become attenuated. The metatarsal head is pushed in a medial direction by the lateral deviation of the proximal phalanx, thereby progressively exposing the sesamoids, which are anchored in place by the transverse metatarsal ligament and the adductor hallucis muscle. As the sesamoid sling slides beneath the first metatarsal head, the hallux gradually pronates. As this dynamic joint deformity occurs the medial eminence often becomes more prominent. Root, Orien and Weed (Root et al., 1977) proposed also that the inverted and dorsiflexed position of the hypermobile first metatarsal, led to articulation of the tibial sesamoid with the osseous intersesamoidal ridge. Erosion of the ridge followed, further destabilising the first metatarsophalangeal joint. Once the hallux had deviated so far laterally that it lay in contact with the second toe, a retrograde force was directed back across the first metatarsophalangeal joint which forced the first metatarsal into metatarsus primus varus, or metatarsus primus adductus as it was called by Root et al. (Root et al., 1977)

4. Etiology

Hallux valgus is certainly a multifactorial disease where extrinsic and intrinsic factors play different roles.

4.1 Extrinsic factors

It is not yet completely clear the relationship between footwear and hallux valgus. Althought hight-fashion footwear has been implicated in the progression of hallux valgus deformities in adults, some studies have suggested that in most cases a juvenile hallux valgus deformity does not appear to be influenced by a history of constricting footwear. But a study conducted on 858 pre-school children (Roddy et al., 2008), has shown that 61% of children wore indoor shoes 2 sizes too short and it was associated with an increase of 37% for the risk of a hallux angle of 4 degrees or more. Furthermore, the risk of a greater hallux angle for children wearing poorly-fitting indoor shoes was markedly higher than for children wearing poorly-fitting outdoor shoes, with a significant relationship between the lengthwise fit of the shoes and the hallux angle: shorter the shoe, higher the value of the hallux angle. Anyway, as the deformity does not develop in many people who wear fashionable or insufficient length footwear, some intrinsic predisposing factors must make some feet more vulnerable to the effect of footwear and likewise predispose some unshod feet to the development of hallux valgus. (Mann & Coughlin, 2010)

4.2 Intrinsic factors

4.2.1 Heredity

The notion that a hallux valgus deformity is inherited has been indeed suggested by many authors. (Mann & Coughlin, 2010) Juvenile hallux valgus deformities have been characterized by their familial tendency and in past different authors proposed that this trait was autosominal dominant with incomplete penetrance (Johnston, 1956) or with maternal trasmission. (Coughlin, 1995) However, this trait can also be associated with x-linked dominant trasmission or polygenic transmission (Mann & Coughlin, 2010).

4.2.2 Pes planus

The association of pes planus with the development of a hallux valgus deformity is controversial. A more than double increased incidence of pes planus has been demonstrated in a adult group with a hallux valgus than in a control group, without evidence of correlation between the hallux valgus angle and pes planus or between pes planus and first ray mobility. (Grebing & Coughlin, 2004) An association was observed, instead, between the hallux valgus angle and both Meary's line and the AP talonavicular coverage angle in those patients with pes planus (King & Toolan, 2004) (Fig. 4). Much more interesting, from a biomechanical point of view, is the observation that a hallux valgus deformity tends to develop in a pronated foot.

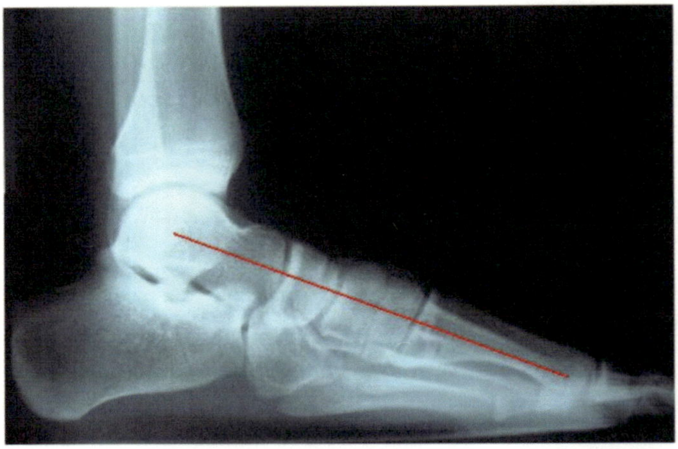

Fig. 4. Normal Meary's angle. The long axis of the talus intersects that of 1st metatarsal. In pes planus, the long axis of the talus is angled plantarward in relation to 1st metatarsal.

Already Jordan and Brodsky in 1951 wrote "We regard the majority of cases of hallux valgus as acquired deformities resulting from pronation of the foot. The role of footwear is secondary, serving to aggravate in mild deformity or produce manifest deformity where only potential hallux valgus previously existed as a result of foot pronation". (Jordan & Brodsky, 1951) Anyway, it is reasonable to think that a hallux valgus deformity will progress more rapid in a patient with pes planus because the foot appears to be less able to withstand the deforming pressures exerted on it by either shoes or weight bearing (Mann & Coughlin 2010).

4.2.3 Hypermobility of the metatarsocuneiform joint

An association between increased mobility of the first MTC joint and hallux valgus was suggested by Lapidus already in 50s. (Lapidus, 1934,1956,1960) Along the years, many authors tried to refine methods to accurately measure first ray mobility, finding a greater flexibility at the MTC joint in patients with hallux valgus. But Grebing and Coughlin showed how the position of the ankle substantially influences the perceived first ray mobility: if the ankle is placed in 30 degrees of plantar flexion, in fact, the rate of hallux valgus considered hypermobile is much higher compared to that with the ankle placed in 5 degrees of dorsiflexion (Grebing & Coughlin, 2004).

Having determined a relationship between hypermobility of the MTC joint and hallux valgus, it's important to understand if the hypermobility is an effect of the deformity or the cause. A follow-up prospective study in which an operative repair to correct hallux valgus deformity was performed on 122 feet, concluded that first ray mobility is an effect of the hallux valgus deformity rather than a cause in most cases. (Coughlin & Jones, 2005) First ray stability is probably a function of first ray alignment and the effectiveness of the intrinsic and extrinsic muscles and the plantar aponeurosis and not an intrinsic characteristic of the first MTC joint.

4.2.4 Ligamentous laxity

Although the findings of ligamentous laxity is probably uncommon in the typical adult patient with hallux valgus, it is instead quite frequently in young patients. In a report on juveniles, Clark et al, noted that 69% of patients in their series had generalized laxity on physical examination. (Clark et al, 1987) Attention should be adressed to ligamentous laxity in any evaluation before correction of hallux valgus. Especially in patients affected by genetic diseases involving mesenchymal tissues, like Marfan or Ehlers-Danlos's syndrome, generalized ligamentous laxity and Down syndrome, the specific laxity and the impairment of the capsuloligamentous structures play a key role about the onset of the disease and the tendency to relapse.

4.2.5 Neurological diseases

Neurological diseases such as spastic paralysis induce the appearance of a hallux valgus deformity by a serious and persistent subtalar pronation, to compensate for muscular equinism. The deformity develops, in these cases too, through a biomechanical impairment, but the different cause justifies their separate classification.

Anyway, in order to find the main cause of the deformity, a complete and accurate biomechanical examination of the lower limbs is important to identify the structural and/or functional defects responsible of the abnormal subtalar pronation of the foot. Causes could concern alterations of the foot, like forefoot varus, not rigid forefoot valgus, osseous ankle equinus, or structural defects over the foot, like tibial and genu varum, tibial and femoral torsional modifications and genu valgum. Also functional defects linked to muscular alterations could have a role in the occurrence of the deformity.

5. Epidemiology

Estimates of the community prevalence of hallux valgus vary widely, ranging from 2%-70% in epidemiologic studies. (Myerson, 2000; Benvenuti et al., 1995; Dunn et al., 2004; Elton & Sanderson, 1986; White & Mulley, 1989; Leveille et al., 1998) This variation is attributable, in part, to different study populations and definitions of hallux valgus used, in particular confusion of the terms hallux valgus and bunion.

In a study on a primary care population of 3868 people, Roddy et al. reported a prevalence of hallux valgus of 31%: bilateral hallux valgus was reported by 16.9% of subjects compared with subjects with unilateral hallux valgus (6.0% in the left foot only, 7.0% in the right foot only).(Roddy et al., 2008) In children, Klein et al. reported only 23.9% of children's feet with a straight position of the great toe; in all the rest, the position of the great toe varied between a hallux angle of 1 degree up to 19 degrees valgus position (14.2% with a valgus deviation of equal to or greater than 10 degrees). (Klein et al., 2009)

A female preponderance of 2:1 was reported in a study of schoolchildren's feet (Wilkins, 1941); the ratio increases up to 3:1 in military recruits (Hewitt, 1953; Marwil & Brantingham, 1943), until to reach approximately the ratio of 15:1 in adult patients (Hardy & Clapham, 1951). Therefore, the prevalence in women increased as patient age increased, also probably due to the use of fashionable female shoes. The reported incidence of females in the juvenile population undergoing surgical correction for hallux valgus deformities varies from 84%to 100%. (Clark et al., 1987; Thompson, 1996)

About the age of onset, most of studies reported that a percentage of 40%-57% of bunion deformities occurred during adolescent year, anyway before the age of 20 (Piggott, 1960; Coughlin, 1995). But, as patients recognize a hallux valgus deformity just when they "feel" the deformity, the symptoms, and the magnitude of the deformity, it's right to think that the development of the hallux valgus probably occurs much earlier than has previously been appreciated.

Of importance is the fact that the late development after skeletal maturity occurs in a foot that at one point most likely had a normal structure, whereas an early onset in the juvenile years occurs before maturation in a foot that most likely "never had a normal structure". (Mann & Coughlin 2010)

6. Anatomic and radiographic consideration

Radiographic examination of the foot has no absolute value and, although crucial, it is not to be separated by a thorough clinical and biomechanics examination of the foot, which must be confirmation and completion at the same time. Only by correlating the results of various radiographic measurements to a correct clinical diagnosis, it's possible choosing the most appropriate surgical technique.

It's interesting to underline that a statistical study found that there was a highly significant difference between the radiographic and the intraoperative assessment of MTP joint congruity (Armanek et al., 1986).

Anyway, during a preoperative evaluation, the following radiographic parameters will always be evaluated (Bartolozzi et al., 2011):

- Hallux valgus angle
- 1-2 intermetatarsal angle
- Proximal Articular Set Angle (P.A.S.A.) or Distal Metatarsal Articular Angle (DMAA)
- Distal Articular Set Angle (D.A.S.A.)
- Joint Congruity
- Relative Metatarsal Protrusion
- First Metatarsocuneiform Joint
- Osteoarthritis
- Rotation of hallux about its long axis

6.1 Hallux valgus angle

On an AP weight-bearing radiograph, hallux valgus angle is created by the intersection of axes drawn on the first metatarsal and proximal phalanx, the first was obtained bisecting the shaft of the metatarsal at two levels, joining the points of bisection and extending the line in both directions; the second was obtained by a line applied by visual estimation, because the irregular outline of the phalanx did not allow of geometrical division at two levels (Fig. 5). While not entirely predictive, Hardy and Clapham's "artificial dividing line" of 15° about hallux valgus angle (Hardy & Clapham, 1951), appears to be supported by the epidemiological studies reviewed. Therefore, a normal angle is less than 15 degrees, mild deformity is less than 20 degrees , moderate deformity is 20 to 40 degrees, and severe deformity is greater than 40 degrees (Coughlin, 1996).

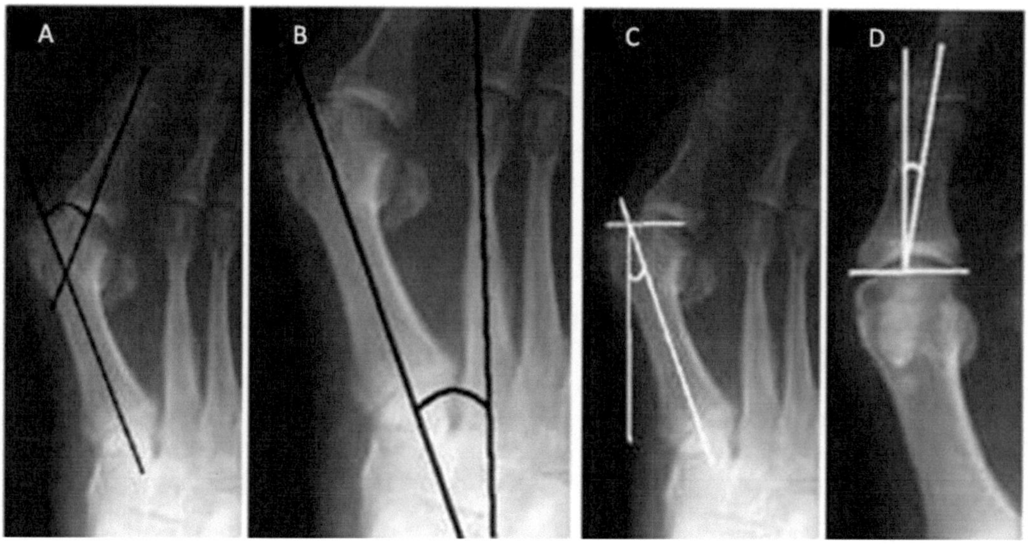

Fig. 5. A, Hallux Valgus Angle; B, Intermetatarsal Angle; C, Proximal Articular Set Angle (P.A.S.A.); D, Distal Articular Set Angle (D.A.S.A.).

6.2 1-2 intermetatarsal angle

On an AP weight-bearing radiograph, this angle is obtained by measuring the angle between the axis of the first and second metatarsals (fig. 5). Normal is less than 9 degrees (Hardy & Clapham, 1951), mild deformity is 11 degrees or less, moderate deformity is greater than 11 and less than 16 degrees, and severe deformity is greater than 16 degrees (Coughlin 1996).

6.3 Proximal Articular Set Angle (P.A.S.A.) or Distal Metatarsal Articular Angle (DMAA)

On an AP weight-bearing radiograph, it is formed by the intersection of the perpendicular line to the line passing through the two medial and lateral end points of the articular surface of the head of the first metatarsal and the longitudinal axis of the first metatarsal (Fig. 5). The measurement of this angle is extremely important when evaluating a patient with a hallux valgus deformity because it will in part determine what type of operative procedure should be performed. Normal angle is regarded as 8 degrees or less of lateral sloping, even if Coughlin observed that in juvenile patients younger than 10 years with hallux valgus, the DMAA was 15 degrees, and in those older than 10 years, it averaged 9 degrees (Coughlin, 1995) .

6.4 Distal Articular Set Angle (D.A.S.A.)

On an AP weight-bearing radiograph, defines the orientation of the proximal phalangeal articular surface in relation to the long axis of the proximal phalanx. Normal is less than 8 degrees, 5 degrees on average (Balding, 1985) (Fig. 5).

6.5 Joint congruity

Congruity is the term used to describe the relationship of the metatarsal and phalangeal articular surfaces. A congruent hallux valgus deformity occurs when the corresponding articular surfaces of the metatarsal and phalanx are concentrically aligned (Coughlin, 1995).

Piggott separated a normal from a hallux valgus foot on the basis of the congruence of the first metatarsophalangeal joint (Piggott, 1960).

In a physiological foot, the first metatarsophalangeal joint remained congruent with the articular surface of the first metatarsal head, and the proximal phalanx of the hallux lying adjacent to one another. Hallux valgus is a deviated joint where the proximal phalanx is moved laterally on the first metatarsal head, leaving the medial side of the metatarsal head exposed. Three groups are identified referred to congruous, deviated and subluxated patterns. In the first, the surfaces are completely congruous as in the normal foot, their central points lying opposite each other. In the second, the distal articular surface is deviated laterally on the proximal articular surface, leaving the medial end of the latter exposed. In the third, the base of the proximal phalanx is subluxated laterally off the metatarsal head.

According to this classification, Piggott considered Hardy and Clapham's dividing line somewhat artificial as he found a number of congruous joints with first metatarsophalangeal joint angles in excess of 15° (Piggott, 1960).

He suggested that mild subluxation of the first MTP joint can progress to significant subluxation and leave the medial metatarsal articular surface uncovered. According to the author, a congruous joint was typically stable and the hallux valgus did not appear to increase with time.

Anyway, a significant hallux valgus that needs surgical intervention, can occur in a patient with a symptomatic deformity and a congruent MTP joint; in some cases, an intraarticular MTP joint realignment could create an incongruent joint, predisposing the patient to a recurrent hallux valgus deformity or to the development of postoperative degenerative joint disease (Coughlin, 1990).

In juveniles, MTP joint congruity is believed to be a significant predisposing factor in the hallux valgus deformity (Coughlin, 1990; Funk & Wells, 1972; Coughlin, 1987; Goldner & Gaines, 1976; Piggott, 1960). Coughlin demonstrated that 47% of juveniles with hallux valgus were noted to have a congruent joint with a laterally sloping DMAA. For those with a subluxated first MTP joint, the average the DMAA was 8 degrees. For congruent joints, the average lateral slope or DMAA was 15 degrees. The DMAA was noted to be significantly higher in patients with a positive family history, in those with early onset of hallux valgus (younger than 10 years), and in those with a long first metatarsal. The DMAA was not affected by the presence of metatarsus adductus. An increased DMAA is the defining characteristic of many juvenile hallux valgus deformities (Coughlin, 1995).

6.6 Relative metatarsal protrusion

The difference of length between first and second metatarsal linked to a possible association with hallux valgus is controversial. It is a somewhat vexed question because definition of terms is difficult and, even when defined, the relevance and iinterpretation of them are obscure.

The axes of the first and second metatarsal are drawn along their long axis; a transverse tarsal line is drawn so as to touch the posterior articular surface of the cuboid and the posterior aspect of the tuberosity of the navicular. At the point of intersection of this line with the axis of the second metatarsal one point of a pair of dividers is placed; arcs were then drawn with the other so as to touch the articular surfaces of the heads of the first and second metatarsal. The radial distance (in millimeters) between the arcs is taken as the measure of relative metatarsal protrusion. Conventionally, the distance between the arcs is preceded by a sign: a positive sign indicates that the first is greater than the second, and a negative sign that the second is greater than the first.

Morton's method using transverse lines is another technique to size the first metatarsal length but is influenced by varying angular deformities (Morton, 1935).

Also measurements in juveniles show short first metatarsals in 28%, first and second metatarsals of equal length in 42%, and long first metatarsals in 30% (Coughlin 1995). According to these data, a short first metatarsal is rarely associated to a hallux valgus deformity.

6.7 First metatarsocuneiform joint

TThe first MTC joint has a key role in the development both of an enlarged 1-2 intermetatarsal angle and an increased hallux valgus angle. The orientation and flexibility of the MTC joint play an important role in development of the deformity at the MTP joint. On an AP radiograph, the angle formed by the intersection of the longitudinal axes of the first and second metatarsals defines the 1-2 intermetatarsal angle. The normal value is 5-10 degrees (La Porta et al., 1974; Weissman, 1989) . If it exceeds 25 degrees, an osteotomy of the first metatarsal base or an arthrodesis of the first MTC joint may be proposed (Lapidus, 1960).

Normally the first MTC joint is deviated medially, but in some cases it may have a marked degree of medial inclination, which is believed to result in joint instability. After anatomic dissection (Haines & Mc Dougall, 1954; Brage et al., 1994) of the MTC joint, it was demonstrated being an association between hallux valgus deformity and an oblique orientation of the first MTC joint. Therefore it's possible to hypothesize (Haines & Mc Dougall, 1954) that an abnormality in the first metatarsal base leads to a metatarsus primus varus deformity and that the first MTC joint is the major actor associated with an increased magnitude of the 1-2 intermetatarsal angle.

DuVries stated that in juveniles, the increased 1-2 intermetatarsal angle was responsible for the development of hallux valgus, whereas in adults, the increased 1-2 intermetatarsal angle was a secondary change following first MTP joint subluxation (DuVries, 1959). It confirms that in juveniles an increased 1-2 intermetatarsal angle is a primary deformity and the hallux valgus deformity is a secondary or acquired deformity.

6.8 Osteoarthritis

Degenerative arthritis of the first MTP joint is rarely associated with a juvenile hallux valgus deformity but is more often associated with an adult bunion.

The altered mechanics of the first MTP joint over time can cause development of arthrosis phenomena.

The first metatarsophalangeal joint is a target joint for osteoarthritis and it was included in Kellgren and Moore's seminal description of generalized osteoarthritis (Kellgren & Moore, 1952). More recently, radiographic evidence of osteoarthritis at the first metatarsophalangeal joint has been shown to be associated with radiographic evidence of osteoarthritis at the knee and hand (Wilder, 2005).

It is therefore interesting that hallux valgus, like an osteoarthritis conseguence, was more frequently found to be a bilateral phenomenon with little difference between the right or left foot. Other components of generalized osteoarthritis (e.g., radiographic knee and interphalangeal joint osteoarthritis) have been found to be asymmetrical with a predominance of disease on the right side (Acheson, 1970; Neame et al., 2004).

This finding has been interpreted in the hands as evidence of the role of biomechanic factors in the development of osteoarthritis. Hence, 2 possible explanations for the symmetry of hallux valgus exist. First, the development of osteoarthritis may relate to constitutional or genetic factors or alternatively, biomechanic factors may apply equally to both feet, in contrast with the hand where use of the dominant side is favored (Roddy et al., 2008).

7. Symptoms

The main symptom is the pain, which occurs initially to the prominence of the metatarsal head because of the conflict with the upper part of the shoe, and it later may be complicated by the appearance of a serious inflammation of the bursa (bursitis). The deviation of the great toe causes a functional failure of the first ray, which causes a shift of weight on the central metatarsal heads with subsequent onset of pain and calluses at this level (metatarsalgia).

The functional overload of central rays leads to a muscular imbalance of the small fingers resulting in the appearance of the *griffe* deformity, sometimes associated to a dorsal subluxation or dislocation of the corresponding MTP joints. Deformities of the small fingers too can lead to pain and callus at the proximal interphalangeal joints, due to the mechanical conflict with the upper part of the shoe. Because of the inadequacy of the first ray, the transfer of the weight may also determine the appearance of Civinini-Morton's neuroma, most often on the third intermetatarsal space.

Besides biomechanical alterations and pain, caused by friction between foot and shoe in a deformed foot, it's important to take account of the tendency to progressive worsening of the deformity with functional and aesthetic impairment.

8. Classification

The main purpose of a classification of hallux valgus deformities is to facilitate the decision-making process on how to treat the deformity. Classification should be used only as a general guide.

In general, hallux valgus deformity is divided into three degrees of severity (Coughlin, 1996):

- **Mild**, if the hallux valgus angle is less than 20 degrees.
- **Moderate**, the hallux valgus angular deformity is 20 to 40 degrees.
- **Severe**, with a hallux valgus deformity greater than 40 degrees of lateral deviation of the hallux

9. Treatment

There are two main modes of treatment: conservative and surgical.

9.1 Conservative treatment

Conservative care is adequate only to relieve symptoms. A custom or prefabricated orthotic device may assist in the treatment of a flexible flatfoot deformity or in a patient with ligamentous laxity and hallux valgus associated with pes planus. A soft leather shoe with a wide toe box and preferably a soft sole may give significant relief of symptoms. The use of bunion pads, night splints, bunion posts, and other commercial appliances may also help in relieving symptoms.

The use of prefabricated or custom orthotics is controversial in the treatment of a patient with hallux valgus. It has not been demonstrated that orthotic devices prevent progression of the deformity. An orthotic device may be uncomfortable for a patient because it occupies space within the shoe. It may place increased pressure against the medial eminence and result in increased symptoms rather than relief of pressure on the first metatarsal head. According to this theory, Kilmartin et al(1991) found that the hallux valgus angle increased more in patients who used orthotics and concluded that orthoses did not prevent progression of a hallux valgus deformity.

Nonsurgical care should also be considered in patients with hyperelasticity, ligamentous laxity, or neuromuscular disorders because of the high recurrence rate.

9.2 Surgical treatment

About surgical treatment, several correction techniques performed on soft tissue and / or bone have been described and the most appropriate method should consider the already described clinical and radiographic factors.

Basically, the corrective actions can be divided as follows:

1. Soft tissues;
2. Arthroplasties
3. First metatarsal osteotomies:
   a. Distal osteotomies
   b. Proximal osteotomies
   c. Metadiaphyseal osteotomies
4. First phalangeal osteotomies
5. Arthrodesises

These techniques, which can be variously combined, aim to correct all the deformities even through the use of fixation devices that may be metallic or absorbable, they may be internal (screws, staples) or external (K-wire) . The internal fixation devices are usually intended to remain, while those outside are removed several weeks after surgery.

In addition to traditional open surgery, which requires large incisions to perform osteotomies and soft-tissue releases, recently the minimally invasive surgery has emerged.

Minimally invasive surgery (MIS) is defined as surgery performed through the smallest incision necessary to perform correctly the surgical technique and with minimal involvement of bony structures, joints, tendons and skin.

For the treatment of hallux valgus deformity with MIS technique, in literature are described Bosch (et al., 1990) technique, the PDO (Percutaneous Distal Osteotomy) (Magnan et al.,1997) and SERI (Simple, Effective, Rapid, Inexepensive) (Giannini et al., 2003); the first two with punctiform percutaneous surgical access, the third with a minimally invasive approach through an incision of 7-10 mm. These three techniques perform essentially a similar distal osteotomy of the first metatarsal with lateral displacement of the epiphyseal fragment of the metatarsal head and stabilization of the correction with a single K-wire located extraperiosteally on the big toe and on the distal epiphyseal fragment, intramedullary the first metatarsal.

As the osteotomy site is fixed temporarily by a K-wire, the relative mobility of fragments allows the consolidation of the osteotomy in the best position under the guidance of the weight bearing. The osteotomy site consolidates in several months as a stress fracture, initially with exuberant callus and with subsequent remodeling of the metatarsal.

These techniques meet the biomechanical principles of traditional distal osteotomies performed with open technique, without requiring any time to release the soft tissues on the lateral side of joint.

Historically distal metatarsal osteotomies have been indicated in cases of mild to moderate deformity with an intermetatarsal angle equal to 15-20°. Distal osteotomies may also be used to correct deformities characterized by deviation of the distal metatarsal articular angle (DMAA) or to address concomitant stiffness.

Many authors over a year described techniques for distal osteotomies, some of them performed percutaneously, and each of them characterized by different approaches, osteotomy and fixation designs. Furthermore, several studies over the years reported more than 80% good results with the use of these techniques.

The MIS technique is indicated to correct mild to moderate reducible deformity when the Hallux Valgus Angle is up to 40° and the Intermetatarsal Angle is up to 20° (Giannini et al., 2003).

The operation is indicated if the MTP joint is either incongruent or congruent or with modification of DMAA, and if mild degenerative arthritis is present. Advantages of these techniques are short operating time required, decreased postoperative discomfort, immediate weight bearing, improvement in postoperative MTP joint motion, fewer local complications and minimal soft-tissue damage.

Regardless of the technique, the indications for surgical treatment are represented by:

1. Pain from conflicts with the use of shoes that does not allow the use of normal shoes;
2. Metatarsalgia;
3. Preventing the aggravation of the deformities in young patients, also asymptomatic, to prevent the development of arthritic degeneration of the first MTP joint;
4. Correction of deformities for cosmetic purposes in selected cases (after appropriate counseling);

The most reliable algorithm of choice of treatment is that proposed by the **American Orthopaedic Foot & Ankle Society** (AOFAS) and by the European **Foot & Ankle Society (EFAS),** modified by the Italian Society of Foot Surgery (SICP) (Fig.6).

10. Our experience and preferred technique by the authors

10.1 Materials and methods

Since 2000 up to now, we treated through S.E.R.I. technique 55 patients (3 males, 52 females; mean age 14,5 years in a range of 13-16 years) with a juvenile hallux valgus deformity always associated with valgus flat foot treated with calcaneo-stop technique.

The surgery for the correction of the hallux valgus deformity was proposed at least two years later calcaneo stop procedure and anyway after the removal of the screw.

All patients were asymptomatic at the moment of the surgery, and the indications for surgical procedure were preventing the aggravation of the deformity and the development of arthritic degeneration of the first MTP joint.

During the preoperative evaluation has been checked all the radiographic parameters above indicated, and in particular the Hallux valgus angle, the 1-2 intermetatarsal angle, the Proximal Articular Set Angle (P.A.S.A.) and the Distal Articular Set Angle (D.A.S.A.).

Target of the surgery was the correction of clinical and radiological parameters which include the right realignment of the great toe, the relocation of sesamoids, the recovery of the inadequacy of 1st radius and the improvement of the valgus angle, the intermetatarsal angle, the proximal articular set angle, and the distal articular set angle.

10.2 Surgical technique

In young patients it is preferable to perform the surgery under general anesthesia, in adults also under local anaesthetic or local anaesthetic with oral sedation.

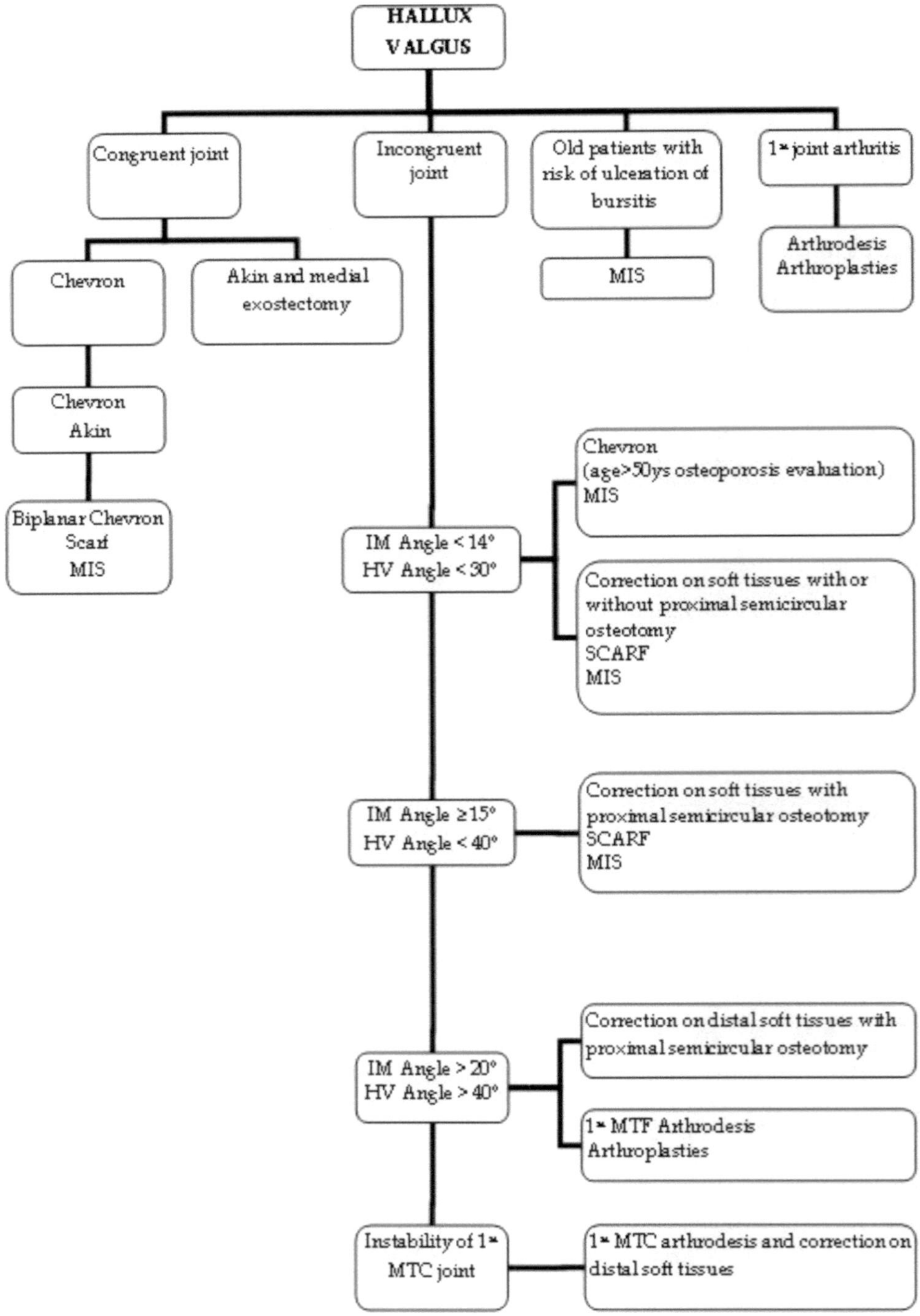

Fig. 6. Algorithm for the hallux valgus deformity treatment proposed by the American Orthopaedic Foot & Ankle Society (AOFAS) and by the European Foot & Ankle Society (EFAS), and modified by the Italian Society of Foot Surgery (SICP). MIS could be used for several types of deformities.

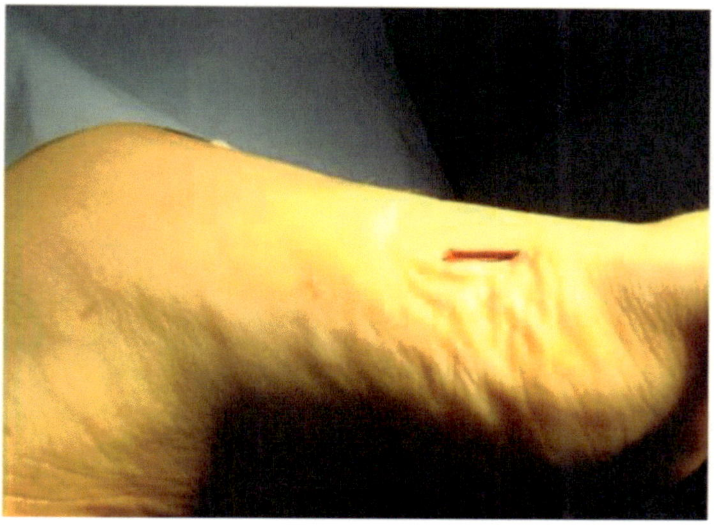

Fig. 7. Surgical incision

A 2 cm incision is made at the subcapital region of the first metatarsal, equidistant between the dorsal and plantar aspects of the bone (Fig. 7). The periosteum is detached dorsally and plantarly with a small elevator, preserving its continuity to protect the soft tissues during the osteotomy.

The transverse osteotomy is made in the first metatarsal subcapital region under fluoroscopic control, using an end cutting burr. The osteotomy is performed perpendicular to the metatarsal shaft in the sagittal plane. In the frontal plane, the mediolateral obliquity of the osteotomy can be varied to shorten or lengthen the first metatarsal according to the preoperative plan. Furthermore, the metatarsal head can be rotated in the axial plane to correct rotational components of the deformity. Once the osteotomy is finished, mobility at the osteotomy site is checked under fluoroscopy.

Through the incision, a 2 mm K-wire is introduced according to a proximal-distal direction until the medial side of the great toe, approximately 5 mm plantar to the proximal edge of the nail; the K-wire must be placed subcutaneously and extraperiosteally to perform the metatarsal head displacement at the osteotomy site. Once the wire has popped up near the nail of the great toe, it was taken from the drill and retracted until it reaches the proximal end of the line of osteotomy.

Next, a bent grooved guide is placed through the proximal incision into the proximal metatarsal bone fragment. The K-wire tip is placed in the concavity of the guide. Using the guide and K-wire as a lever, the metatarsal head lateral displacement and rotation is achieved and maintained during the wire progression into the medullary canal. While holding the hallux in a varus position, the wire is driven with smooth blows of the mallet to the base of the metatarsal. Fluoroscopy is used to confirm the lateral displacement of the head, and overlap of the proximal and distal fragments (Fig. 9). The probe is taken out and the wire is cut, leaving 1 cm outside the skin .

The incision is sutured and a short leg cast is packed. The weight-bearing is allowed with "walking" cast after 10 days.

Through this technique, the release of soft tissue is not required because their detensioning is obtained with the lateral displacement of the metatarsal head. However, it is advisable to perform a manual stretching of the adduttor hallucis, forcing the great toe in varus.

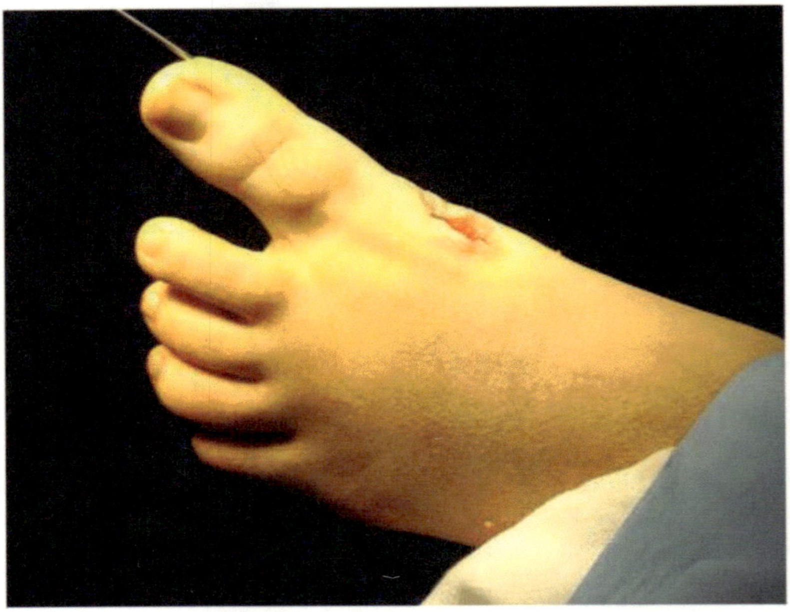

Fig. 8. Through the incision, the K-wire is introduced until the medial side of the great toe.

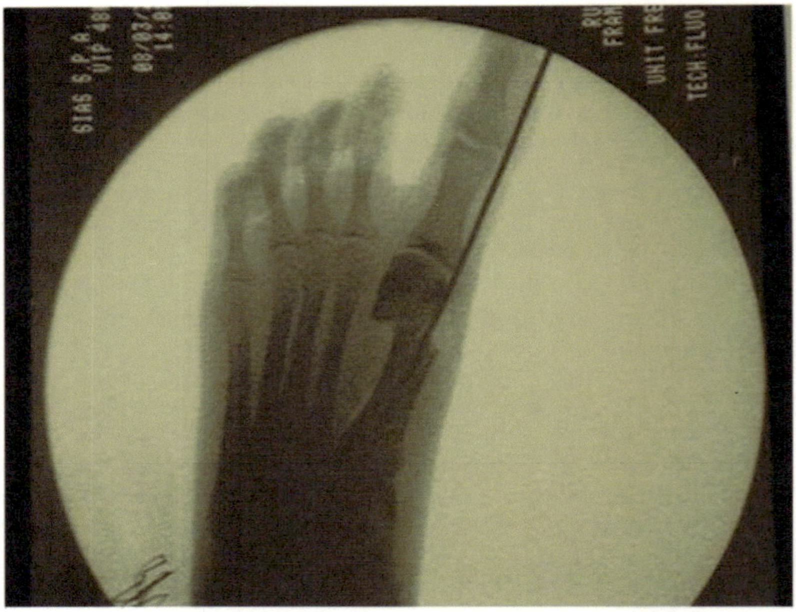

Fig. 9. Using a bent grooved guide the guide into the proximal metatarsal bone fragment and K-wire as a lever, the metatarsal head lateral displacement and rotation is achieved and maintained during the wire progression into the medullary canal.

The choice of the quadrant, according to the transverse direction (inferior-medial or superior-medial), of the first ray for the insertion and progress of the K-wire along the phalanx and the distal epiphysis of metatarsal is very important. The choice affects the subsequent positioning of the osteotomized epiphysis compared to the diaphysis. The wire is inserted into the superior-medial quadrant determining thus a plantar displacement of the head of the metatarsal (Fig. 10). An insertion of the wire into the inferior-medial quadrant should be avoided because it determines dorsal displacement of the great toe.

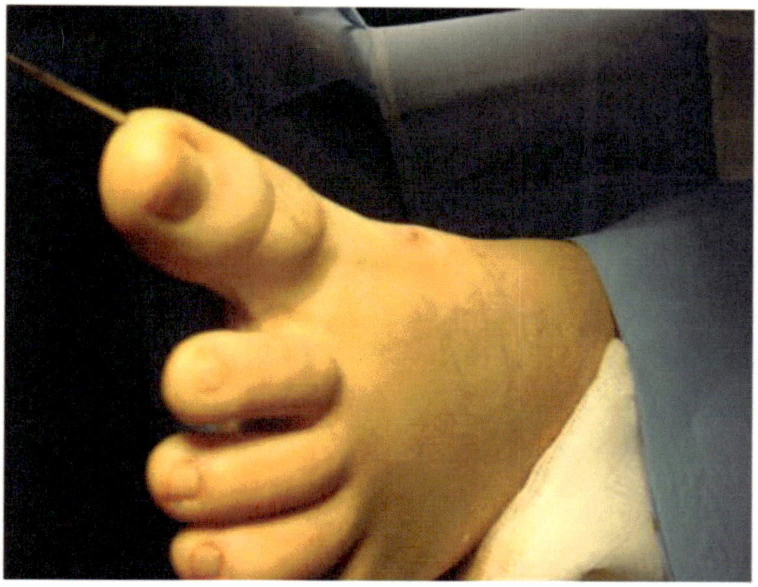

Fig. 10. The wire is inserted into the superior-medial quadrant determining a plantar displacement of the head of the metatarsal.

10.3 Post-operative care

The wire and the cast are kept for 30 days. After their removal, the patient can wear a "talus" shoe that distributes the weight-bearing on the hindfoot. Clinical and radiographic controls were performed at 1, 3, 6 and 12 months.

11. Results

There were no intraoperative complications. At a mean follow-up of 3 years (min. 1, max 5), radiographic parameters were evaluated and all showed values within normal range.

The radiographic follow-up showed a complete consolidation of the osteotomy and a great metatarsal bone remodeling. Clinical results showed an excellent aesthetic and multiplanar correction of the deformity. The translocation of the metatarsal head causes a normalization of the intermetatarsal angle and a realignment of sesamoids, extensor and flexor apparatus of the great toe. Only in 3 patients a varus osteotomy of the base of the proximal phalanx of the finger (Akin) was necessary due to a severe alteration of the phalangeal axis. All patients were satisfied according to the obtained aesthetic and functional results.

There were no cases of avascular necrosis of the metatarsal head or nonunion of the osteotomy. In the indicated follow up period, we have not observed loss of correction and no foot has developed hallux varus (Fig. 11-12).

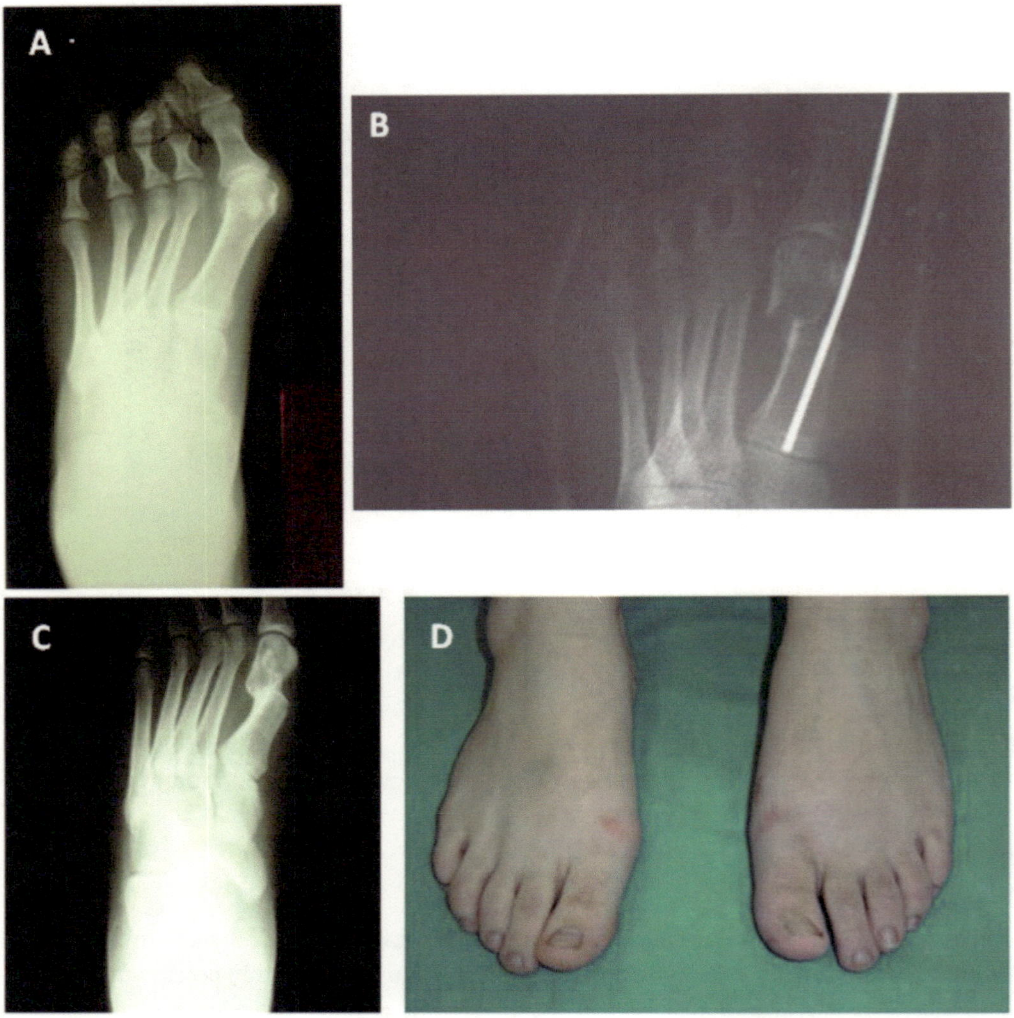

Fig. 11. 13 years old female with hallux valgus deformity of the left foot. The patient had been treated for flatfoot 2 years before. A, preoperative X-ray; B, Postoperative X-ray; C –D, X-ray and Clinical Control after 1 year.

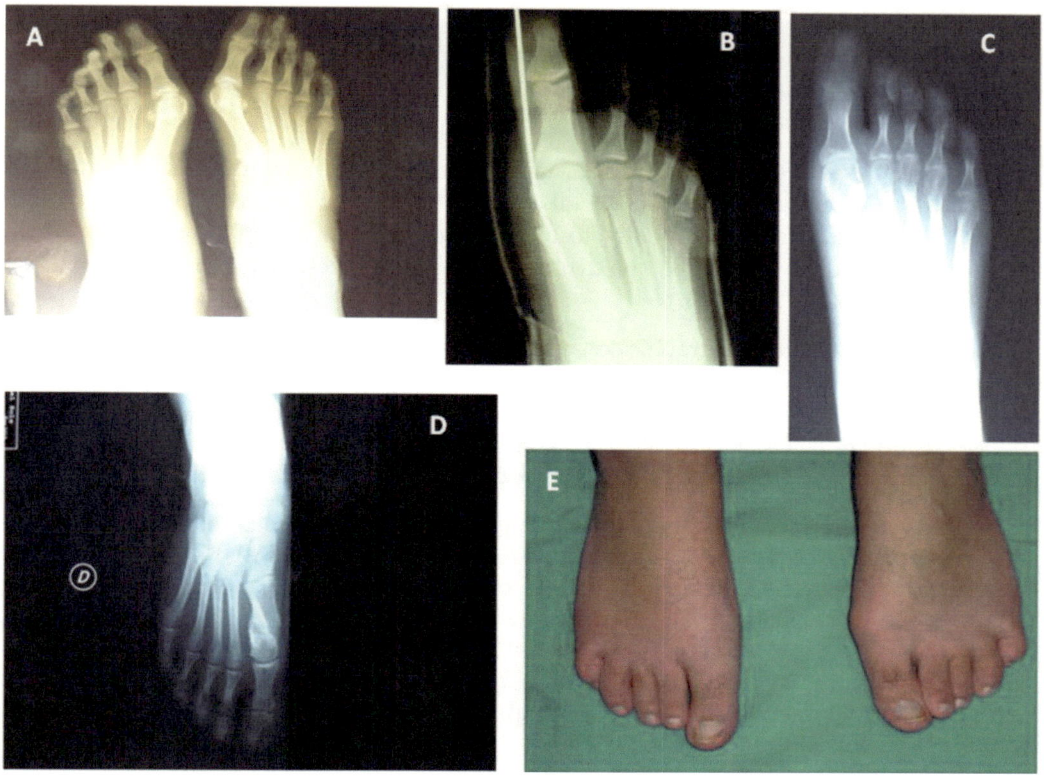

Fig. 12. 14 years old female with bilateral hallux valgus deformity. The patient had been already treated for flatfoot. A, preoperative X-ray; B, Postoperative X-ray; C, X-ray control 4 weeks later; D-E, X-ray and Clinical Control after 1 year.

12. Discussion

Minimally invasive surgical technique (MIS) for the treatment of the hallux valgus deformity has been described for the first time by Bosch in 1990 with his "distal linear osteotomy with temporary fixation with a single Kirschner wire". Bartolozzi and Magnan in 1997 described, than, the P.D.O. (Percutaneous Distal Osteotomy) and Giannini in 2003 the "S.E.R.I." (Simple, Effective, Rapid, Inexpensive).

These three techniques involve a distal first metatarsal osteotomy with a minimally invasive access and stabilization with K-wire. They differ only in surgical times and in the K-wire direction. Bosh technique involves incision, osteotomy and stabilization with a K-wire applied according to a distal-proximal direction; in the PDO, the application of the wire according to a distal-proximal direction comes before the incision and the osteotomy; SERI proposed by Giannini, consists of incision, osteotomy and K-wire according to proximal-distal direction through the skin incision already made.

Authors that have proposed surgical techniques for distal osteotomy with internal fixation, indicated like limit of a medium lateral shift of the metatarsal epiphysis 30-50% of the transverse diameter of the metatarsus, to allow an optimum stability of the synthesis.

Whereas potentially the correction of a distal osteotomy is about 1° per each mm of lateral displacement (Johnson 1994), traditional protocols provide like indication as an upper limit of a distal metatarsal osteotomy, a varus deformity of the first metatarsal not greater than 15-18 degrees of the intermetatarsal angle.

The minimally invasive technique with K-wire fixation, allows a lateral shift up to 90% of the transverse diameter of the metatarsal ("cortex on cortex") with a correction of the deformity which can be up, potentially, to 10-12 degrees, also including some cases in which traditional protocols would have opted for different techniques, as a proximal metatarsal osteotomy (Magnan et al., 1998).

All osteotomies reached radiographic consolidation within 6 months with abundant periosteal callus. This needed time could be considered entirely physiological for the healing of a metatarsal osteotomy, especially with a elastic type stabilization, with an evolution like to a "stress" fracture (Magnan et al., 1998). Although 1% of nonunion in osteotomies treated with a K-wire is reported in literature (Bosch, 1990), we did not observe nonunions in our experience.

Even if in literature the association of pes planus with the development of a juvenile hallux valgus deformity is controversial, in our experience and in the series we described there is a 100% association between hallux valgus and pes planus valgus, so with a pronated foot. Therefore, we can conclude that especially in the etiology and pathophisiology of hallux valgus, a defect in pronation of the foot plays a key role in the development of a metatarsus varus and therefore of a bunion, as described by Jordan and Brodsky in 1951. In addition, many of these young patients are overweight and this could affect the structural and biomechanical changes of the foot.

So if the pronation of the foot is a predisposing condition for the hallux valgus deformity, it is essential first of all to correct the valgus flat foot, especially to avoid recurrences that a wrong weight transfer on the forefoot could cause.

95% of young patients with hallux valgus deformity in the described series were females. This suggests a natural predisposition of women to this type of deformity, not influenced by the use of deforming fashionable women's shoes.

As younger patients poorly tolerate pain during the first postoperative days and, considering the age, they are not careful to protect the forefoot, we prefer not to allow the weight-bearing for about 7 days after surgery and immediately apply a short leg cast that allows walking, but protecting the osteotomy and synthesis site.

13. Conclusions

Since 2000, we treated 55 young patients with juvenile hallux valgus deformity always associated with valgus flat foot, performing a transverse osteotomy below the head of 1st metatarsal with minimally invasive surgical technique (S.E.R.I.). In our experience, it is a condition more common in young girls and it's often associated to valgus flat foot.

Surgery was indicated to restore the correct aesthetic and functional anatomy of the foot. It's important correcting it before deformity is structured, using the repair capability of the bone during adolescence, to prevent morphological more serious alterations in future and difficulty in walking.

As also indicated by the algorithm suggested by AOFAS, minimally invasive technique for the correction of the hallux valgus deformity allows to correct about 80% - 90% of all deformities without the need to remove the medial prominence or to run lateral release, but doing just the manipulation of the great toe with good or excellent results.

With this technique, we can obtain a plantar displacement of the first metatarsal head and a redistribution of weight on the other metatarsal heads, thereby reducing metatarsalgia.

The complete avoidance of surgical procedures on soft tissue, eliminates risks linked to this type of surgery, responsible sometimes of overcorrection.

Anyway, it's necessary for a correct timing surgery, an accurate clinical and radiological evaluation of the foot on weight-bearing with the analysis of the radiological angles linked to the hallux valgus deformity.

In all treated cases, correction of the hallux valgus deformity was performed about 2 years later the calcaneo stop surgical treatment for the flatfoot.

This technique can be applied safely in children. But, first of all, it is very important to correct the biomechanical imbalance in pronation of the foot predisposing the formation of the hallux valgus deformity.

For this reason it is advisable to carry out the surgery only when the pronation of the foot is corrected to obtain a right transmission of the weight on the metatarsals and to avoid recurrences in the growth phase.

Moreover, especially in children, the osteotomy area must be prevented from trauma and post-operative pain may be poorly tolerated by juveniles much more than adults. This is why we recommend to deny the weight-bearing for the first week and apply a short leg cast for 4 weeks.

In all cases, the treated metatarsals showed a remodeling even in case of significant displacement of the osteotomy with only few millimeters of bone contact. The consolidation of the osteotomy and the metatarsal bone remodeling capacity are not related to the displacement of the osteotomy, although an even minimal contact between the two bone fragments is necessary.

X-rays performed postoperatively, appear to be sufficient for proper clinical evaluation only after 3 months. In fact, this is the minimum period in order to obtain significant information regarding the healing of a metatarsal osteotomy. X-rays performed before that period, reassure the surgeon about the relationship of bone segments, but give no information about the clinical course.

Compared with conventional osteotomy (Scarf) (Mafulli et al., 2009), the minimally invasive technique has demonstrated comparable efficacy and a reduction in surgical time and hospital stay. Moreover it is inexpensive because it does not require any special tools, but only a K-wire for the stabilization, and has a minimal incidence of complications.

14. Acknowledgment

We gratefully acknowledge the assistance of Dr. Letizia Averna, University of Palermo.

15. References

Acheson RM, Chan YK, Clemett AR. (1970). New Haven Survey of joint diseases. Distribution and symptoms of osteoarthritis in the hand with reference to handedness. *Ann Rheum Dis;* Vol,12. No,29. Pp.275-285.

Amarnek DL, Jacobs AM, Oloff LM. (1985). Adolescent hallux valgus: an etiology and surgical management. *J Foot Surg* No,24. Pp.54-61.

Amarnek DL, Mollica A, Jacobs A, Oloff LA. (1986). A statistical analysis on the reliability of the proximal articular set angle; *J. Foot Surgery.* No,25. Pp.39-43.

Balding MG, Sorto LA jr. (985). Distal Articular Set Angle. Etiology and X-Ray Evaluation; *J.A.P.M.A.* No,75. Pp.648-652.

Bamel F, Canovas F, poiree G, Dusserre F, Vergnes C. (1999). Radiological results of scarf osteotomy for allux valgus related to distal metatarsal articular angle. *Rev Chir Orthop Reparatrice App Mot.* No,85. Pp.381-386.

Bartolozzi P. et al. (2011). Chirurgia mininvasiva dell'alluce valgo; *GIOT.* No,37. Pp.92-112.

Bartolozzi P., Magnan B. (2000). *L'osteotomia distale percutanea nella chirurgia dell'alluce valgo.* (Timeo). Bologna.

Benvenuti F, Ferrucci L, Guralnik JM, Gangemi S, Baroni A. (1995). Foot pain and disability in older persons: an epidemiologic survey. *J Am Geriatr Soc.* No,43. Pp.479–84.

Bosch P., Markowski H., Rannicher V. (1990). Technik und erste ergebnisse der subkutanen distalen metatarsale - I - osteotomie. *Orthopaedische Praxis.* No,26. Pp.51-6.

Bosch P., Wanke S., Legenstein R. (2000). Hallux valgus correction by the method of Bosch: a new technique with a seven-to-ten-year follow-up. *Foot and Ankle Clinics.* Vol.5, No.3, pp.485-98.

Brage ME, Holmes JR, Sangeorzan BJ. (1994). The influence of x-ray orientation of the first metatarsocuneiform joint angle. *Foot Ankle Int.* No.15, pp.495-497.

Clark HR., Veith RG. & Hansen STJr.(1987). Adolescent bunions treated by the modified Lapidus procedure. *Bull HospJt Dis Orthop Inst.* No.47, pp.109-122.

Coughlin MJ, Jones CP: Hallux valgus. (2005). Demographics, radiographic assessment and clinical outcomes. A prospective study, *Proceedings of 21st annual summer meeting of the American Orthopedic Foot and Ankle Society,* July 17, 2005.

Coughlin MJ. & Mann RA. (1987). The pathophysiology of the juvenile bunion. *Instr Course Lect.* No.36, pp.123-136.

Coughlin MJ. (1990). President's Forum:evaluation and treatment of juvenile hallux valgus. *Contemp Ortoph.* No.21, pp.169-203.

Coughlin MJ. (1996). Hallux valgus. *J Boone Joint Surg Am.* No.78, pp.932-966.

Coughlin MJ: Roger A. Mann Award. (1995). Juvenile hallux valgus: Etiology and treatment. *Foot Ankle Int.* No.16, pp.682-697.

Dunn JE, Link CL, Felson DT, Crincoli MG, Keysor JJ, Mc-Kinlay JB. (2004). Prevalence of foot and ankle conditions in a multiethnic community sample of older adults. *Am J Epidemiol.* No.159, pp.491–498.

DuVries H (Ed.). (1959). Surgery of the foot. CVmosby St. Louis. pp. 346-442.

Elton PJ, Sanderson SP. (1986). A chiropodial survey of elderly persons over 65 years in the community. *Public Health* No.100, pp.219–222.

Funk FJ Jr, Wells RE. (1972).Bunionectomy-with distal osteotomy. *Clin Orthop* No.85, pp.71-74.

Giannini S, Ceccarelli F, Bevoni R, et al. (2003). Hallux valgus surgery: the minimally invasive bunion correction. *Tech Foot Ankle Surg.* No.2, pp.11-20.

Giannini S, Vannini F, Faldini C, Bevoni R, Nanni M, Leoneni D. (2007). The minimally invasive hallux valgus correction (S.E.R.I.). *Interact Surg.* No.2, pp.17-23.

Glasoe WM, Alen MK, Saltzman CL. (2001). First ray dorsal mobility in relation to hallux valgus deformity and first intermetatarsal angle. *Foot Ankle Int.* No.22, pp.98-101.

Goldner JL. & Gaines RW. (1976). Adult and juvenile hallux valgus:analysis and treatment. *Orthop Clin North Am.* No.7, pp.863-887.

Grebing BR, Coughlin MJ. (2004). The effect of ankle position on the exam for first ray mobility. *Foot Ankle Int.* No.25, pp.467-475.

Grebing BR. & Coughlin MJ. (2004). Evaluation of Morton's Theory of second metatarsal hypertrophy. *J Bone Joint Surg Am.* No.86, pp.1375-1386.

Haines RW. & Mc Dougall AM. (1954). The anatomy of hallux valgus. *J Bone Joint Surg Br.* No.36, pp.272-293.

Hardy RH, Clapham JCR. (1951). Observations on hallux valgus; based on a controlled series J. *Bone Joint Surgery.* No.33B, pp.376-391.

Hardy RH. & Clapham JC. (1952). Hallux valgus; predisposing anatomical causes. *Lancet.* No.1, pp. 1180-1183.

Hohmann G. (1925). Der Hallux valgus und die uebrigen Zchenverkruemmungen. *Egerb Chir Orthop* No.18, pp.308-348.

Hueter C. in Kelikian H. (1965). Hallux valgus. Allied deformities of the forefoot and metatarsalgia; *Philadelphia & London.* pp. 10.

Johnson KA. (1994). Master techniques in orthopaedics surgery, in: *the foot and the ankle,* No.4, pp.31-48.

Johnston O. (1956). Further studies of the inheritance of hand and foot anomalies. *Clin Orthop.* Vol.8, pp. 146-160.

Jones A. (1948). Hallux valgus in the adolescent. *Proc R Soc Med.* No.41, pp.392-393.

Jordan HH, Brodsky AE. (1951). Keller operation for hallux valgus and hallux rigidus; *A.M.A. Arch Surg.*No.62, pp.586-596.

Kelikian H. (1965). Hallux valgus. Allied deformities of the forefoot and metatarsalgia; *Philadelphia and London: Saunders Company.*

Kellgren JH, Moore R. (1952). Generalised osteoarthritis and Heberden's nodes. *Br Med J.* No.1, pp.181-187.

Kilmartin TE. (1994). The Orthotic Treatment of Juvenile Hallux Valgus. *Submitted to the University of Nottingham for the Degree of Doctor of Philosophy.*

King DM & Toolan BC. (2004). Associated deformities and hypermobility in hallux valgus: an investigation with weightbearing radiographs. *Foot Ankle Int.* Vol. 25, pp. 251-255.

Klaue K, Hansen ST, Masquelet AC. (1994). Clinical, quantitative assessment of first tarsometatarsal mobility in the sagittal plane and its relation to hallux valgus deformity. *Foot Ankle Int.* No.15, pp.9-13.

Klein C, Groll-Knapp E, Kundi M, Kinz W. (2009). Increased hallux angle in children and its association with insufficient length of footwear: A community based cross-sectional study. *BMC Musculoskeletal Disorders.* No.10, p.159.

La Porta G, Melillo T, Olinsky D. (1974). X-Ray evaluation of hallux abducto valgus deformity. *J.A.P.A.* Vol.64, No.8, pp.544-566.

Lapidus PW. (1934). Operative correction of metatarsus varus primus in hallux valgus. *Surg Gynecol Obstet.* No.58, pp.183-191.

Lapidus PW. (1956). A quarter of a century of experience with the operative correction of the metatarsus varus primus in hallux valgus. *Bull Hosp Jt Dis.* No.17, pp.404-421.

Lapidus PW. (1960). The author's bunion operation from 1931 to 1959. *Clin Orthop.* No.16, pp.119-135.

Leveille SG, Guralnik JM, Ferrucci L, Hirsch R, Simonsick E, Hochberg MC. (1998). Foot pain and disability in older women. *Am J Epidemiol,* No.148, pp.657–665.

Mafulli N, Longo UG, Oliva F, et al. (2009). Bosch osteotomy and scarf osteotomy for hallux valgus correction. *Orthop Clin North Am,* No.40, pp. 515-524.

Magnan B, Montanari M, Bragantini A, Fieschi S, Bartolozzi P. (1997). Trattamento dell'alluce valgo con tecnica "mini-invasiva" percutanea (P.D.O.: Percutaneous Distal Osteotomy). *Progressi in Chirurgia del Piede,* No.6, pp.91-104.

Magnan B. Et al. (1998). Trattamento chirurgico dell'alluce valgo con osteotomia distale percutanea del primo metatarsale. Note di tecnica. G.I.O.T., Vol.XXIV, No.4, (dicembre 1998), pp.473-487.

Mann RA, Coughlin MJ. (2010). Hallux Valgus. In Coughlin M, Mann RA, Saltzmann CL (eds.): *Surgery of the foot and ankle,* 8th edition. Philadelphia, Elsevier, No7, pp. 184-354.

McHale K, McKay D. (1986). Bunions in a child: Conservative versus surgical management. *J Musculoskel Med,* No.3, pp.56-62.

Myerson MS. (2000). Hallux Vaulgus, in: *Foot and ankle disorders.* Saunders WB, Philandelphia, pp. 213-289.

Neame R, Zhang W, Deighton C, Doherty M, Doherty S, Lanyon P, et al. (2004). Distribution of radiographic osteoarthritis between right and left hands, hips, and knees. *Arthritis Rheum,* No.50, pp.1487-1494.

Piggot H. (1960). The natural history of hallux valgus in adolescence and early adult life. J Bone Joint Surgery; No.42-B, pp. 749-760.

Roddy E, Zhang W, Doherty M. (2008). Prevalence and Associations of Hallux Valgus in a Primary Care Population. *Arthritis & Rheumatism (Arthritis Care & Research)* Vol. 59, No. 6, pp.857–862.

Root ML, Orien WP, Weed JR. (1971). Biomechanical Examination of the foot; Clinical Biomechanics Corp. Los Angeles.

Root ML, Orien WP, Weed JR. (1977). Normal and abnormal function of the foot. Vol II Clinical Biomechanics Corp. Los Angeles.

Scranton PE Jr (1982). Adolescent bunions: Diagnosis and management. *Pediatr Ann,* No.11,.

Sim-Fook L, Hodgson AR. (1958). A comparison of foot forms among the non-shoe and shoe-wearing Chinese population. *J Bone Joint Surg Am,* No.40, pp.1058-1062.

Thompson GH. (1996). Bunions and deformities of the toes in children and adolescents. *Instr Course Lect.* No.45, pp.355-367.

Weissman SD. (1989). *Radiology of the foot* – 2nd Ed., Wiliam and Wilkins, Baltimore.

White EG, Mulley GP. (1989). Footcare for very elderly people: a community survey. *Age Ageing,* No.18, pp.276–278.

Wilder FV, Barrett JP, Farina EJ. (2005). The association of radiographic foot osteoarthritis and radiographic osteoarthritis at other sites. *Osteoarthritis Cartilage,* No.13, pp.211-215.

14

Minimally Invasive Distal Metatarsal Osteotomy for Mild-to-Moderate Hallux Valgus

Ahmed Enan
Mansoura University,
Egypt

1. Introduction

Hallux valgus is a common disorder of the forefoot that results from medial deviation of the first metatarsal and lateral deviation and / or rotation of the great toe (hallux) with or without medial soft-tissue enlargement of the first metatarsal head (bunion) (1).

2. Potential etiology

The pathogenesis of hallux valgus has been described as being due to muscle imbalance.

A. Extrinsic factors

Hallux valgus occurs almost exclusively in shoe - wearing societies. Coughlin and Thompson (2) noting the extremely high prevalence of bunions in American women in the fourth, fifth or sixth decade of life, implicated constricting footwear as a cause of hallux valgus. Likewise, in Japan, Kato and Watanabe (3) noted that the prevalence of hallux valgus in women increased dramatically following the introduction of high - fashion footwear after World War II.

B. Intrinsic factors

While constricting footwear appears to be the major extrinsic cause of hallux valgus, intrinsic factors play a role as well. Inman (4) and Hohmann (5) both suggested pronation of the hindfoot as a major cause of bunion formation, while Mann and Coughlin (6) as well as others (7,8) reported that pes planus plays a minor role in this process. An increased angle between the first and second metatarsals (metatarsus primus varus) is often associated with hallux valgus deformity. (9) Other intrinsic causes of Hallux valgus may include contracture of the Achilles tendon, generalized joint laxity, hypermobility of the first metatarso - cuneiform joint, and neuromuscular disorders (including cerebral palsy and stroke). (10) Heredity is thought to influence the development of hallux valgus in many individuals. Hardy and Clapham noted that 63 % of the patients in their series had a parent who had hallux valgus. (9) The primary symptom of hallux valgus is pain over the medial eminence. Pressure from footwear is the most frequent cause of this discomfort.

2.1 Measurements of the deformity

Two angles frequently are used to describe the anatomical deformity and the effects of a surgical procedure: the first intermetatarsal angle (IMA) and the hallux valgus angle (HVA).

Authors classify mild as an IMA < 13°, moderate as IMA 13 - 20°, and severe as an IMA > 20°. Generally, a HVA > 40° is considered severe. (11)

2.2 Surgical treatment

The condition is widely reported in the Western literature. The incidence of hallux valgus was as high as 50 % in a study in South Africans (12) and as low as 2 % in a study on barefoot population. (13) Nonoperative treatment is always the first option for a patient with hallux valgus deformity. Surgery is proposed when the painful hallux valgus is not adequately controlled by the nonoperative treatment. Over the past century, around 150 surgical procedures have been developed to reduce the deformity, and the continued development of new techniques would suggest that previous techniques are not completely successful. Poorly planned or executed surgery may lead to high levels of patient dissatisfaction. In the last few years, several new osteotomies have been described, but often it is difficult to ascertain what the best choice for a given patient is, as evidence-based guidelines are lacking.(1) The main goal of surgical correction of hallux valgus is the morphologic and functional rebalance of the first ray, correcting all other characteristics of the deformity. Historically, distal metatarsal osteotomies have been indicted in cases of mild or moderate deformity with an intermetatarsal angle as large as 15°. Using certain osteotomies, it is possible to correct intermetatarsal angles as large as 20°. Distal osteotomies may also be used to correct deformities characterized by deviation of the distal metatarsal articular angle (DMAA) or to address concomitant stiffness.(14) Since the first operation published by Revenrdin (15) in 1881, many authors have reported their experience using different operations, each of them characterized by different indications, approaches, designs, and fixation.(16-24) There is an increasing concern among orthopaedists towards the potentials of minimally invasive procedures. Applied to foot surgery, minimally invasive surgery (MIS) can be accomplished is shorter time respect of a conventional surgery, together with less distress and problems to the soft tissues. In addition, the operation can be done bilaterally; it allows use of distal anaesthetics blocks and early weight-bearing. In 1986, Van Enoo defined the minimum-incision surgery as an operation done through the smallest incision required for a proper procedure, and the percutaneous surgery as that performed within the smallest possible working incision in a closed fashion. (25) A percutaneous MIS requires the use of dedicated instruments and frequently a fluoroscopy. Lui and other colleagues from Hong Kong have described arthroscopic and endoscopic assisted correction of hallux valgus deformities. (26, 27) Morton Polokoff, a podiatric physician, in 1945 tried to use fine chisels, rasps and spears to perform subdermal surgery. Years later, Leonard Britton accomplished the first osteotomy on bunion deformities with percutaneous exposure of the first metatarsal, a closing wedge osteotomy, and the Akin procedure. North American podiatrists started to adopt MIS of the foot in 1970.(28) The technique percutaneous surgery for hallux valgus correction that we use derives from that described by Lamprecht-Kramer-Bösch in 1982.(16,29) These authors based the procedure on the subcapital metatarsal linear osteotomy of Hohmann.(30) In 1991, Isham described a minimally invasive distal metatarsal osteotomy without implantation.(31) The results of recent French studies showed that patients treated with minimally invasive surgery for hallux valgus needed less hospitalization time and recovered earlier.(32) Minimum incision techniques, by allowing limb safety with reduced damage of soft tissue or bones trauma should be a first choice indication to patients at high risk of ulceration.(33,34) The characteristics of this technique can be summarized with the abbreviation SERI (simple, effective, rapid, inexpensive).

3. Indications

The SERI technique is indicated to correct mild to moderate reducible deformity when the hallux valgus angle is as large as 40° and the intermetatarsal angle is as large as 20°. The operation is indicated if the metatarsophalangeal joint is either incongruent or congruent, or with modification of the DMAA, and if mild degenerative arthritis is present. The technique is indicated even in cases of recurrent deformity.

4. Contraindications

Specific contraindications of the SERI technique are patients older than 75 years, severe deformity with the intermetatarsal angle larger than 20°, severe degenerative arthritis or stiffness of the metatarsophalangeal joint, and severe instability of the cuneometatarsal or metatarsophalangeal joint. The technique is not indicated in hallux rigidus and in patients in whom a Keller's procedure unsuccessful .(35,36)

5. Preoperative assessment

The preoperative plan includes acquiring a complete history of the patient plus physical and radiographic examination. The patient's complaints of pain, limitation in the use of footwear, and cosmetic concerns should be considered. Moreover, the severity of the prominent medial eminence and the hallux valgus deformity, as well as the great toe mobility at the metatarso - phalangeal joint and the reducibility of the deformity should be evaluated. The latter is tested by pushing laterally the metatarsal head with one hand, and simultaneously the great toe medially with the other hand. Stability of the metatarso - phalangeal and metatarso - cuneiform joints must be assessed. Combined rotational deformity of the great toe or callosities under the first or second and third metatarsal heads must be considered, as well as any associated deformities of the lesser toes. A standard radiographic examination, including anteroposterior and lateral weight-bearing views of the forefoot, allows the assessment of the arthritis and congruency of the joint; measurement of the hallux valgus angle and intermetatarsal angle. The hallux valgus angle was measured by the method of Piggot. (37) The intermetatarsal angle by the method of Coughlin et al . (38) (fig. 1). The relative length of the first metatarsal was measured by the method of Morton. (39) (fig. 2)

6. Surgical technique

This technique was described by the author in the study that was published in Acta Orthopædica Belgica, Vol. 76 - 4 - 2010. The patient is placed in the supine position, with a below knee wedge bracket allowing 90° of knee flexion and a plantigrade position of the foot on the operating table. Pneumatic tourniquet was applied in all cases. The operation is performed with either general or ankle - block anesthesia. The fluoroscopic image intensifier must be positioned to the side of the patient while the surgeon stands in front of the patient at the end of the table. Normally with this technique, soft - tissue release is not needed because attenuation is achieved with the lateral offset of the metatarsal head itself. If a slight stiffness of the metatarsophalangeal joint is present, manual stretching of the adductor hallucis is performed, forcing the big toe into a varus position.

Step 1. Wire insertion. Under image intensifier a 2.0 mm K - wire is inserted starting from the proximal medial corner of the nail of the great toe. (fig. 3- A) The pin is manually driven along the medial border of the proximal phalanx in a distal – to – proximal direction to end distal to the site of the planed osteotomy. It is mandatory to place the wire in an extraperiosteal position in order to allow lateral displacement of the capital fragment at the osteotomy site. (fig. 3- B) The wire must be midway between the dorsal and plantar aspect of the great toe in order to engage the metatarsal head correctly. This represents one of the most important biomechanical aspects of the technique. If the metatarsal head should be shifted plantarward, the pin has to be inserted more dorsally. If the metatarsal head should be shifted dorsally, the K – wire has to be inserted more plantarward. Plantar translation is done more often.

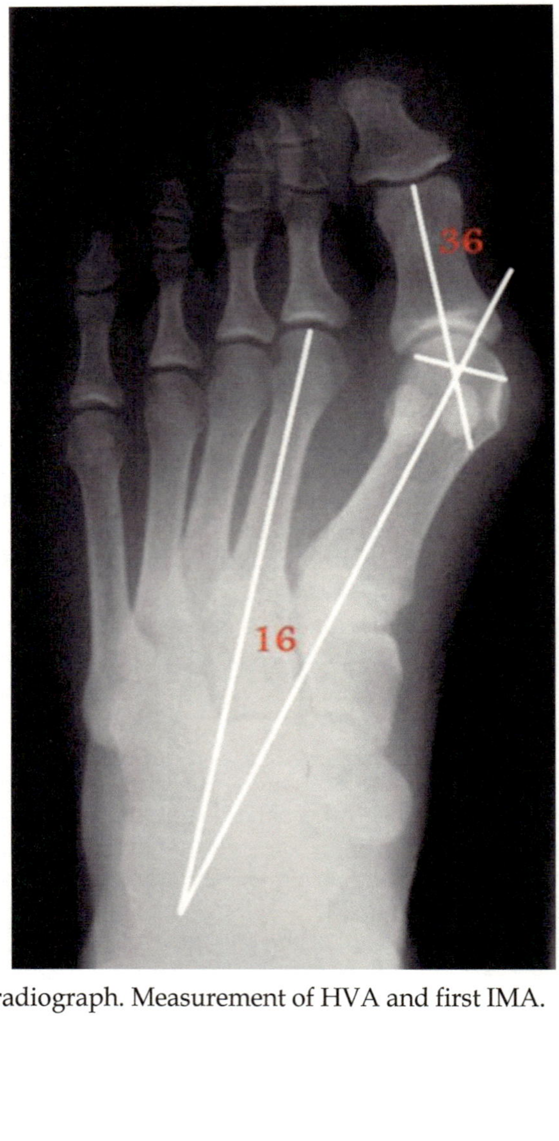

Fig. 1. A-P standing radiograph. Measurement of HVA and first IMA.

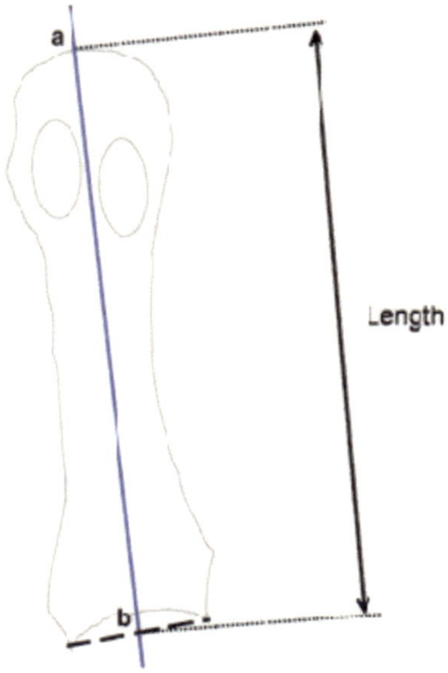

Fig. 2. Method of measuring the length of the first metatarsal. (a) Distal end of the first metatarsal head. (b) Point of intersection of the first metatarsal longitudinal axis with a line connecting the proximal-medial and proximal-lateral ends of the metatarsal base.

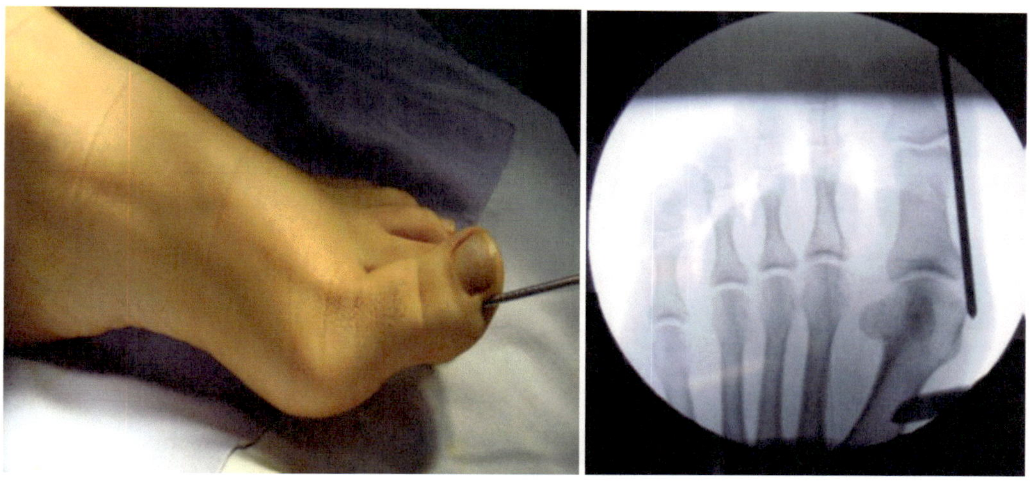

A B

Fig. 3. A. 2 mm Kirschner wire is inserted in the medial corner of the nail of the great toe. B. Extraperiosteal position of the K- wire along the medial border of proximal phalanx

Step 2. Skin incision. A 1.5 cm skin incision was made and centered over the medial aspect of the first metatarsal neck. (fig. 3- C) The incision was carried directly to the bone, cutting the periosteum, with care being taken to remain in the midline equally between the dorsal and plantar aspects of the metatarsal neck in order to avoid the neurovascular bundle.

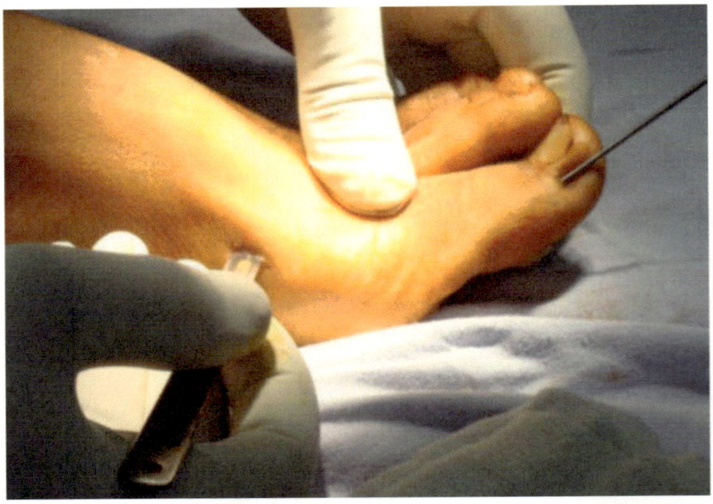

Fig. 3. C. 1.5 cm skin incision centered over the medial aspect of the first metatarsal neck.

Step 3. Periosteal detachment. Next, the periosteum around the osteotomy site is detached dorsally and then plantarly, with use of small scissors inserted through the skin incision. (fig. 3- D) In this way, the soft tissues surrounding the metatarsal shaft can be kept away from the bone cutter (saw).

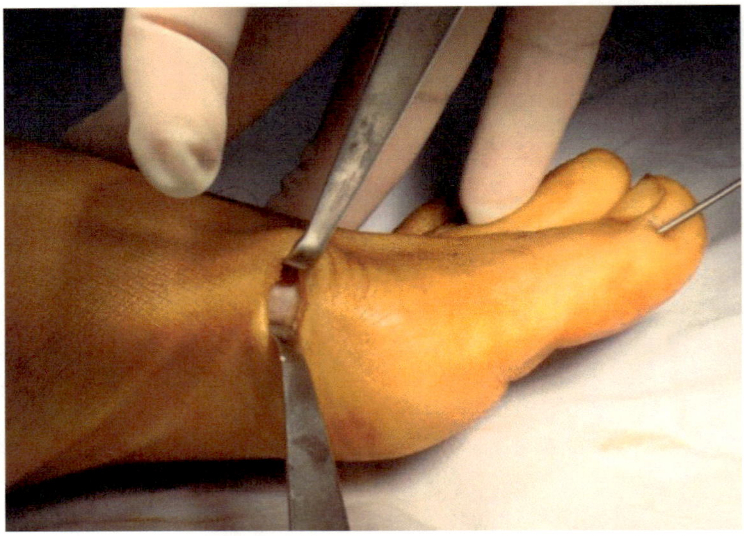

Fig. 3. D. Periosteum around the osteotomy site is detached dorsally and then plantarly

Step 4. Osteotomy. The osteotomy is then performed through the subcapital region of the first metatarsal with an oscillating saw. (fig. 3- E) The level of the cut is first checked under fluoroscopy. The osteotomy is made perpendicular to the long axis of the shaft of the first metatarsal in the sagittal plane. (fig. 3- F) In the frontal plane, the osteotomy should be performed with slight mediolateral obliquity to facilitate lengthening or shortening as dictated by the preoperative plan. Generally, a slight lengthening is recommended in order to avoid metatarsal shortening. Finally, the osteotomy site is checked manually and under fluoroscopy to confirm sufficient mobility of the metatarsal head.

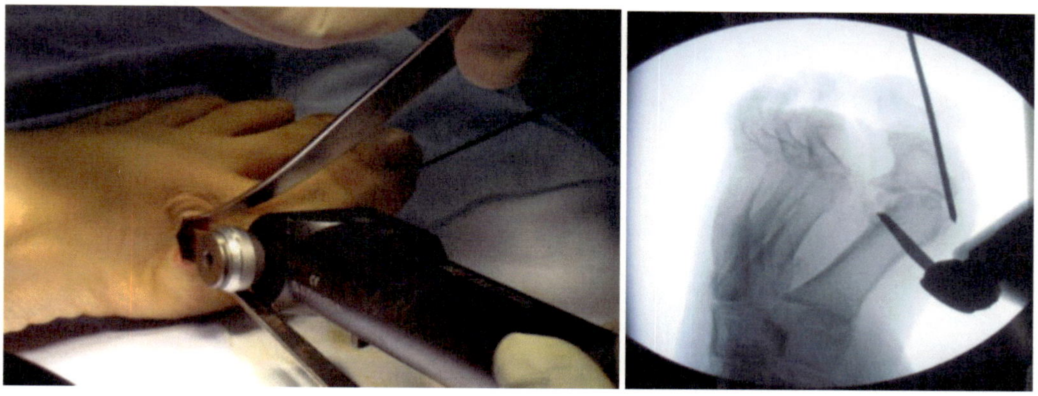

Fig. 3. E. The osteotomy performed through the subcapital region of the first metatarsal with an oscillating saw. F. The level of the cut is checked

Step 5. Metatarsal displacement and correction. The proximal part of the first metatarsal is then displaced medially with the aid of a curved small artery forceps introduced in the medullary canal in order to facilitate the insertion of the K - wire. (fig. 3- G) After lateral translation of the metatarsal head, the wire was introduced under direct vision into the medullary canal of the metatarsal shaft. (fig. 3- H) The correction of the big toe was determined grossly. If pronation of the first metatarsal bone is present, the correction is obtained with a derotation of the big toe up to the neutral position.

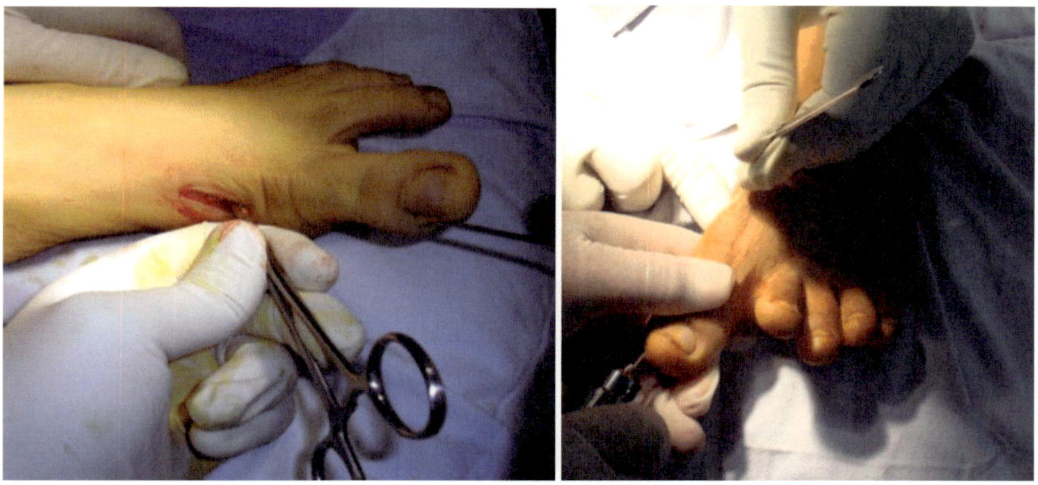

Fig. 3. G. Using a curved small artery forceps the proximal part of first metatarsal is displaced medially. H. Lateral displacement of the head and correction of hallux achieved with the Kirschner wire introduced under direct vision into the medullary canal

Step 6. Advancement of the wire through the mid tarsals. The wire was driven through the first tarsometatarsal joint for greater stabilization. (fig. 3- I)

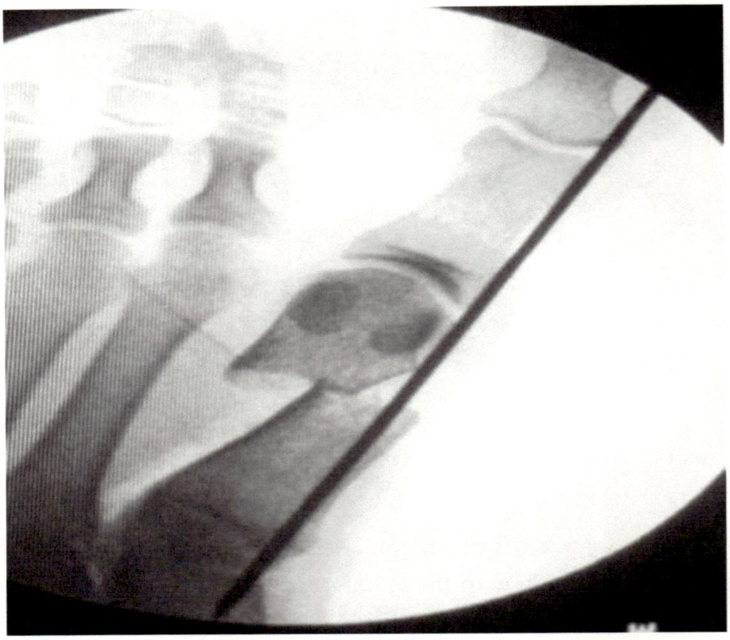

Fig. 3. I. The kirshner wire is driven through the first tarsometatarsal joint for greater stabilization.

Step 7. Closure. The skin is sutured with two 2 - 0 prolene stitches. The distal extremity of the K - wire is curved and cut out of the tip of the toe. (fig. 3- J) A plantar pad was placed under the operated foot to reduce weight - bearing pressure under the first metatarsal head area. An elastic bandage was used as a postoperative dressing to hold the big toe in alignment . It was taped in a supination manner to counteract pronation of the big toe. (fig. 3- K)

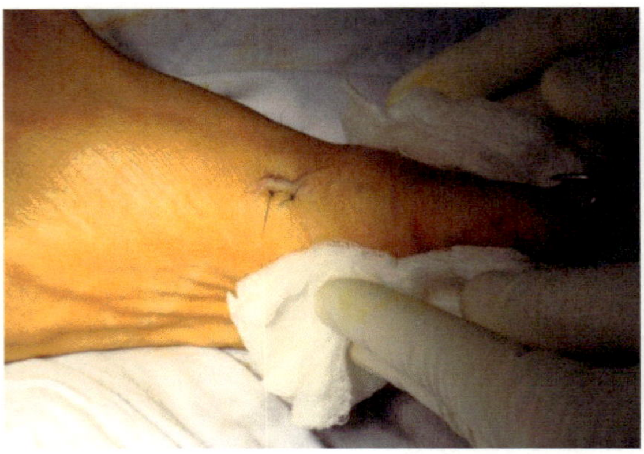

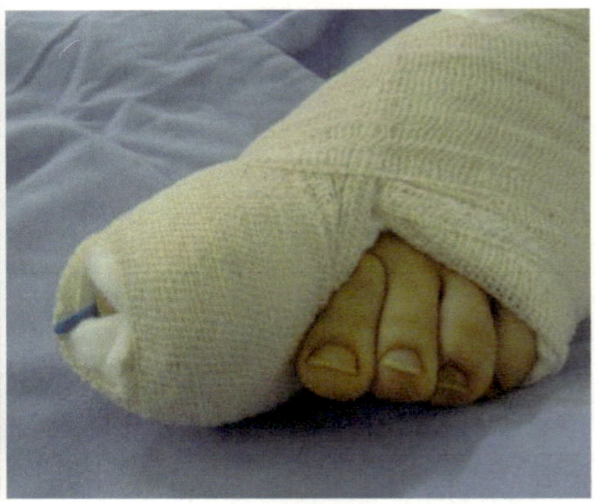

Fig. 3. J. Skin is closed with two 2-0 prolene stitches and the wire bend and cut. K. Elastic bandage was used as a postoperative support to hold the big toe in alignment.

7. Follow-up

Postoperatively, Patients can walk immediately in a flat, rigid sole postoperative shoe, which allows not to put weight through the osteotomy, though in the beginning they are advised to walk for short times only, and to rest with the foot raised while supine or sitting.

The stitches were removed two weeks after surgery, while the K - wire was removed 6 weeks postoperatively.

Patients were allowed to bear weight with normal shoes, and range of motion exercises of the first metatarsophalangeal joint was carried out from then on.

The postoperative examinations included X - ray next day postoperative and then six weeks after the operation. The patient is then reviewed between two and three months later for the third radiological and clinical control. The future follow - up frequency is variable, and usually every 6 months.

Clinically the patients on each follow - up were questioned about the cosmetic appearance of the foot, pain over the metatarsal head and shoe - wear problems. Thorough clinical examination was done looking for appearance, calluses under second and third metatarsal heads (transfer lesions), sensory abnormalities, and the range of motion of first MTP joint.

Furthermore, the clinical rating system for foot and ankle function, established by Kitaoka et al (40) [American Orthopaedic Foot and Ankle Society (AOFAS) Hallux - Metatarsophalangeal - Interphalangeal Score] was used as a quantification of the clinical and subjective evaluation at follow - up. Additionally the patients have been asked whether they were satisfied with the result of the operation or not. During the examination, special attention was paid to the aspect of metatarsalgia. The assessment of the passive range of motion (ROM) of the first metatarso - phalangeal joint was performed according to Okuda et al. (41)

The preoperative and the follow - up radiographs were made with the patient in the weight - bearing position.

Quantitative data were described by mean ± standard deviation (SD) or if more appropriate by median and range. Statistical analyses were performed using SPSS software V. 16.0 (SPSS Inc., Chicago, IL, USA).

8. Results of our study

Twenty - six patients with symptomatic mild - to - moderate hallux valgus deformities were operated using minimally invasive distal metatarsal osteotomy. Two patients were lost to follow - up and could not complete the minimum follow - up period of 12 months. The study describes the results of 36 feet in 24 patients comprising 20 female and 4 male patients. Twelve patients had a bilateral involvement. The age of the patients ranged from 17 to 52 years, the mean age being 37.8 years. The average follow - up period was 21 months (range 12 - 36 months).

9. Clinical results

Hallux - Metatarsophalangeal - Interphalangeal Scale proposed by the American Orthopaedic Foot and Ankle Society (AOFAS) was used for the clinical assessment. This system provides a score ranging from 0 to 100 points, which takes into consideration both subjective and objective elements such as pain (maximum score, 40 points), functional capacity (maximum score, 45 points), and hallux alignment (maximum score, 15 points). For all patients were seen at the time of final follow - up, there was no case of worsening of pain and no patient who presented with shoe - wear restriction as primary symptom had such pain after surgery. Eighteen patients (thirty feet; 83.3 %) reported total disappearance of the pain, four patients (four feet; 11.1 %) had only mild occasional pain, two patients (two feet; 5.6 %) had daily moderate pain, and no patient had severe or constant pain. The mean overall pain score was 37.3 ± 4.7 points of the 40 point maximum on the AOFAS.

The functional capacity of the hallux, which was graded by summing the scores for the six different aspects of functional performance on the hallux - metatarsophalangeal - interphalangeal scale, averaged 40.9 ± 3.6 points (maximum score on the scale, 45 points). The maximum score for hallux alignment (15 points, indicating excellent or good alignment) on the hallux - metatarsophalangeal - interphalangeal scale was recorded for thirty feet (83.3%) in 20 patients; mild, asymptomatic malalignment (a score of 8 points) was recorded for six feet (16.7%) in four patients; and symptomatic malalignment (a score of 0 points) was not recorded in our study. The overall mean score for hallux alignment was 12.9 ± 4.2 points.

The total scores at the time of final follow - up according to the system of the American Orthopaedic Foot and Ankle society was 91.2 ± 6.8 points. Motion of the first metatarsophalangeal joint was limited to < 30° in three feet (8.3%). Patients were satisfied with the results of 31 (86%) of the 36 procedures and dissatisfied with the results of five (14%). Satisfaction was evaluated as the patient's willingness to undergo surgery again or not.

10. Radiographic results

According to radiographic results of the 36 consecutive MIDMOs the mean HVA decreased from 27.7° preoperatively to 14.6° at the final follow - up ($p < 0.001$). The first IMA decreased from an average of 11.2° preoperatively to 5.8° at the final follow - up ($p < 0.001$).

Plantar displacement of the first metatarsal head (mainly a plantar translation, with some degree of plantar angulation) was found at the time of follow - up in 17 (47.3%) of the 36 feet, dorsiflexion of the head (mainly angular deformity) was seen in three feet (8.3%), and a position that can be defined as neutral (essentially similar to the preoperative position) was observed in sixteen feet (44.4%). The extent of lateral displacement of the first metatarsal head was 56.2% ± 18.4% of the diameter of the first metatarsal shaft in the immediate postoperative period and 36.1% ± 15.9% at the time of follow - up. The relative shortening of the first metatarsal was measured in 11 feet (30.6%). In the remaining 25 feet the shortening was not measured. The mean first metatarsal shortening was 2.2 ± 2.8 mm (range: -8 to 3.4 mm). All of the osteotomies healed well, with callus evidence after an average of 3 months. All of the metatarsal bones remodeled themselves over time (fig. 4) even in cases with marked offset at the osteotomy (several millimeters of bony contact). In our experience, the healing of the osteotomy and remodeling capability of the metatarsal bone are not related to the offset at the osteotomy, but it is preferable to obtain a bony contact not less than one third of the metatarsal section.

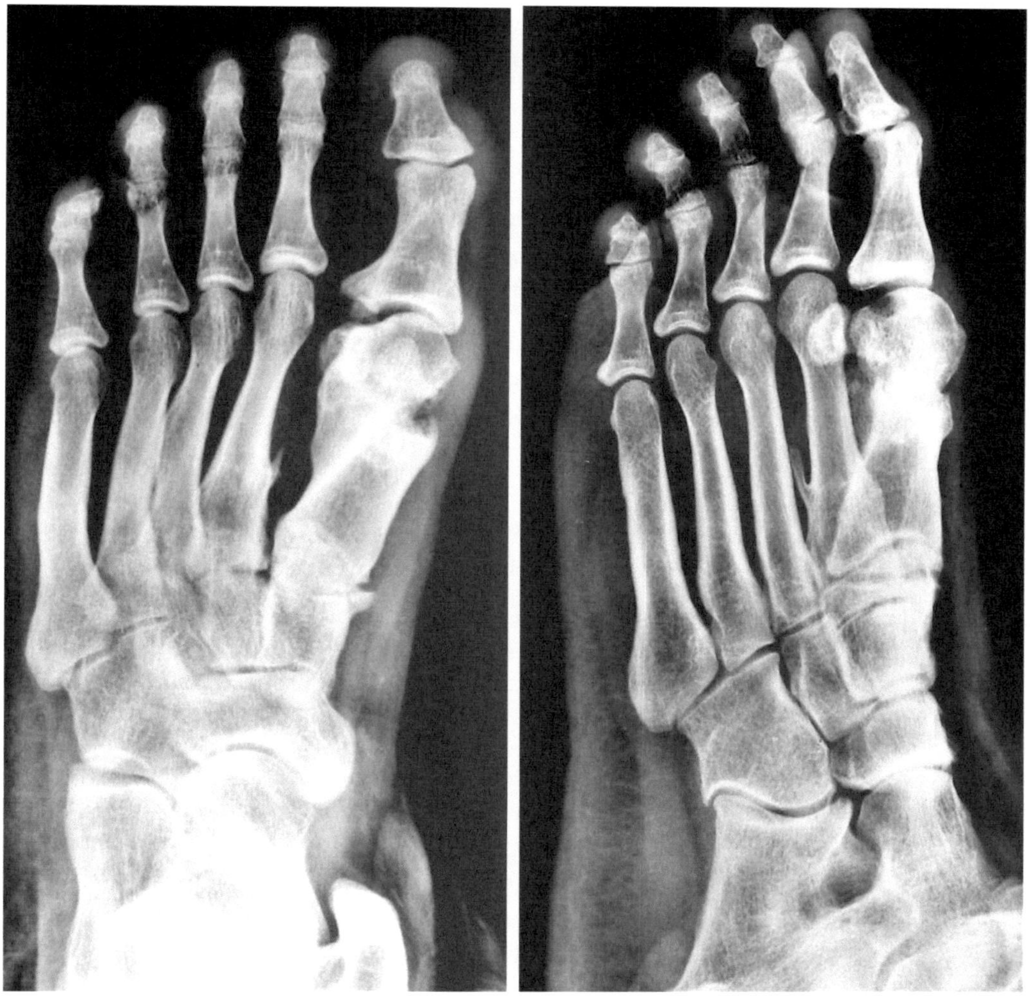

Fig. 4. A-P and oblique standing radiograph, showing remodeling of the First MTP 24 months postoperative.

11. Complications

No intraoperative complications occurred in our study except in one foot some comminution occurred at the osteotomy site but did not affect either the stability of fixation or the union of the osteotomy. After dressing removal, in 3 feet a mild skin inflammatory reaction was present around the outlet of the K - wire at the tip of the toe. There was no need to remove the K - wire before the scheduled time. There were no episodes of nonunion, malunion, transfer metatarsalgia or avascular necrosis of the metatarsal head. No cases of secondary hallux varus were observed despite the slight overcorrection that had been consistently achieved at the time of stabilization of the osteotomy site. No patient underwent a deep venous thrombosis.

12. Discussion

The goal of operative treatment is to offer relief of pain, correction of forefoot deformity and a biomechanically functional foot. For a long time, bunion surgery had a reputation for being very painful with a lengthy recovery period. Indeed, many people put up with their bunions for years rather than face surgery. This was because older techniques involved cutting the bone and not using any form of fixation. Newer techniques introduced during the past decade enabled surgeons to fix the bones into the correct position, reducing pain and promoting a better and more controlled recovery.

However, we are constantly exploring ways of moving from open surgery to minimally invasive techniques, replacing large incisions with small 'ports' through which the surgeon works. In doing so, we offer important benefits for the patient, removing or damaging less tissue, reducing scarring and the subsequent risk of infection.

Minimally invasive distal first metatarsal osteotomy with a percutaneous technique was first described by Bösch et al in 1990 , and a satisfactory result was reported in a 7 - 10 year follow - up study. (30) Portaluri (42) achieved 89% satisfaction rate with the Bösch method and stated that the advantages of this technique included short operation time and low incidence of complications. Sanna and Ruiu (43) reported excellent results in a long - term follow - up study of percutaneous distal first metatarsal osteotomies. Magnan et al (44) reported that the patients were satisfied following 107 (91%) of 118 percutaneous distal first metatarsal osteotomies.

Numerous studies have revealed that minimally invasive hallux valgus surgery can achieve a good satisfaction rate similar to other open techniques. (45,46) The distal metatarsal osteotomy in our study was a minimally invasive, simple bony procedure without other advanced soft tissue procedures. We did not perform bunion resection, formal capsulorrhaphy, lateral release or capsulotomy.

Our study involved twenty - four adult patients (36 feet) in the age range of 17–52 years with mild - to - moderate hallux valgus managed with the minimally invasive distal metatarsal osteotomy (MIDMO). The mean overall pain score was 37.3 ± 4.7 points of the 40 point maximum on the AOFAS. These results are comparable to other series that have reported satisfactory improvement in pain in 80–95% patients using open techniques. In a study of 91 Mitchell osteotomies, in which painful bunion justified surgery in 92% of patients; Desjardins et al (47) achieved satisfactory improvement of pain in 92% of patients. Johnson et al (48) published their results comparing distal chevron osteotomy to the modified McBride bunionectomy in a retrospective study. Ninety - two percent of patients in the chevron group and 88% of patients in the modified McBride group responded that they were totally satisfied or improved regarding pain relief after surgery.

The results of other series using minimally invasive techniques also reported comparable results to that of our study as the mean overall pain score reported by Magnan et al (44) was (36.3 ± 6.2 points) and that reported by Yu-Chuan Lin et al (49) was (35.7 ± 5 points).

In our study, the mean HVA and first IMA corrections were 13.1° and 5.4° respectively compared with 17.8° and 5.1° in Magnan et al's study and 11.8° and 6.3° in the study by Yu-Chuan Lin et al.

Our results indicate that this minimally invasive technique can achieve angular correction that is as good as that achieved using traditional techniques. It has been demonstrated that the mean HVA correction ranged from 8.8° to 26°, and the mean first IMA correction ranged from 3.8° to 11° in studies that used open techniques. (6, 50, 51)

A limitation of this minimally invasive approach is that we were unable to control the magnitude of lateral translation. This method simply relied on the stiffness of the K - wire and the size of the capital fragment to achieve lateral translation. We believe that the magnitude of angular correction might limit the use of our approach to treat more severe hallux valgus deformities. This explains why the inclusive criterion in our study was set at first intermetatarsal angle ≤ 18°.

The absence of lateral release or formal capsulorrhaphy might explain the absence of hallux varus after surgery. In Magnan et al's and our studies, there were no episodes of hallux varus (overcorrection).

The valgus deformity recurrence rate reported by Magnan et al was 2.5%. In our study there was no cases of recurrence this may be explained by the smaller number of cases (36 feet) compared with (118 feet) operated by Magnan et al, also due to good selection of the cases according to the inclusion criterion.

The lack of soft tissue surgery does not appear to affect the prevalence of recurrent hallux valgus deformity, perhaps because reorientation of the metatarsal head and reduction of the head on the sesamoids were the consistently achieved primary surgical objectives. In other studies that used open techniques in association with soft tissue procedures, the recurrence rate ranged from 0% to 10%. (17,51,52,53)

Although some of our cases had an increase in HVA after K - wire removal, the HVA and first IMA were significantly decreased at final follow - up. The Kirschner wire insertion level in the study of Yu-Chuan Lin et al was at the middle of the proximal phalanx. In our study and that of Magnan et al, the more distal percutaneous insertion level of the K - wire, might achieve a greater correction of the hallux valgus angle because of a longer level arm to abduct the big toe.

The mean extent of lateral displacement of the first metatarsal head in our study was 56.2% of the diameter of the first metatarsal shaft in the immediate postoperative period and 36.1%

at the time of full consolidation of the osteotomy site. This seems similar to that reported by Magnan et al (52.6%, 32.8% respectively). The action of the long extensor and long flexor tendons on the hallux during the plasticity phase of the healing callus probably offset the slight hypercorrection obtained at the time of surgical stabilization.

In our study the relative length of the first metatarsal was measured by the method of Morton. (39) Morton's method has two advantages: First, it detects the "biomechanical length" of the first metatarsal (medial deviation of the first metatarsal leads to a functional shortening). Second, the probability of a measuring fault caused by perspective distortion of the radiographs is reduced. In our study the relative shortening of the first metatarsal was measured in 11 feet (30.6%). In the remaining 25 feet the shortening was not measured. The mean first metatarsal shortening was 2.2 ± 2.8 mm (range: - 8 to 3.4 mm). The measured lengthening in some cases can be explained by the reduction of the first IMA and the consequent functional lengthening of the first metatarsal.

Transfer metatarsalgia, which might affect clinical outcomes, is a serious complication after first metatarsal osteotomy. Transfer metatarsalgia occurred with a range from 0% to 40% in studies that used other open techniques. (52) It may be found as a sequelae of dorsalization of the first metatarsal head or significant shortening of the first metatarsal. Transfer metatarsalgia was not reported in our series, and it was not mentioned by Magnan et al . This may be explained by that the osteotomy performed in MIDMO was in a single perpendicular plane, which was unable to cause over shortening of the first metatarsal. Also there was mild dorsiflexion of the capital fragment in the lateral radiographic image after surgery in only 3 feet out of the 36 feet in our study.

Stiffness of first metatarsophalangeal joint was reported to range from 0% to 37.8% using open techniques with capsulotomy. (52,54) This may be explained by lengthening of the first metatarsal through an oblique distally oriented osteotomy (dorsal arm) and excessive medial capsular tightening may lead to impaired range of motion of the MPI joint. However, this problem can be treated by early passive mobilization of the MPI joint. Postoperative stiffness of the first metatarsophalangeal joint in our study was calculated as 8.3% while was 6.8% in Magnan et al and 4.26% in that done by Yu-Chuan Lin et al . This problem was related to poor mobilization of the hallux following removal of the tape. However, these patients did not regard the joint motion deficit as disabling, and the rigidity did not cause pain during walking.

We did not have any case of postoperative avascular necrosis of first metatarsal head. This is probably due to the preservation of soft tissues on the lateral side of the metatarsal. These structures on the lateral side are important for the blood supply of the distal fragment. In our study, there were no episodes of nonunion, malunion or deep infection.

13. Conclusions

The results of our study demonstrate that MIDMO with a percutaneous K - wire stabilization under fluoroscopic control, without removal of the eminence and without open lateral release, performing only a manipulation of the great toe is an effective, reliable method of treating mild - to - moderate hallux valgus deformity in adult patients. The results appear to be comparable with those reported following traditional open techniques. Good satisfaction, functional improvement, and low complication rates were achieved with this technique. Nevertheless, we think that this technique requires a long learning curve and should be learned through both theoretical and practical courses. A well - designed prospective randomized controlled study with long - term results of a large study population is needed to support general use of this minimally invasive technique.

Figure 5 and 6 represent examples of some cases in our series.

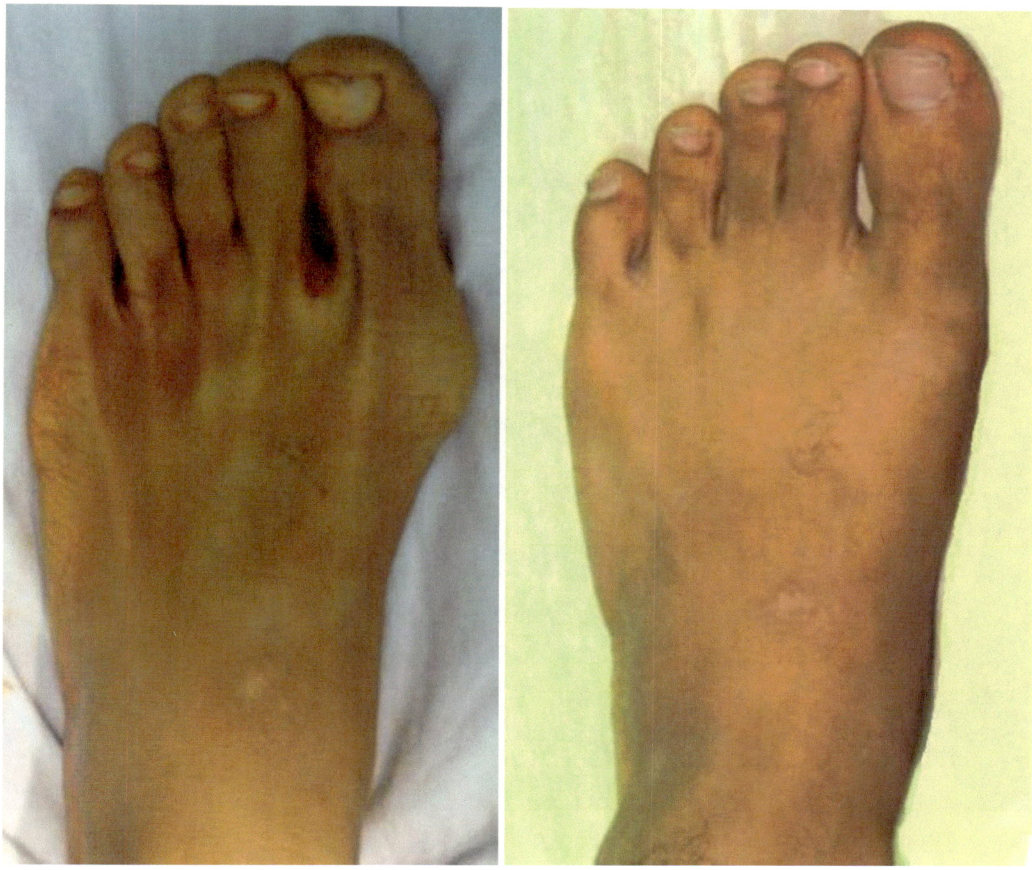

Fig. 5. A & B. Clinical preoperative and six months postoperative photos in 18 y. male patient with moderate hallux valgus deformity.

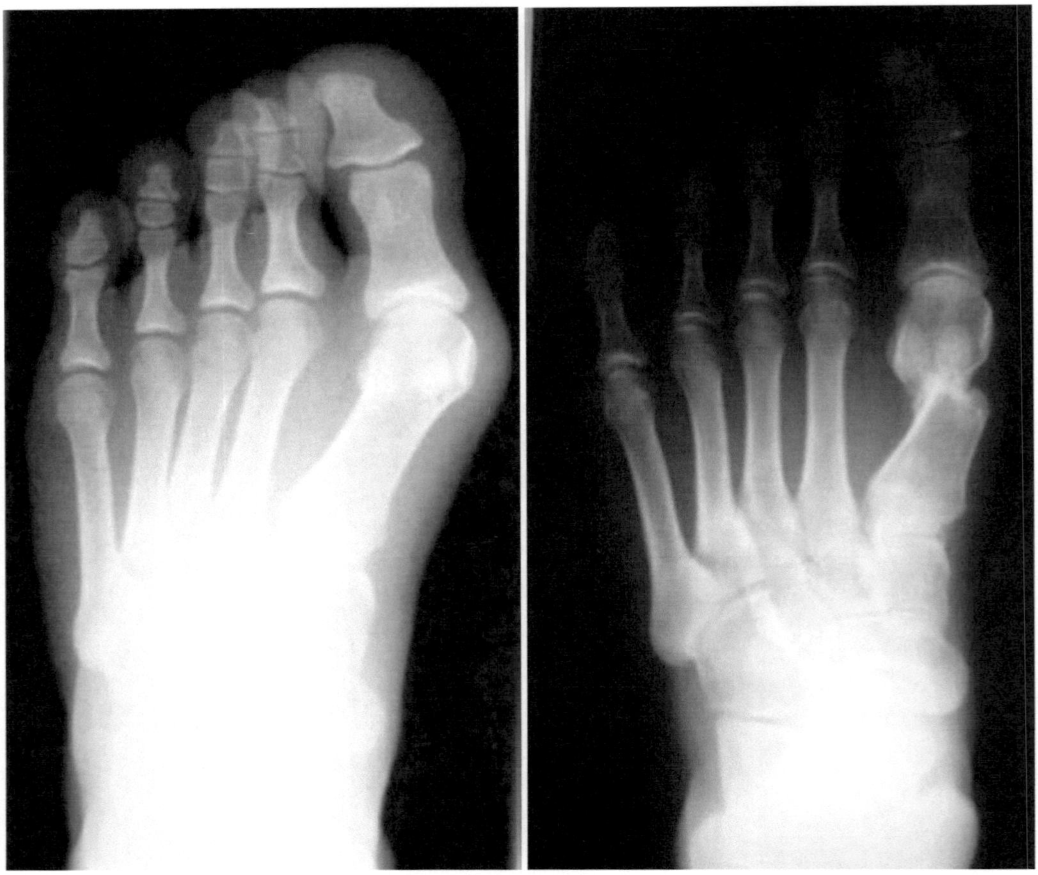

Fig. 5. C & D. Radiological preoperative and 6 months postoperative photos of the same patient

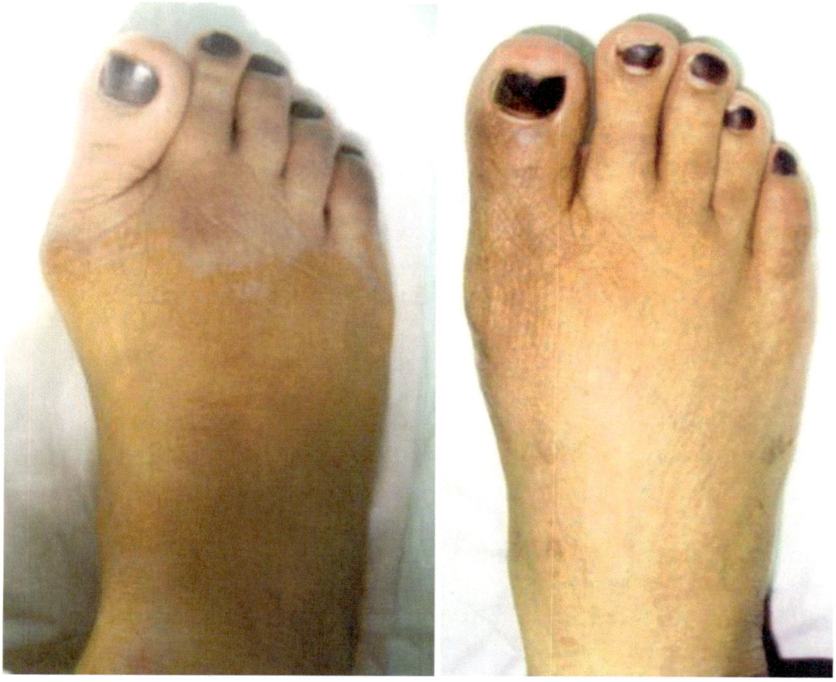

Fig. 6. A & B. Clinical preoperative and 18 months postoperative photos in 45 y. female with moderate hallux valgus.

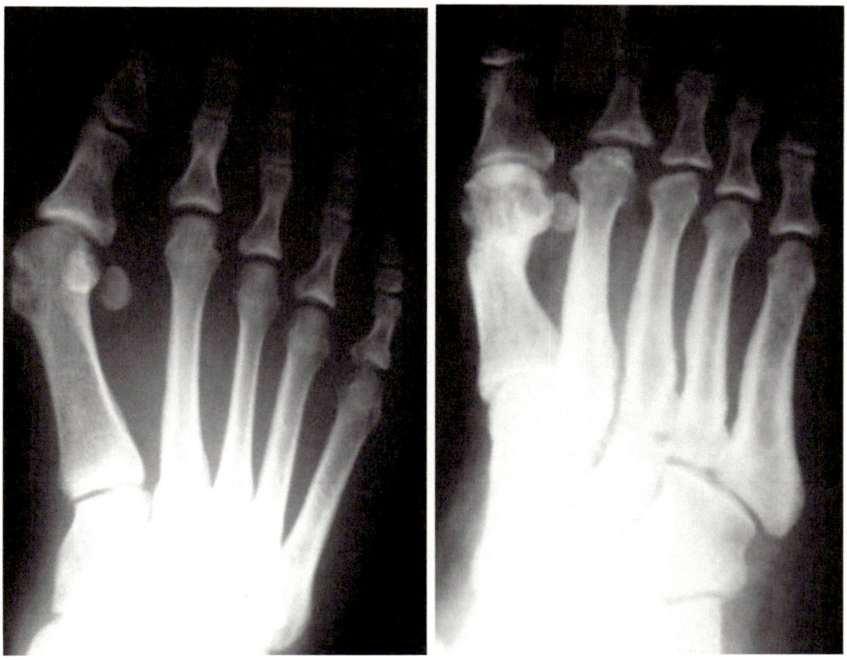

Fig. 6. C & D. Radiological preoperative and 18 months postoperative photos of the same patient

14. References

[1] Mann RA, Coughlin MJ. Hallux valgus – etiology, anatomy, treatment and surgical considerations. Clin Orthop Relat Res. 1981 ; 157 : 31- 41

[2] Coughlin MJ, Thompson FM. The high price of high - fashion footwear. In Instructional Course Lectures, Rosemont, Illinois, the American Academy of Orthopaedic Surgeons. 1995 ; Vol. 44, pp. 371-377.

[3] Kato T, Watanabe S. The etiology of hallux valgus in Japan. Clin. Orthop. 1981 ; 157 : 78-81.

[4] Inman VT. Hallux valgus : a review of etiologic factors. Orthop. C/in. North America. 1974 ; 5 : 59- 66.

[5] Hohmann G. The hallux valgus and the remaining Toes straightness. Results. Chir. Orthop. 1925 ; 18 : 308-376.

[6] Mann RA, Coughlin MJ. Hallux valgus – etiology, anatomy, treatment and surgical considerations. Clin Orthop Relat Res. 1981 ; 157 : 31- 41

[7] Coughlin MJ. Juvenile hallux valgus : etiology and treatment. Foot Ankle Int. 1995 ; 16 : 682- 697.

[8] Kilmartin TE, Wallace WA. The significance of pes planus in juvenile Hallux valgus. Foot and Ankle. 1992 ; 13 : 53- 56.

[9] Hardy RH, Clapham JC. Observations on hallux valgus ; based on a controlled series. J Bone Joint Surg Br. 1951 ; 33 : 376- 391.

[10] Mann RA, Coughlin MJ. Hallux valgus in adults. In : Coughlin MJ, Mann RA, editors. Surgery of the foot and ankle. 7th ed. St Louis: Mosby. 1999 ; p 147- 264

[11] Robinson AHN, Limbers JP. Modern concepts in the treatment of hallux valgus. J Bone Joint Surg [Br]. 2005 ; 87-B : 1038–1045.

[12] Gottschalle FAB, Sallis JG, Beighton PH. A comparison of prevalence of hallux valgus in three South African populations. S Afr Med Jr. 1980 ; 57 : 355-357

[13] Shine I. Incidence of hallux valgus in a partially shoe - wearing Chinese population. BMJ. 1965 ; 1 : 1648-1650.

[14] Chang JT. Distal metaphyseal osteotomies in hallux abducto valgus surgery. In: Banks AS, Downey MS, Martin DE, et-alet al.et-al (eds.), McGlamry's comprehensive textbook of foot and ankle surgery. Philadelphia: Lippincott, 2001:505–27

[15] Revenrdin J. De la deviation en dehors du gros orteil (hallux valgus. Vulg. "oignon" "bunions" "ballen") et de son traitment chirurgical. Trans Int Med Congr 1881;2:406–12

[16] Hohmann G. Symptomatische oder Physiologische Behandlung des Hallux Valgus? Munch Med Wochenschr 1921;33:1042–5

[17] Mitchell CL, Fleming JL, Allen R, et al. Osteotomy bunionectomy for hallux valgus. J Bone Joint Surg Am 1958;40:41–60

[18] Wilson JN. Oblique displacement osteotomy for hallux valgus. J Bone Joint Surg Br 1963;45:552–6

[19] Austin DW, Leventen EO. A new osteotomy for hallux valgus: a horizontally directed "V" displacement osteotomy of the metatarsal head for hallux valgus and primus varus. Clin Orthop Relat Res 1981 Jun;157:25–30

[20] Youngswick FD. Modifications of the Austin bunionectomy for treatment of metatarsus primus elevatus associated with hallux limitus. J Foot Surg 1982;21:114–6

[21] Magerl F. Stabile osteotomien zur Behandlung des Hallux valgus und Metatrsale varum. Orthopade 1982;11:170–80
[22] Kalish SR, Spector JE. The Kalish osteotomy: a review and retrospective analysis of 265 cases. J Am Podiatr Med Assoc 1994;84: 237–49
[23] Lair PO, Sirvers SH, Somdhal J. Two Reverdin-Laird osteotomy modifications for correction of hallux abducto valgus. J Am Podiatr Med Assoc 1988;78:403–5
[24] Elleby DH, Barry LD, Helfman DN. The long plantar wing distal metaphyseal osteotomy. J Am Podiatr Med Assoc 1992;82:501–6
[25] Van Enoo RE, Cane EM. Minimal incision surgery: a plastic technique or a cover-up? Clin Podiatr Med Surg. 1986;3:321–335.
[26] Lui TH, Ng S, Chan KB. Endoscopic distal soft tissue procedure in hallux valgus surgery. Arthroscopy. 2005;21:1403.e1–1403.e7.
[27] Lui TH, Chan KB, Chow HT et al. Arthroscopy-assisted correction of hallux valgus deformity. Arthroscopy. 2008 Aug;24:875–880.
[28] De Lavigne C, Guillo S, Laffenêtre O, De Prado M. The treatment of hallux valgus with the mini-invasive technique. Interact Surg. 2007;2:31–37.
[29] Bösch P, Markowski H, Rannicher V. Technik und erste Ergebnisse der subkutanen distalen Metatarsale-I-Osteotomie. Orthop Praxis. 1990;26:51–56.
[30] Bösch P, Wanke S, Legenstein R. Hallux valgus correction by the method of Bösch: a new technique with a seven-to-ten year follow-up. Foot Ankle Clin. 2000;5:485–498.
[31] Isham SA. The Reverdin-Isham procedure for the correction of hallux abducto valgus. A distal metatarsal osteotomy procedure. Clin Podiatr Med Surg. 1991;8:81–94.
[32] Leemrijse T, Valtin B, Besse JL. Hallux valgus surgery in 2005. Conventional, mini-invasive or percutaneous surgery? Uni- or bilateral? Hospitalisation or one-day surgery? Rev Chir Orthop Reparatrice Appar Mot. 2008;94:111–127.
[33] Weitzel S, Trnka H-J, Petroutsas J. Transverse medial slide osteotomy for bunionette deformity: long-term results. Foot Ankle Int. 2007;28:794–798.
[34] Roukis TS, Schade VL. Minimum-incision metatarsal osteotomies. Clin Podiatr Med Surg. 2008;25:587–607.
[35] Magnan B, Samaila E, Viola G, Bortolazzi P. Minimally invasive retrocapital osteotomy of the first metatarsal in hallux valgus deformity. Oper Orthop Traumatol. 2008;20:89–96.
[36] Giannini S, Vannini F, Faldini C et al. The minimally invasive hallux valgus correction (S.E.R.I.) Interact Surg. 2007;2:17–23.
[37] Piggott H. The natural history of hallux valgus in adolescence and early adult life. J. Bone and Joint Surg. 1960 ; 42-B (4): 749-760.
[38] Coughlin MJ, Saltzman CL, Nunley II JA. Angular measurements in the evaluation of hallux valgus deformities : a report of the Ad Hoc Committee of the American Orthopaedic Foot & Ankle Society on angular measurements. Foot Ankle Int. 2002 ; 23 : 68–74.
[39] Morton DJ. The human foot. New York : Columbia University Press; 1935
[40] Kitaoka HB, Alexander IJ, Adelaar RS et al. Clinical rating systems for the ankle - hindfoot, midfoot, hallux, and lesser toes. Foot Ankle Int. 1994 ; 15 : 349-353.
[41] Okuda R, Kinoshita M, Morikawa J, Yasuda T, Abe M. Proximal metatarsal osteotomy : relation between 1- to greater than 3-years results. Clin Orthop Relat Res. 2005 ; 435 :191-196.

[42] Portaluri M. Hallux valgus correction by the method of Bösch : a clinical evaluation. Foot Ankle Clin. 2000 ; 5 : 499-511.
[43] Sanna P, Ruiu GA. Percutaneous distal osteotomy of the first metatarsal (PDO) for the surgical treatment of hallux valgus. Chir Organi Mov. 2005 ; 90 : 365–369.
[44] Magnan B, Pezze L, Rossi N, Bartolozzi P. Percutaneous distal metatarsal osteotomy for correction of hallux valgus. J Bone Joint Surg Am. 2005 ; 87 : 1191–1199
[45] Schneider W, Knahr K. Keller procedure and chevron osteotomy in hallux valgus : five - year results of different surgical philosophies in comparable collectives. Foot Ankle Int. 2002 ; 23 : 321–329.
[46] Torkki M, Malmivaara A, Seitsalo S et al. Surgery vs orthosis vs watchful waiting for hallux valgus : a randomized controlled trial. JAMA 2001 ; 285 : 2474–2480.
[47] Desjardins AL, Hajj C, Racine L, Fallaha M, Bornais S. Mitchell osteotomy for treatment of hallux valgus. Ann Chir. 1993 ; 47 : 894-899.
[48] Johnson JE, Clanton TO, Baxter DE, Gottlieb MS. Comparison of chevron osteotomy and modified McBride bunionectomy for correction of mild to moderate hallux valgus deformity. Foot Ankle. 1991 ; 12 : 61–68.
[49] Lin YC, Cheng YM, Chang JK, Chen CH, Huang PJ. Minimally invasive distal metatarsal osteotomy for mild -to- moderate hallux valgus deformity. Kaohsiung J Med Sci. August 2009 ; Vol 25 : No 8.431-437.
[50] Caminear DS, Pavlovich JR, Pietrzak WS. Fixation of the chevron osteotomy with an absorbable copolymer pin for treatment of hallux valgus deformity. J Foot Ankle Surg. 2005 ; 44 :203–210.
[51] Schneider W, Knahr K. Keller procedure and chevron osteotomy in hallux valgus : five - year results of different surgical philosophies in comparable collectives. Foot Ankle Int. 2002 ; 23 : 321–329.
[52] Kuo CH, Huang PJ, Cheng YM et al. Modified Mitchell osteotomy for hallux valgus. Foot Ankle Int. 1998 ; 19 : 585–589.
[53] Oh IS, Kim MK, Lee SH. New modified technique of osteotomy for hallux valgus. J Orthop Surg (Hong Kong) 2004 ; 12 : 235– 238
[54] Klosok JK, Pring DJ, Jessop JH, Maffulli N. Chevron or Wilson metatarsal osteotomy for hallux valgus. A prospective randomized trial. J Bone Joint Surg Br. 1993 ; 75 : 825–829.

15

Joint Salvage Techniques for Stage III/IV Hallux Rigidus

Lawrence M. Oloff, Colin Traynor and Shahan R. Vartivarian
Sports Orthopedic and Rehabilitation
USA

1. Introduction

Hallux rigidus is a disorder of the first metatarsophalangeal joint, characterized by diminished range of motion and progressive degeneration of the joint [Vanore et al, 2003]. It was first described by Davies-Colley who named the disorder "hallux flexus" [Davies-Colley, 1887], then the same condition was reported later by Cotterill and the term "hallux rigidus" was introduced [Cotteril, 2003]. It can occur as a result traumatic injury, congenital or acquired structural deformities, metabolic diseases, biomechanical abnormalities, neuromuscular disorders, or iatrogenic causes.

There is a high prevalence of hallux rigidus in the general population; it is the most common form of osteoarthritis of the foot affecting approximately 2.5% of the adult population, second only to hallux valgus [Keiserman et al, 2005; Padanilam, 2004].

Traumatic causes occur from injuries that result in forced hyperextension or plantar flexion which may create compressive and shear forces that result in chondral or osteochondral injury. The resultant joint damage leads to progressive arthritic changes over time [Shurnas, 2009]. Non-traumatic etiologies alter the normal biomechanics of the first metatarsophalangeal joint. Normal range of motion of the first metatarsophalangeal joint has been defined as being greater then 65 degrees of dorsiflexion and 15 to 20 degrees of plantar flexion [Chang & Camasta, 2001]. Hallux rigidus is a limitation of the normal range of motion. While systemic disease may cause direct degeneration of the articular cartilage, mechanical causes generally result in deterioration through eccentric forces with resultant wear and tear.

Mechanical causes which include metatarsus primus elevatus, congenitally long first metatarsal, hypermobile first ray, pes planus, hallux equinus, hallux valgus and hallux varus [Nilsonne, 1930; Bonney & Macnab, 1952; Bingold & Collins, 1950; Lambrinudi, 1938]. These structural abnormalities alter the axis of motion of the first metatarsophalangeal joint. Elevation of the first metatarsal does not allow the base of the proximal phalanx of the hallux to freely move over the metatarsal head during propulsion. The base of the proximal phalanx instead creates a forced bone on bone interface, jamming the first metatarsophalangeal joint. The dorsal jamming of the joint results in a decrease in dorsiflexion and leads to articular impingement causing abnormal stresses to the dorsal articular surface, promoting osteophytic formation. This further limits joint range of motion, leading to continued development of periarticular hypertrophic changes and progressive cartilage loss. Continued eccentric wear of the articular surface may progress to anklyosis of the joint. An abnormally long first metatarsal also results in limited dorsiflexion and dorsal eccentric joint overload by preventing plantar flexion of the first metatarsal which improves motion.

2. Clinical evaluation

Patients usually present with complaints of pain localized to the first metatarsophalangeal joint or joint stiffness. Onset may be insidious, often times with a history of an arthritic condition, or associated to a specific injury. Patients that describe acute onset need to be evaluated for acute gout, calcium pyrophosphate dehydrate deposition disease, septic arthritis, stress fracture of the sesamoids, soft tissue masses such as ganglion cysts, capsulitis and tendonitis etiologies. Symptoms of hallux rigidus are usually associated with increased activity or by irritation from shoe gear. Casual athletes will note gradual increased pain with trail and hill running in comparison to training on level surfaces. Female patients may state that the height of their heeled shoes has decreased over time due to inability to walk without pain in the great toe joint.

The most common finding on physical exam is the dorsal bunion. Dorsiflexion is generally limited from the jamming of the joint and may or may not be painful [Vanore et al 2003]. Early stage hallux rigidus has pain only at the end range of motion, while in contrast, end stage hallux rigidus may be pain free due to ankylosis of the first metatarsophalangeal joint. Crepitus during range of motion of the joint may also be present. Plantar flexion of the hallux reveals a more pronounced dorsal bump. The patient may experience pain with direct palpation of the dorsal surface of the joint. Gait analysis may reveal compensation leading to lateral metatarsalgia and formation of plantar hyperkeratoses. Gait changes to accommodate the limited motion in the big toe joint. This may manifest as a shortened stride, inverted posture of the foot, or as circumduction of the entire extremity. It is important to note that there may not be a direct correlation between the severity of the disease and the severity of the patient's symptoms.

3. Radiographic evaluation

Radiographic evaluation is critical and should include weight bearing Anterior Posterior (AP) and lateral views of the foot. An oblique view can be complementary. The AP view will commonly show eccentric narrowing of the joint, flattening or widening of the joint. Osteophytic changes can be seen and can obscure evaluation of the joint. It is important to evaluate the parabola of the metatarsals and length of the first metatarsal. Lateral view will show a more accurate assessment of the joint without overlying osteophytes. The extent of dorsal osteophytic spurring can be evaluated, however the radiograph tends to underestimate size. The lateral view is also important in evaluating for elevatus of the first metatarsal. Computed tomography or magnetic resonance imaging (MRI) can be helpful for evaluating for osteochondral injuries; however, MRI tends to overestimate severity [Vanore et al 2003].

There are clinical symptoms and radiographic signs that indicate stage and severity of disease. There have been multiple published classification systems for the evaluation of hallux rigidus. The American College of Foot and Ankle Surgeons have adopted a 4-stage classification, evaluating the disease process by radiographic and clinical findings [Vanore et al, 2003] (Table 1).

Hallux Rigidus Grade	Radiographic Findings	Clinical Findings
I-Functional Limitus	metatarsus primus elevatus, plantar subluxation of the proximal phalanx, no radiographic evidence of degenerative joint disease	Pain at end range of motion
II-Joint adaptation	Dorsal spurring, subchondral eburnation, sclerosis, periarticular lipping, flattening of first metatarsal head, possible development of osteochondral defects	Limited passive range of motion
III-Established joint destruction	Subchondral bone cyst, severe flattening of joint, severe spurring asymmetrical joint space loss, first metatarsal head OCD, articular cartilage loss	Grade II plus joint crepitation, pain with full range of motion
IV-Ankylosis	Obliteration of joint space, intraarticular loose bodies	Grade III plus less than 10 degrees of first metatarsophalangeal joint, possible total ankylosis (asymptomatic)

Table 1. Hallux Rigidus classification.

4. Non-operative treatment

Treatment must be tailored to each patient depending on the extent of arthritis, patient preferences, patient lifestyle and progression of symptoms [Shurnas, 2009]. Initial treatment of hallux rigidus is usually non-operative and is aimed at reduction of inflammation and the painful range of motion of the metatarsophalangeal joint [Keiserman et al, 2005]. Non-surgical management of hallux rigidus focuses on mechanical and systemic intervention. Patients should avoid activities that aggravate their symptoms. Shoe education is a must. Patients need to avoid flexible non-supportive shoes and those with a heel. Rocker bottom shoes allow for a propulsive gait with limited dorsiflexion of the metatarsophalangeal joints. Shoe gear with a wider toe box will help to accommodate an enlarged first metatarsophalangeal joint. A simple over the counter insert with a semi-flexible arch can be beneficial in transferring weight to the arch and decrease medial column loading, allowing the first ray to plantar flex thereby resulting in greater motion. Custom, more rigid orthoses improve mechanics and allow for forefoot modifications. A patient with pain only at end range of motion can benefit with an extension under the lesser metatarsal joints allowing plantar flexion of the first ray and an increase in dorsiflexion. Patients who have pain throughout range of motion because of more extensive and severe arthritic changes will not be able to tolerate an increase in motion. These patients require either a Morton's extension under the hallux, which will limit the motion, or a completely rigid extension, known as a gait plate, which blocks most motion in the joint. With the progression of the disease and irritation caused by shoegear, orthoses in later stages of hallux rigidus may not be so readily tolerated due to extent of space occupation [Shurnas, 2009]. Oral, as well as topical nonsteroidal anti-inflammatory drugs (NSAIDs) can be beneficial in decreasing the inflammatory response and reduce associated pain. If unrelieved by NSAIDs, corticosteriods may be considered in the form of intra-articular injections or tapered doses orally [Vanore et al, 2003]. Physical therapy can be helpful in the application of iontophoresis, and mobilization of the joint through distraction techniques.

5. Operative treatment

Surgical approach towards hallux rigidus can be grouped into two categories: joint sparing or joint destructive procedures. Traditionally, proposed surgical intervention for Stage I and II hallux rigidus has been geared toward joint salvage procedures. These include cheilectomy, chondroplasty, and/or decompressional osteotomy. Stage III and IV rigidus have been directed toward a joint destructive approach, such as resectional arthroplasty, total joint replacement, and arthrodesis.

5.1 Joint salvage procedures

Joint salvage procedures usually use cheilectomy alone or in combination with additional procedures such as a metatarsal or phalangeal osteotomy, and chondroplasty.

5.1.1 Cheilectomy

Cheilectomy is essentially the resection of the dorsal osteophytic formation and the degenerative portion of the articular surface of the metatarsal. It has become a popular procedure for treatment of hallux rigidus, offering the advantage of relieving pain while preserving some motion, propulsive power, and stability [Keiserman et al, 2005]. It also avoids lengthy healing times, allows immediate weight-bearing, doesn't require internal fixation, and doesn't "burn bridges" affording secondary or definitive procedures at a future date if necessary. Typically 25-33% of the metatarsal head are removed [Coughlin & Shurnas, 2004; Mann & Clanton, 1988] with the goal to achieve increased dorsiflexion of the joint, however, the amount of bone to be removed depends on the size of the bony proliferation, damage to the articular cartilage, and intraoperative degree of dorsiflexion achieved during the procedure [Keiserman et al, 2005].

A study on the outcome of cheilectomy on high level athletes demonstrated 95% good or excellent results, and found the procedure to be reliable in this population because it increases joint motion, maintains stability, avoids loss of purchase power, and permits an early return to sport activity [Mulier et al, 1999]. Mann and Clanton reported 90% patient satisfaction with the procedure and an average 20° of dorsiflexion improvement [Mann & Clanton, 1988]. Feltham et al reported good results in 53 feet, most of which had grade II or III radiographic changes, suggesting radiographic classification does not correlate with surgical outcome [Feltham et al, 2001]. A long term follow-up study, average of 9.6 years, showed significant improvement in dorsiflexion, total motion, and post-operative pain following cheilectomies, with a 92% success rate in terms of function and pain relief [Coughlin & Shurnas, 2003]. The authors showed predictable success in Grade I and II, as well as selected Grade III cases, but recommended arthrodesis in patients with <50% articular cartilage remaining on the metatarsal head. The authors also reported good to excellent outcomes that did not correlate with radiographic appearance of the joint at final follow-up.

Many studies have shown satisfactory results clinically and subjectively in mild to moderate cases of hallux rigidus with cheilectomy. Care must be taken to identify those patients whose complaints are localized to the dorsal exostosis and no pain throughout the midrange of first metatarsophalangeal motion [Seibert et al, 2009].

5.1.2 Metatarsal osteotomy

There are several described metatarsal osteotomies that are designed to correct the structural abnormality of either the first ray, or the metatarsophalangeal joint itself. Metatarsal osteotomies shorten and/or plantar flex the first metatarsal and may be performed at the distal or proximal segments of the metatarsal. The degree of dorsiflexion or elevatus determines the required location of the osteotomy [Vanore et al 2003]. If hypermobility is identified, a first metatarsal cuneiform arthrodesis with the first metatarsal fused in a plantar flexed position may be considered. Plantar flexion allows for improved range of motion through an increase in dorsal clearance of the joint. Shortening, or decompressional, osteotomies result in a relative increase in the joint space, hence, increasing dorsiflexion. All of the described osteotomies are commonly done in conjunction with a cheilectomy. The combination of these two treatments allow for a greater effect on the dorsiflexion of the joint. A recent study looked at 57 references in a review of metatarsal osteotomies for hallux rigidus and found a mean increase of 10.4 degrees in dorsiflexion of the first metatarsophalangeal joint [Roukis, 2010]. Healing time is prolonged with all of the osteotomy procedures when compared to an isolated cheilectomy, however immediate weight bearing is tolerated when distal osteotomies are performed. Decompressional osteotomies also allow for future revisional surgery if deemed necessary.

5.1.2.1 Metatarsal osteotomy surgical technique

The first metatarsal osteotomy is performed with a dorsal linear incision centered over the first metatarsophalangeal joint. The extensor hallucis longus tendon is identified and moved laterally to allow visualization of the first metatarsophalangeal joint. A dorsal linear incision is then made through the joint capsule to expose the first metatarsophalangeal joint. The dorsal and medial bony prominences are then resected along with any additional periarticular spurring. The articular cartilage of the first metatarsal head is then evaluated and any isolated and well-defined areas of cartilage loss are debrided to a stable perimeter of cartilage, followed by microfracture with a 0.035 inch K-wire. The osteotomy is the final step in the surgical approach. A chevron-type osteotomy is created from medial to lateral with the apex of the osteotomy within the head of the first metatarsal. A wedge typically 2-3 mm is then resected from the dorsal arm of the osteotomy. The capital fragment is then impacted onto the shaft of the first metatarsal. A guide wire for a 3.0mm cannulated screw is placed under fluoroscopic guidance. Passive range of motion is then evaluated. If satisfactory, the osteotomy is then fixated with a 3.0mm cannulated short-thread cortical screw (Fig. 1-4).

5.1.2.2 Postoperative management

An isolated decompressional osteotomy of the first metatarsal is allowed to be weight bearing in a postoperative shoe. The DARCO® wedge shoe is preferred for the first three weeks, limiting forefoot loading and possible ground reactive forces that could displace the osteotomy. After week three the patient is then transitioned to a flat stiff soled postoperative shoe for an additional three weeks. Eliminating the propulsive phase of gait with a postoperative shoe is advantageous to the healing of the osteotomy; it does however tend to lead to stiffing of the first metatarsophalangeal joint. To counter the negative affects of a prolonged apropulsive gate, it is critical to start early passive range of motion of the first metatarsophalangeal joint as early as postoperative day three. If chondroplasty of the joint was performed it is absolutely imperative that gentle passive range of motion of the first metatarsophalangeal joint is started early to prevent hemarthrosis, which could also lead to stiffening of the joint (Fig 5).

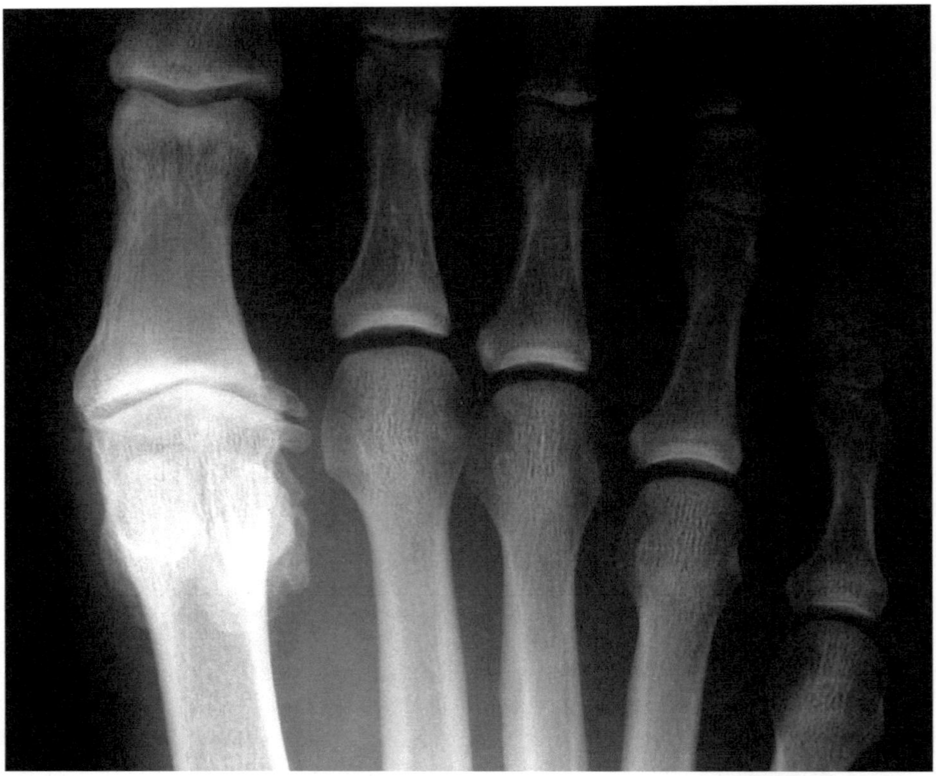

Fig. 1. Late Stage III Hallux Rigidus. Pre-operative AP radiograph with clear evidence of joint narrowing and osteophytic formation.

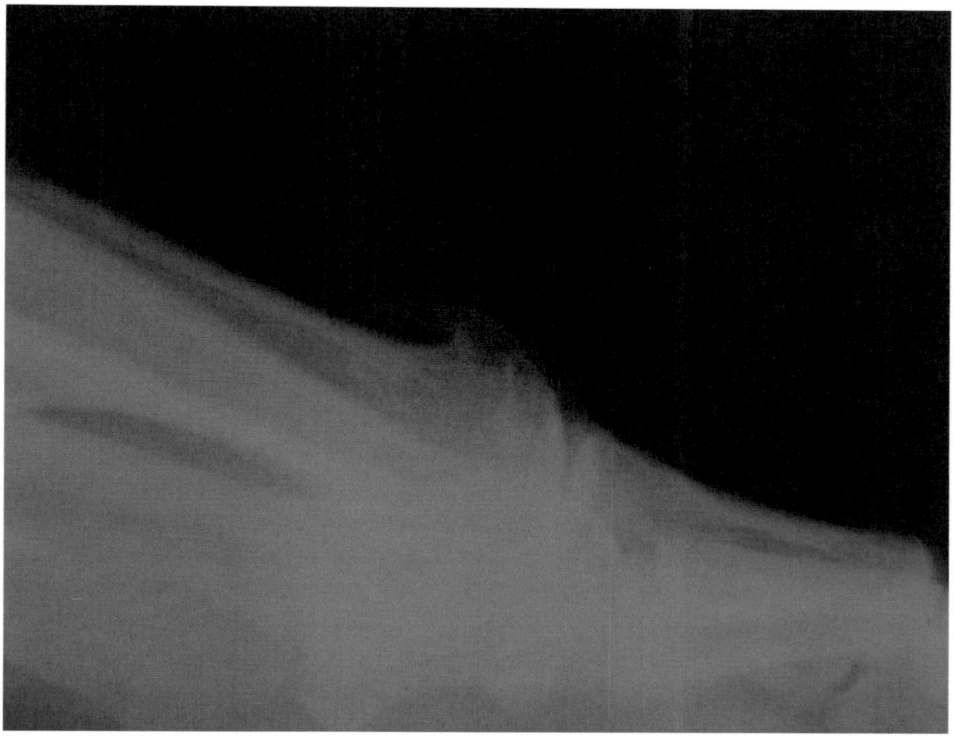

Fig. 2. Pre-operative lateral image of the same patient in Fig 3 with late Stage III Hallux Rigidus. Note the dorsiflexion of the first metatarsal, as well as the large dorsal osteophytic formation to the head of the metatarsal.

5.2 Joint destructive procedures

Joint destructive procedures include, arthrodesis, arthroplasty and implant arthroplasty of the first metatarsophalangeal joint. Traditionally joint destructive are reserved for stage III and IV hallux rigidus.

5.2.1 Arthrodesis

Arthodesis of the first metatarsophalangeal joint is a satisfactory procedure for many pathological processes, including hallux rigidus. The optimal position of the hallux after fusion should be 10° to 15° of dorsiflexion in relation to the floor, 10° to 20° of valgus, and neutral rotation [Keiserman, 2005]. These recommended numbers should strictly be used as a relative guideline, and each individual patient should be taken into consideration during the preoperative planning [Brage & Ball, 2002].

It is critical to avoid malalignment after the arthrodesis. Overcorrecting or under-correcting is not without consequence. Too little valgus can place the interphalangeal joint at risk of degenerative arthritis [Fitzgerald, 1969], while excessive valgus may cause shoeing difficulties. Overzealous dorsiflexion can cause irritation to the hallux, whereas inadequate dorsiflexion may create pressure and source of pain to the distal aspect of the toe [Coughlin & Shurnas, 2004]. Meticulous joint preparation is essential as well to avoid nonunion and enable a successful fusion. Disadvantages of arthrodesis include possibility of nonunion or malunion, interphalangeal arthritis, prolonged postoperative time, transfer metatarsalgia, and the possible need for a second procedure to remove hardware. The loss of joint motion is not without potential problems, particularly in the more active patient.

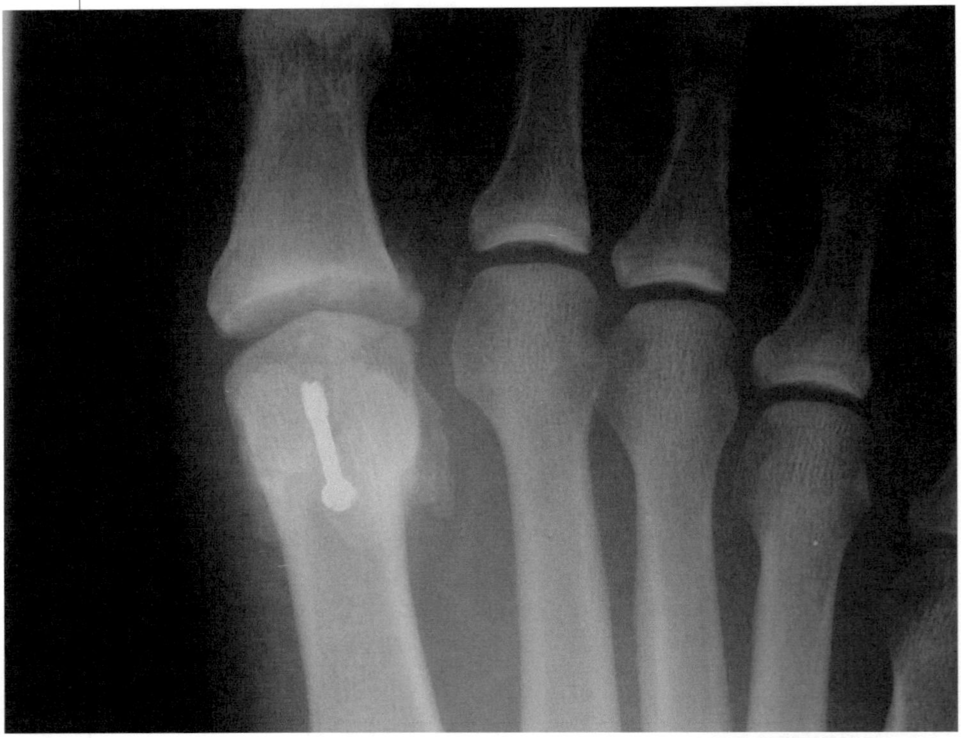

Fig. 3. Post-operative images of the same patient following decompressional osteotomy of the first metatarsal with cheilectomy. Note the significant increase to the first metatarsophalangeal joint space status post decompression. This patient exhibited improved range of motion post-operatively.

5.2.2 Arthroplasty and hemi/total implant arthroplasty

Resectional arthroplasty creates increased space between the first metatarsal and proximal phalanx allowing for motion of the hallux without pain, but without function. The hallux, as a result, is shortened. Hemi and total implants also allow for the increased motion; however, they have not proven stable over extended periods of time as have knee and hip arthroplasty. Due to the lack of function as a result of these procedures, patient selection is crucial. It is important to remember that reaction synovitis is still a concern for implants, as well as increase in lateral column pressure, implant loosening, and cost [Gibson & Thomson, 2005]. The ideal candidate is mostly sedentary with the treatment goal of improving symptoms enabling patients to perform activities of daily living [Vanore et al 2003]. The degree of permitted unrestrictive lifestyle following implants remains questionable. However, the biggest problem following joint replacement remains the ability to convert failed implants to arthrodesis. When these implants fail, primary fusion becomes difficult and the resultant tissue loss often requires importing bone to facilitate fusion.

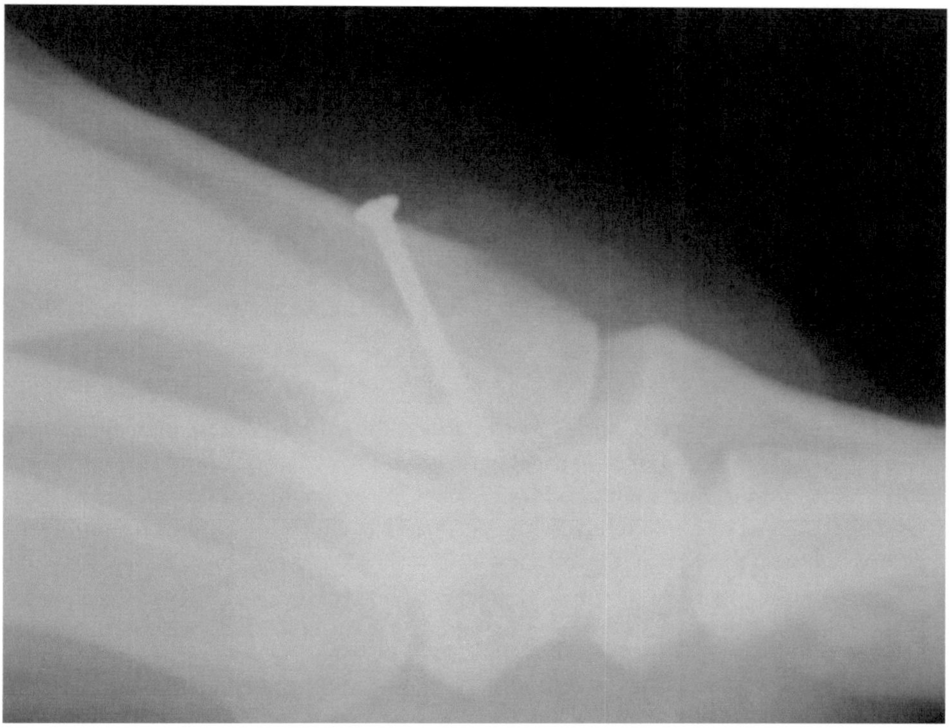

Fig. 4. Lateral radiographic image of the same patient revealing resection of the osteophyte from the dorsal first metatarsal. The increase in joint space can be appreciated in this image as well. Fixation of the osteotomy was provided with a single 3.0 mm short thread cortical screw.

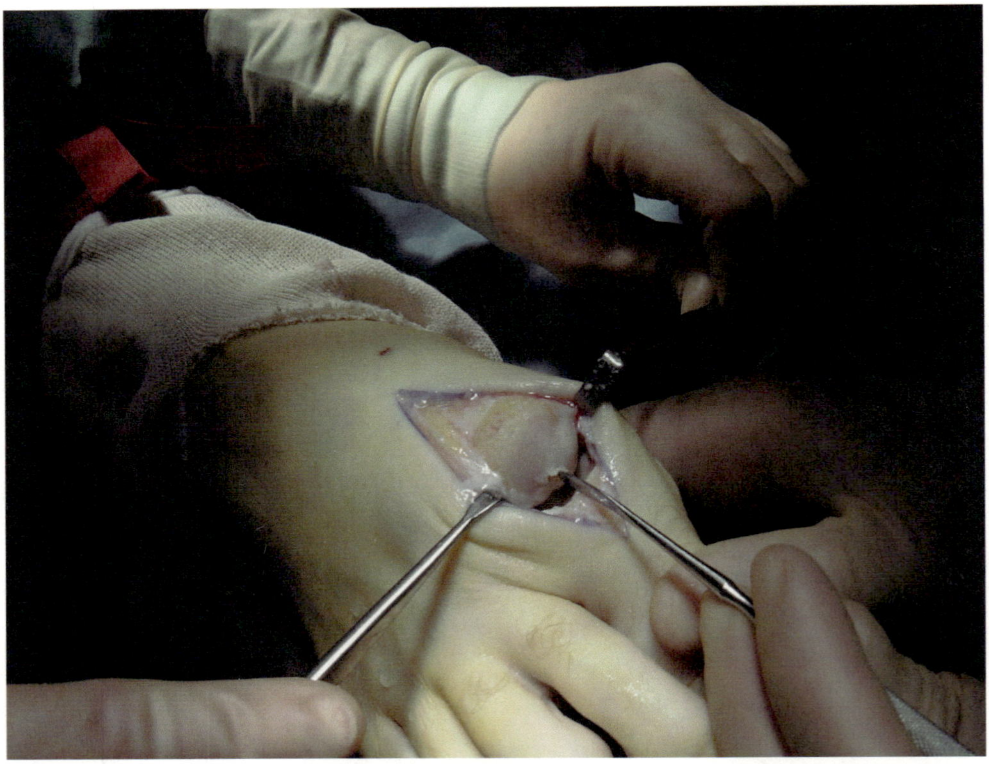

Fig. 5. Intra-operative image revealing degeneration of the dorsal articular surface cartilage. Also note the loosely adhered, friable cartilage toward the center of the joint. This is typical wear pattern found in patients with Hallux Rigidus. At this point chondroplasty of the articular defect should be considered. When performimg chondroplasty, early mobilization is important to lessen the chance for ankylosis.

6. Discussion

Joint destructive procedures have traditionally been the mainstay of treatment for hallux rigidus stage III and IV patients. The treatment options for joint destruction are not equivalent and require the surgeon to thoroughly evaluate the patient. Traditionally the patient's age dictated the treatment option; however, this has become less important. The patient's function and activity level must be assessed. Patients are living longer and thus staying more active in later stages of life. Arthroplasty of the first metatarsophalangeal joint along with hemi and total implants were traditionally reserved for elderly patients with sedentary lifestyles. It is important to note that implants of the first metatarsophalangeal joint are non-functional and provide nothing more than a spacer preventing shortening of the hallux. This creates a foot that is easier to shoe and provides a more cosmetic appearance. Highly active individuals regardless of age are poor candidates for implant or resectional arthroplasty.

Systemic disease must also be considered. Patients with inflammatory arthritic conditions are poor candidates for implants secondary to an increased risk of failure and may be inappropriate for joint preservation. Traditionally the accepted treatment for such patients was resectional arthroplasty or arthrodesis. The approach to systemic inflammatory diseases continues to change with the fairly recent introduction of disease modifying anti-rheumatic drugs (DMARDs). These classes of drugs can limit the joint destruction and allow the consideration of joint preservation (Fig. 6-7) [Drago et al, 1984; Niki et al, 2010].

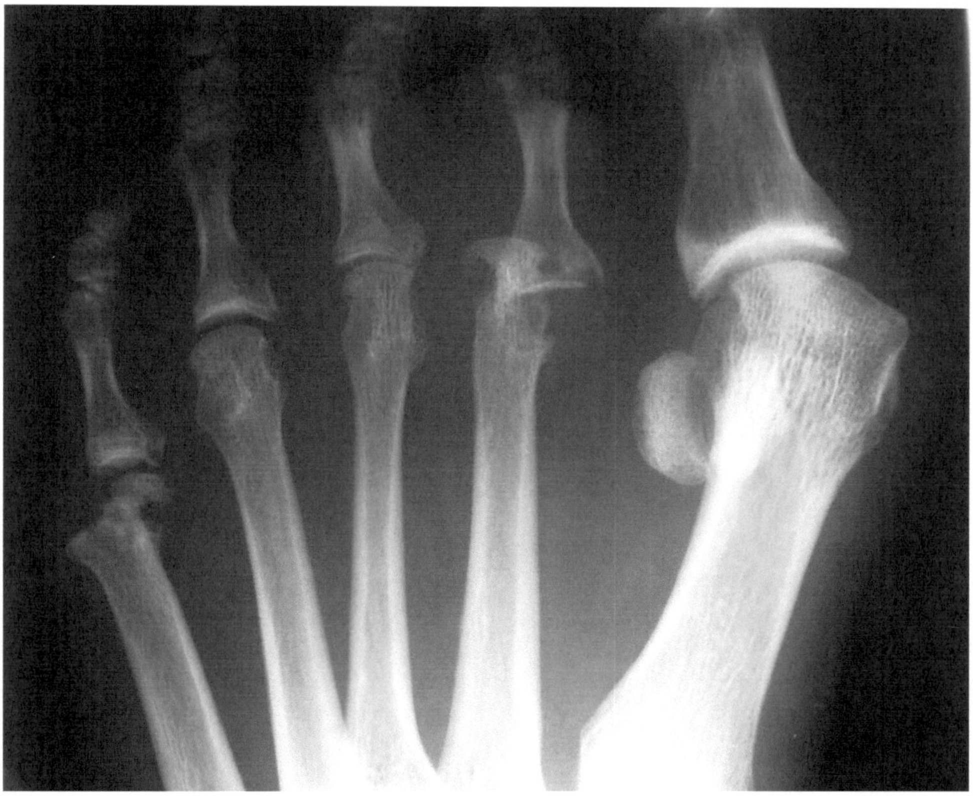

Fig. 6. Pre-operative AP image of a rheumatoid arthritic patient with Hallux Rigidus.

Inability to be non-weight bearing due to lack of care at home, atrophy or deconditioning of upper body muscles, obesity and of course poor compliance are deleterious to arthrodesis of the first metatarsophalangeal joint. While some literature suggests earlier weight bearing is allowable for arthrodesis [Hunt et al, 2011], typically patients are kept non-weight bearing for 4 weeks postoperatively with a transition to protected weight bearing for an additional 2 weeks.

The lead author performed a retrospective analysis of all patients that underwent decompressional osteotomies for stage III and IV hallux rigidus from 1994 to 2004. The inclusion criteria required the patient diagnosis of stage III or IV hallux Rigidus by the senior author, at least 1 year of postoperative follow-up, surgical treatment consisting of first metatarsal decompressional head osteotomy with or without cheilectomy and/or chondroplasty, and the ability to return for the long term follow-up evaluation. The retrospective analysis of all medical records and foot radiographs revealed that 23 patients

(28 feet) met the inclusion criteria. All of the returning patients were asked to complete a subjective 9-item questionnaire. No patients were reported as being worse or without any improvement. The mean AOFAS score was 25.9 preoperatively to 52 postoperatively out of a maximum 70. Of the patients 21 of 28 feet stated a 90% improvement with only 1 patient stating less then 50% improvement [Oloff & Jhala-Patel, 2008].

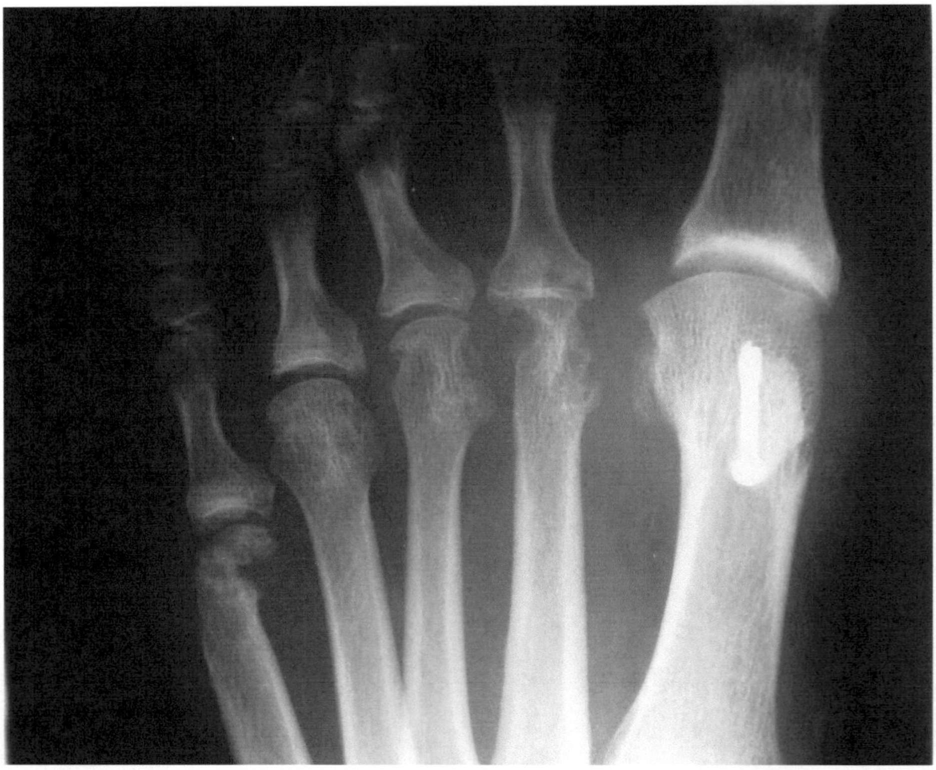

Fig. 7. Post-operative images following decompressional osteotomy of the first metatarsal in the same rheumatoid arthritis patient. In this case a joint preservation procedure was chosen because the patient's long standing rheumatoid arthritis came under control and there was reasonable cartilage remaining in her first metatarsophalangeal joint.

7. Summary

Hallux rigidus is a progressive, degenerative osteoarthrosis of the first metatarsophalangeal joint with numerous etiologic factors [Vanore et al 2003]. Historically, surgical procedures have been discussed with the nature of the progression of the arthritis in the joint, based on radiographic classification.

Treatment for this condition should be approached with the goal to reduce pain and improve function of the foot as a whole [Vanore et al 2003]. The choice of procedure for a particular patient often is difficult and depends on clinical findings, radiographic staging, and patient lifestyle. It is necessary to approach treatment with the mind set on joint salvage when rationally appropriate.

If decompression alone does not relieve a patients symptoms, autologous osteochondral transplantation may be considered prior to a joint destructive procedure. The lead author believes that joint salvage can be approached as a two staged procedure. The first stage would be to perform the decompressional osteotomy with possible cheilectomy and chondroplasty followed by autologous osteochondral transplantation as the second stage, which should only to be considered after the osteotomy has completely healed radiographically. It is also important to note that current research suggests that we may have additional alternatives to arthrodesis and implants with the advancement of cartilage regeneration. Mesenchymal stem cells could possibly allow for viable cartilage regeneration and repair with positive results in animal models [Dashtdar et al, 2011].

The proposed decompressional osteotomy procedure, with or without cheilectomy and/or chondroplasty has been shown to be an effective procedure even in cases of severe, late stage hallux rigidus. It keeps the door open for new and potentially regenerative techniques on the horizon. Such later stage reconstruction is not feasible after arthrodesis or joint replacement.

8. References

Bingold AC, Collins DH. Hallux rigidus. *J Bone Joint Surg* Vol. 32-B (1950), pp 214–22.

Bonney G, Macnab I. Hallux valgus and hallux rigidus: a critical survey of operativeresults. *J Bone Joint Surg Br* Vol. 34(3) 1952, pp 366–85.

Brage M, Ball S. Surgical options for salvage of end-stage hallux rigidus. *Foot Ankle Clin N Am,* Vol. 7 (2002), pp 49-73.

Chang TJ, Camasta, CA. (2001) Hallux Limitus and Hallux Rigidus. In: *Downey MS, Martin DE, Miller SJ, eds. McGlamry's Comprehensive Textbook of Foot and Ankle Surgery, 3rd ed.*, Banks AS, pp 679-711, Lippincott Williams & Wilkins, Philadelphia.

Cotteril JM. Stiffness of the great toe in adolescents. *British Med J,* 1888;1:158.

Coughlin MJ, Shurnas PS. Hallux rigidus: grading and long-term results of operative treatment. *J Bone Joint Surg* Vol. 85-A(11), (2003), pp 2072–2088.

Coughlin M, Shurnas P. Hallux Rigidus: Surgical Techniques (Cheilectomy and Arthrodesis). *J Bone Joint* Surg Vol. 86-A (2004), pp 119-130.

Dashtdar H. et al. A preliminary study comparing the use of allogenic chondrogenic pre-differentiated and undifferentiated mesenchymal stem cells for the repair of full thickness articular cartilage defects in rabits. *J Orthop Res* Vol. 29-9, (2011), pp 1336-1342.

Davies-Colley M. Contraction of the metatarso-phalangeal joint of the great toe. *British Med J,* 1887, pp 1-728.

Drago JJ, Oloff L, Jacobs AM. A comprehensive review of hallux limitus. *J Foot Ankle Surg* Vol. 23 (1984), pp. 213-220.

Feltham G, Hanks SE, Marcus RE. Age-based outcomes of cheilectomy for the treatment of hallux rigidus. *Foot Ankle Int* Vol. 22-3 (2001),192–197.

Fitzgerald JAW. A review of long-term results of arthrodesis of the first metatarso-phalangeal joint. *J Bone Joint Surg,* Vol. 51-B (1969), pp 488–493.

Gibson JN, Thomson C. Arthrodesis or Total Replacement Arthroplasty for Hallux Rigidus: A randomized controlled trial. *Foot Ankle Int,* Vol. 26, No. 9 (2005), pp 680-690.

Hunt KJ, Ellington JK, Anderson RB, Cohen BE, Davis WH, Jones CP. Locked Versus Nonlocked Plate Fixation For Hallux MTP Arthrodesis. *Foot Ankle Int* Vol. 32-7 (2011), pp 704-709.

Keiserman L, Sammarco J, Sammarco GJ. Surgical Treatment of the Hallux Rigidus. *Foot Ankle Clin N Am,* Vol. 10 (2005), pp 75-96.

Lambrinudi C. Metatarsus primus elevatus. *Proc R Soc Med* Vol. 31 (1938), pp 1273.

Mann RA, Clanton TO. Hallux rigidus: treatment by cheilectomy. *J Bone Joint Surg* Vol. 70-A(3), (1988), pp. 400–406.

Mulier T, Steenwerckx A, Thienpont E, et al. Results after cheilectomy in athletes with hallux rigidus. *Foot Ankle Int* Vol. 20-4, (1999), pp 232–237.

Niki H et al. Combination joint-preserving surgery for forefoot deformity in patients with rheumatoid arthritis. *J Bone Joint Surg (Br)* Vol. 92-B (2010), pp 380-386.

Nilsonne H. Hallux rigidus and its treatment. *Acta Orthop Scand,* Vol. 1 (1930), pp 295– 302.

Oloff LM, Jhala-Patel G. A retrospective analysis of joint salvage procedures for grades III and IV hallux rigidus. *J Foot Ankle Surg* Vol. 47-3 (2008), pp 230-236.

Padanilam, T. (2004). Disorders of the First Ray. In: *Orthopaedic Knowledge Update: Foot and Ankle, 3rd ed,* Richardson EG, pp 17-20, Rosemont, American Academy of Orthopaedic Surgeons.

Roukis T. Clinical outcomes after isolated periarticular osteotomies of the first metatarsal for hallux rigidus. *J Foot Ankle Surg,* Vol. 49, (2010), pp 553-560.

Seibert, Nicholas R. Kadakia, Anish R. Surgical Management of Hallux Rigidus: Cheilectomy and Osteotomy (Phalanx and Metatarsal). *Foot Ankle Clin N Am* Vol. 14, (2009), pp 9-22.

Shurnas, P. Hallux Rigidus: Etiology, biomechanics, and nonoperative treatment. *Foot Ankle Clin N Am,* Vol. 14 (2009), pp 1-8.

Vanore J, Christensen J, Kravitz S, Schuberth J, Thomas J, Weil L, Zlotoff H, Couture S. Diagnosis and Treatment of First Metatarsophalangeal Joint Disorders. Section 2: Hallux Rigidus. *Journal Foot Ankle Surg,* Vol 42, No. 3 (2003).